The Weider System Of Bodybuilding

Joe Weider

with Bill Reynolds

Contemporary Books, Inc.
Chicago

Library of Congress Cataloging in Publication Data

Weider, Joe.
    The Weider system of bodybuilding.

    Includes index.
    1. Bodybuilding—Training.   I. Reynolds, Bill.
II. Title.
GV546.5.W46   1983   646.7′5   83-1814
ISBN 0-8092-5561-8
ISBN 0-8092-5559-6 (pbk.)

All photos courtesy of the International Federation of Bodybuilders.
Principal Photographers: Bill Reynolds, John Balik, Mike Neveux,
Robert Gardner, Craig Dietz, Russ Warner, Jimmy Caruso, Pete Brenner,
Bill Dobbins.

Principal Models: Tom Platz, Lou Ferrigno, Frank Zane, Franco
Columbu, Chris Dickerson, Dennis Tinerino, Roy Callender, Tony
Pearson, Tony Emmott, Ken Waller, Tim Belknap, Carlos Rodriguez,
Casey Viator, Samir Bannout, Ed Corney, Andreas Cahling, Bill Grant,
Mohamed Makkawy, Larry Scott, Mike Mentzer, Ray Mentzer, Boyer
Coe, Bertil For, Lance Dreher, Steve Davis, Robby Robinson, Roger
Walker, Greg DeFerro, Ken Passariello, Ed Giuliani, and Bob Birdsong.

Published by Contemporary Books, Inc.
180 North Michigan Avenue, Chicago, Illinois 60601
Manufactured in the United States of America
Library of Congress Catalog Card Number: 83-1814
International Standard Book Number: 0-8092-5561-8 (cloth)
                                     0-8092-5559-6 (paper)

Published simultaneously in Canada by
Beaverbooks, Ltd.
150 Lesmill Road
Don Mills, Ontario M3B 2T5
Canada

Contents

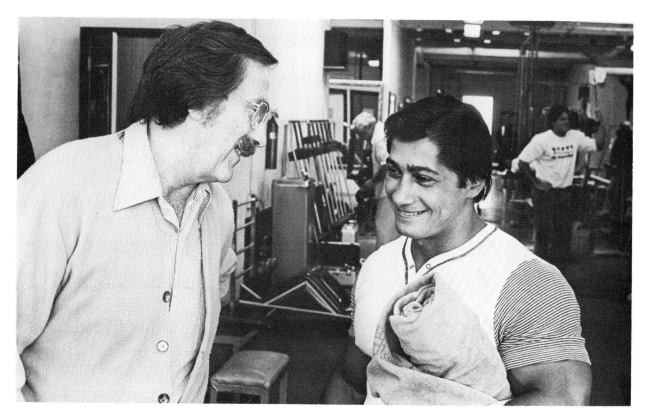

Joe Weider with Danny Padilla (above) and Robby Robinson (below).

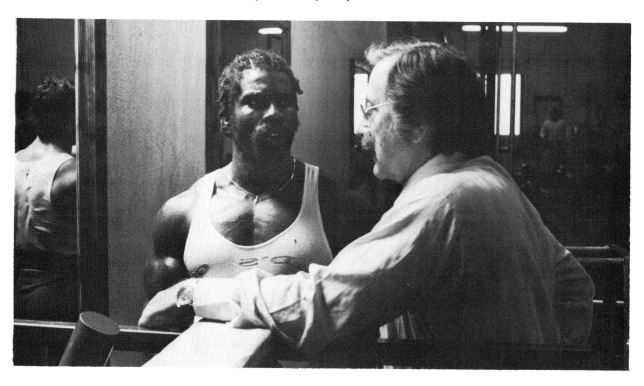

Introduction

Before I get down to the business of training and inspiring you to pump iron til you puke, I want you to seriously consider the limited aspects of a career in bodybuilding. Above all else, I urge you to continue training hard, but please avoid making bodybuilding your entire life. Such a move is counterproductive, since it limits you to existence as a unidimensional person. All of the great IFBB champions—Schwarzenegger, Ferrigno, Zane, Columbu, Scott, *et al.*—are well-rounded individuals, and I am convinced unidimensional bodybuilders just don't make it to the top.

Don't throw all of your eggs into the bodybuilding basket, since many are called and few chosen as bodybuilding champions. You could end up shooting snakeyes in the bodybuilding game and have nothing to fall back on when you are older and should be enjoying the fruits of a lifetime of work.

Jack Neary, a former editor of my *Muscle & Fitness* magazine, wrote eloquently about the role bodybuilding *should* play in the life of a young athlete: "A bodybuilder's success is not determined by desire alone; the factor which decides how far a bodybuilder will go is something over which he

has no control: genetic potential. Every man can train to his yearning heart's content, but only a fraction of a percent will reach the top.

"The number of young men who want to leave school, quit jobs, tear themselves away from familiar ground to head west to the supposed 'Mecca' of bodybuilding, Los Angeles, and to train under Joe Weider's guidance is appalling. Every day we receive letters from teenagers assuring us they will be the greatest bodybuilders of all time.

"Sometimes young men will eschew writing as a way of introduction and actually come west on a hope and a prayer. I remember the day when a bedraggled kid of 21 visited us. He had left his home in Ohio on a Greyhound bus with only $40 in his pocket. He spent his nights in a church. He wanted to be a champion bodybuilder. His delusion was so great that he told us in two years he would have 25-inch arms and 23-inch calves. We could only shake our heads and urge the kid to hop on the next bus back to Ohio.

"Then there was the boy from Oklahoma who dropped out of high school so he could train at Gold's Gym. He came west with

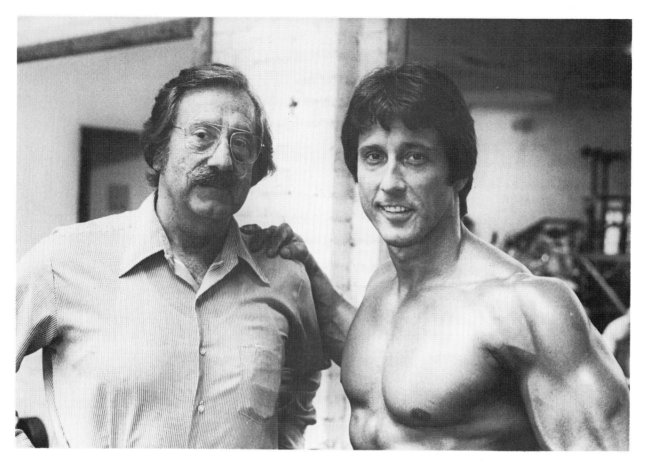

The Master Blaster and Frank Zane.

$2,000, but for fear of his money dwindling, he slept on park benches and subsisted on coffee and doughnuts. He trained hard, but at Gold's he was just a small fish in a big pond; his life was going nowhere.

"It takes many years of hard work to become a champion, and hard work alone doesn't mean you'll make it. So if there's one bit of advice from the Weider Research Clinic a young bodybuilder should heed, it's this: stay at home, finish school, go to college, get a job, and keep training. If, along the way, you become a promising title-winner, don't worry. *You needn't come to us, because we will come to you.*

"The worst thing you can do is throw it all away on the slim chance you'll one day be Mr. Olympia and cash in on your fame. You just can't fight the odds. For every man who makes it, thousands don't."

Jack Neary has focused perfectly on this issue—don't throw all reason and prudence to the wind by moving to L.A. to train under me. I simply don't have the time to train more than a handful of the world's elite bodybuilders, so I focus my personal attention on the men who already are the sport's superstars. If you live in Seattle, Miami, San Diego, Brooklyn, or Katmandu, you can learn all you need to know from reading my books and digesting every issue of *Flex* and *Muscle & Fitness*.

There aren't any "secrets" in bodybuilding other than choosing the right parents and dedicating yourself to putting in enough time and effort to maximize your genetic physical potential. And you can do that where you live now, even if you work out in a home gym. There's no difference in the composition of the oxygen and food here in L.A. compared to where you live. And the champion bodybuilders here still put their pants on one leg at a time.

Set your goals, then go for them hard. But, do it realistically, leaving yourself an escape hatch and parachute in case your rocket to the moon goes off course. You can provide yourself this escape hatch and parachute by continuing with your education until you have the skill or academic credentials necessary to land a good job. And you can maintain your parachute in good order by holding on to this job once you get it.

Never sacrifice your vocation, family, friends, social life, spiritual life, or morals just on one roll of the dice. Life's enough of a crapshoot as it is, so you needn't aggravate the situation by playing with loaded dice. *Always* live a normal life, with bodybuilding as a valuable supplement to it. In this way *you will be a winner* in the game of life, even if no one happens to give you a tin pot for your efforts.

Good luck with your workouts, and **keep on pumping iron!**

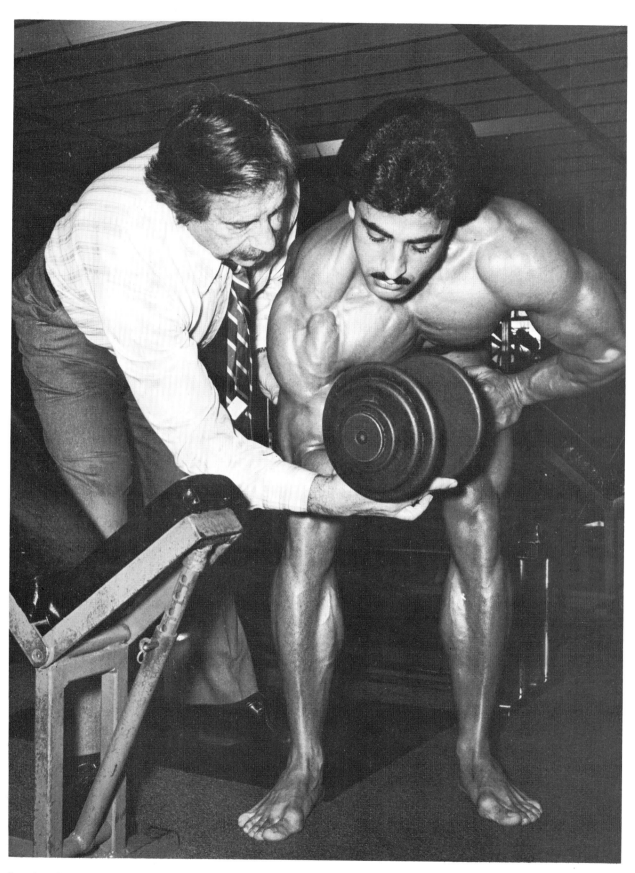

Joe gives Samir Bannout a tip on Concentration Curling.

Foreword

In a way this book is a sequel to *Bodybuilding: The Weider Approach*, since it would not have been possible to write it had my first book not proven to be so overwhelmingly popular with serious bodybuilders in America and the rest of the world. *The Weider System of Bodybuilding* builds upon and augments the knowledge of training and nutrition propounded in *Bodybuilding: The Weider Approach*.

Over and above being a sequel, however, *The Weider System of Bodybuilding* stands on its own as a landmark book on the art and sport of bodybuilding. There are nearly 100 individual routines of the sport's superstars, plus scores of exercise descriptions that will immediately assist you in your own workouts. From my discussions you'll gain more knowledge of the techniques, exercises, and routines that can turn you into a champion bodybuilder.

The Weider System of Bodybuilding has been constructed and written as a companion piece to *Bodybuilding: The Weider Approach*. These two books are like book ends to my Joe Weider Muscle Library—you can't have one without the other.

I also firmly believe that you will profit greatly from reading my six "Best of Muscle & Fitness" anthologies:

- *Training Tips and Routines*
- *Bodybuilding Nutrition and Training Programs*
- *The World's Leading Bodybuilders Answer Your Questions*
- *Champion Bodybuilders' Training Tips and Routines*
- *More Training Tips and Routines*
- *More Bodybuilding Nutrition and Training Programs;*

You should also read my two magazines, *Muscle & Fitness* and *Flex*, which present up-to-the-minute developments in bodybuilding methods on a regular basis. And, don't forget to pick up a *Muscle & Fitness Training Diary*, so you can keep accurate training records.

In conclusion, always remember that I am concerned about your progress as a bodybuilder. Feel free to write to me in care of *Muscle & Fitness* magazine, 21100 Erwin Street, Woodland Hills, CA 91367 and tell me about your progress. And, if you have made exceptional progress, send me details of your training philosophy with "before" and "after" photos of yourself. Perhaps I will publish your story.

Joe Weider

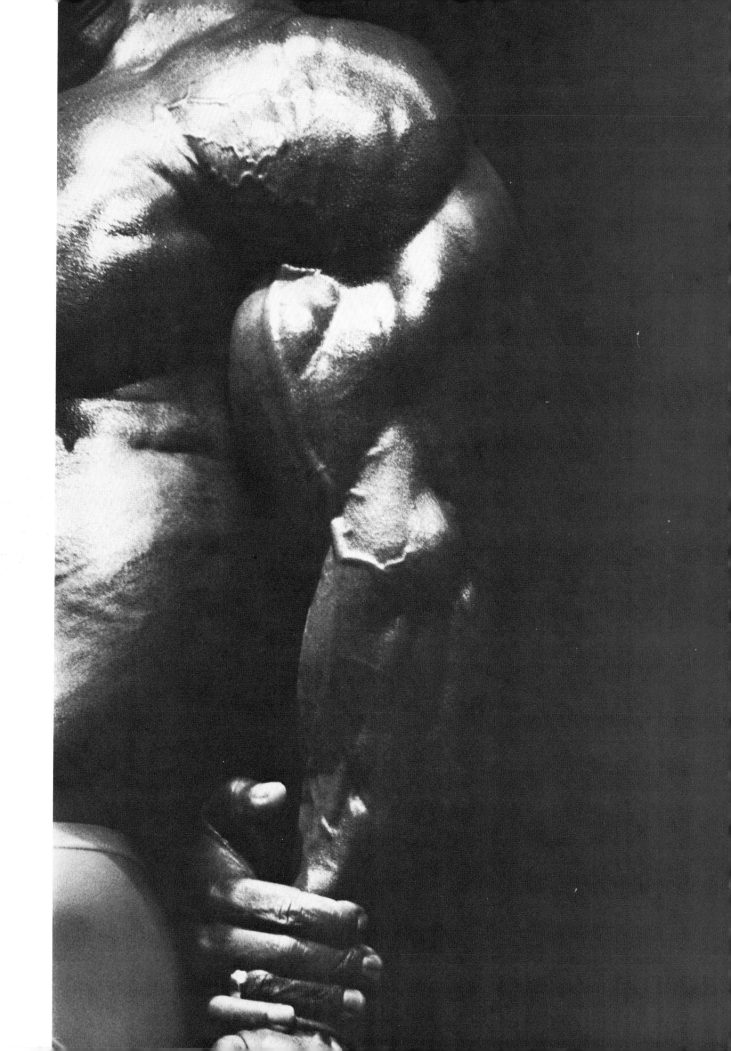

Part I:
Principles and Techniques

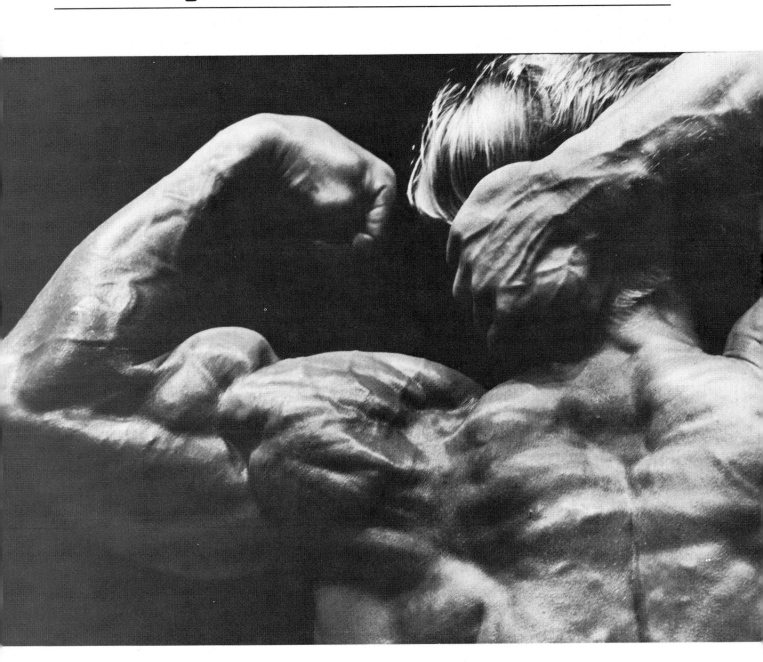

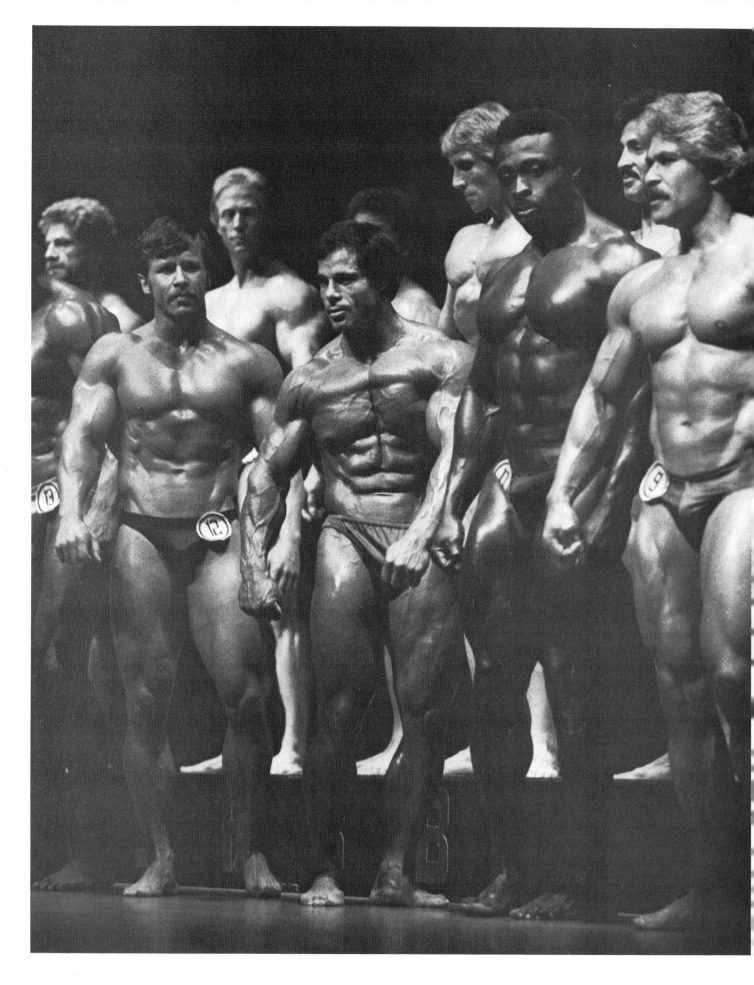

The Weider Cycle Training Principle

World records in all sports have soared during the past 20 years, and the physiques of bodybuilders today would literally shock the bodybuilders of 20 years ago. This explosive growth in bodybuilding and other sports during the past two decades has come as a result of a variety of factors: improved mental, training, and dietary techniques; increased use of pharmacology in sport; and the fact that vastly more athletes are training for competition, increasing the chances that genetically gifted individuals are entering every sport.

Over and above all this, the explosive growth of sports records and bodybuilding standards over the past 20 years is largely due to the use of *cycle training*. And this is the reason why the Weider Cycle Training Principle has become one of the newest weapons in the bodybuilder's arsenal for achieving success.

Very literally, bodybuilders and other athletes formerly trained the same year-round. They went all out in every workout, and as a result they didn't make much progress from year to year. They became chronically overtrained and had frequent disabling injuries, or often burned out completely.

Just as one example of this, one of the heroes of "Chariots of Fire," the Academy Award winner for Best Picture during 1981, was a British sprinter named Harold Abrahams, who was the surprise winner of the 100-meter dash at the 1924 Olympics. But the real-life Abrahams had become so chronically overtrained that his career was ended soon afterward when he *badly broke his leg* merely demonstrating his sprinting technique to the British press following the Olympic Games.

Today, athletes have come to realize that two types of training—an off-season building phase and a precompetition sharpening phase—with transitional phases between are necessary for the development of maximum athletic prowess. And, thus, has slowly developed the concept of cycle training in athletics, as well as in bodybuilding.

The crux of the Weider Cycle Training Principle lies in the fact that a bodybuilder trains heavily and with lower repetitions primarily on basic exercises in the off-season to build up muscle mass. Then during a precontest sharpening cycle, he trains differently—as will be discussed in detail in later chapters—for a period of time in order to sharpen up the newly gained muscle mass for competition.

Alternating off-season and precontest cycles in bodybuilding over a period of years will result in the relatively quick development of a championship physique. Athletes in other sports have also used the Weider Cycle Training Principle just as successfully. But, unlike those other athletes, we bodybuilders also use the Weider Cycle Training Principle in our diets.

In the off-season, champion bodybuilders consume a diet at or slightly above their caloric maintenance level for several months. They eat a relatively high amount of protein to help build muscle mass, as well as a lot of simple and complex carbohydrate foods to allow sufficient training energy to handle the heavy off-season workouts that build muscle mass. And, the combination of heavy training and a high-protein/high-carbohydrate diet results in the acquisition of new muscle mass as quickly as possible.

As a competition approaches, a champion bodybuilder gradually makes a transition from his off-season building cycle to a muscle-sharpening precontest cycle. During this precontest cycle, he follows a calorie-restricted diet as low in fats as possible. By consuming a number of calories under his daily maintenance level for a period of time—combined with special precontest training—he can strip away all surface body fat while losing as little muscle mass as possible to reveal the muscles acquired during the off-season in sharp relief. The champ becomes totally ripped to shreds, almost as though someone had taken a straight razor and sliced off all superfluous body fat!

During precontest training, a bodybuilder concentrates more on isolation exercises to carve all possible muscle details into his physique. Still, at least one basic exercise per muscle group is performed to maintain a maximum degree of muscle

mass while training down for extreme muscular definition. The IFBB superstars also use a variety of other Weider Training Intensification Principles during their precontest cycle in order to further sharpen up their physiques.

Some of the Weider Training Intensification Principles and other intensification techniques that are used include the Weider Quality Training Principle (or reducing the length of rest intervals between sets, even though this practice results in a drop in training poundages); adding total sets to the training programs for each muscle group; using the Weider Continuous Tension and Peak Contraction Training Principles; switching to the use of supersets, trisets, and/or giant sets; adopting the Weider Descending Sets Training Principle; use of the Weider Staggered Sets Training Principle; training most body parts more frequently; using the Weider Double-Split System Training Principle; practicing the Weider Iso-Tension Contraction Training Principle; and increasing the volume of aerobic training done each day.

Overall, I want you to understand that the Weider Cycle Training Principle will allow you to most quickly develop a championship physique. For the first two or three years of your training, you will be on one long off-season training and dietary cycle in order to build up sufficient muscle mass to be a viable physique competitor in your first bodybuilding competition. And for that competition you will follow a precontest diet and training phase to totally sharpen up for competition.

The lengths of your off-season and precontest cycles will vary. For Olympian competitors who compete only once per year—men like Frank Zane, Tom Platz, Chris Dickerson, Danny Padilla, and Samir Bannout—the off-season cycle will last approximately nine months and the precontest cycle will continue for the remaining three months of the year. With such a plan in which you compete only once per year and follow a long off-season cycle, you can make dramatic progress in developing muscle mass, muscle quality, and physical proportions from year to year.

Many lower-level competitive body-builders tend to become "trophy hunters." They remain in a precontest training and dietary phase for months at a time, competing almost every weekend and adding substantially to their trophy collections. But it's impossible to add muscle mass to your body—and thus improve your physique—when on a long-term precontest cycle. So, these trophy hunters look the same contest after contest, or (horrors!) even gradually lose muscle mass.

To both improve your physique at a rapid rate of speed and gain enough contest experience to become a great competitor later in your career, I strongly recommend that, at the lower levels of competition, you should enter only two competitions per year. Compete each six months, which will allow you a 4–4½-month off-season building cycle and a 6–8-week precontest sharpening phase.

By alternating these longer off-season phases with shorter periods of intense precontest training, you will be able to use the Weider Cycle Training Principle to its best advantage in building a championship physique. And, cycle training is the way to most quickly reach superstar status in bodybuilding.

BASIC AND ISOLATION EXERCISES

To fully understand the difference between off-season and precontest training, you must understand the differences between basic movements and isolation exercises. This is because you will use primarily basic movements in the off-season and primarily isolation exercises during a precontest phase.

Basic exercises are those that work the large muscle groups of the body (e.g., the thighs, back, chest) in conjunction with smaller muscle groups (e.g., biceps and triceps). You will be able to use very heavy weights in such basic exercises as the Squat, Bench Press, and Seated Pulley Row. Many Weider-trained champs Squat for reps with 600+ pounds, Bench Press

450+ pounds for reps, and do reps in the Seated Pulley Row with 350+ pounds.

Here is a comprehensive list of basic exercises for each major muscle group:

Thighs (front)—Squats, Leg Presses
Thighs (hamstrings)—Stiff-Leg Deadlifts
Lower Back—Deadlifts, Stiff-Leg Deadlifts
Lats—Barbell Bent Rowing, Seated Pulley Rowing, Dumbbell Bent Rowing, Chins, Pulldowns
Traps—Upright Rowing, Barbell Shrugs
Delts—Military Presses, Presses Behind Neck, Machine Presses, Dumbbell Presses, Parallel Bar Dips, Upright Rowing
Chest (upper)—Incline Barbell Press, Incline Dumbbell Press
Chest (lower)—Parallel Bar Dips, Decline Barbell Presses, Decline Dumbbell Presses
Chest (general)—Barbell Bench Presses, Dumbbell Bench Presses
Biceps—Barbell Curls, Dumbbell Curls, Preacher Bench Barbell Curls, Chins, Rows (all forms)
Triceps—Parallel Bar Dips, Presses (all forms), Lying Barbell Triceps Extension
Forearms—Barbell Reverse Curls, Barbell Wrist Curls, Standing Barbell Wrist Curls
Calves—Standing Calf Machine Toe Raises, Seated Calf Machine Toe Raises
Abdominals—Sit-Ups, Leg Raises

Since you work at least one large muscle group and one small body part with heavy weights in each basic exercise, you will be able to build a great deal of muscle mass with these basic movements. As a result, basic exercises are best used in the off-season when you should be building most of your muscle mass. Still, you will need to perform at least one basic exercise per body part prior to a contest to maintain muscle mass as you are training down for competition.

Isolation exercises work single muscle groups—and often even parts of muscle groups—in relative isolation from the rest of the body. Usually you will be restricted to using relatively lighter weights on isolation exercises, and they are meant to shape and fully define each muscle group. Therefore, isolation movements are intended primarily for use during a precontest training cycle.

To eliminate confusion, here is a list of isolation movements corresponding to the one I just gave you for basic exercises:

Thighs (front)—Leg Extensions, Sissy Squats
Thighs (hamstrings)—Leg Curls
Lower Back—Hyperextensions
Lats—Pullovers
Traps—Dumbbell Shrugs, Machine Shrugs
Delts—Dumbbell/Cable Side Laterals, Dumbbell/Cable Bent Laterals, Dumbbell/Barbell/Cable Front Raises
Chest (upper)—Incline Dumbbell/Cable Flyes
Chest (lower)—Decline Dumbbell/Cable Flyes, Cable Crossovers
Chest (general)—Flat-Bench Dumbbell/Cable Flyes
Biceps—Dumbbell/Barbell/Cable Concentration Curls, Incline Dumbbell Curls, One-Arm Dumbbell Preacher Curls
Triceps—Pulley Pushdowns, One-Arm Dumbbell/Cable Triceps Extensions, Dumbbell Kickbacks
Forearms—Barbell/Dumbbell Reverse Wrist Curls, One-Arm Dumbbell Wrist Curls (supported)
Calves—Donkey Calf Raises, One-Leg Dumbbell Calf Raises
Abdominals—Crunches (various types)

Generally speaking, you will use mainly basic exercises in the off-season and primarily isolation movements prior to a competition.

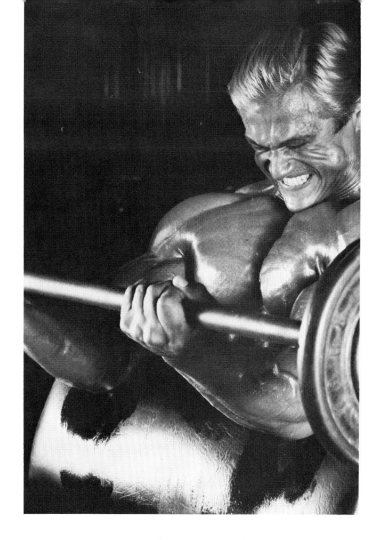

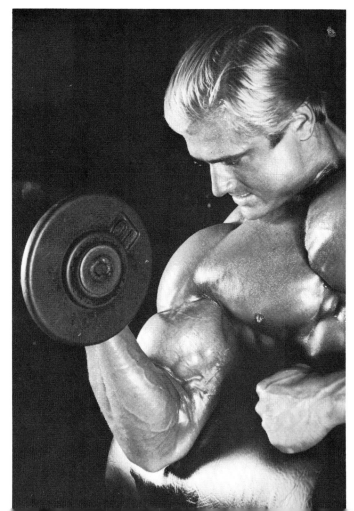

Tom Platz performs a basic, off-season exercise such as a Preacher Bench Curl (top right), then an isolation exercise such as a Preacher Bench Concentration Curl (bottom right) before a contest.

OFF-SEASON GOALS

Your primary goal in the off-season will be to build up general muscle mass, and particularly to build up lagging body parts. It's impossible to build muscle mass and especially to bring up a lagging body part during a precontest cycle when you are training fast with light weights and following a diet lower in calories than your caloric maintenance level (your maintenance level is that number of calories that you must consume to maintain a stable body weight).

Another of your off-season goals will be to keep your body weight within 8–10 pounds of your previous competitive weight at all times. Many bodybuilders foolishly use the off-season as a pig-out cycle, eating everything that isn't nailed down and gaining 20–30 pounds of useless body fat. Then they find it difficult during a precontest cycle to lose the great deal of weight they've accumulated in the off-season. Therefore, you're far better off holding your weight down during an off-season cycle.

PRECONTEST GOALS

During a precontest cycle you must totally refine the new degree of muscle mass and better physical proportions that you acquired during the off-season. And, you can do this by using the Weider Intensification Training Principles and a restricted diet, as mentioned earlier. This will rip your physique to shreds, leaving every muscle group with a good degree of mass and a maximum number of striations across it.

Next, you must prepare yourself mentally to have the body language of a winner and then *be* a winner. You will learn how to do this through a technique called "visualization," which is explained in detail by Tom Platz in Chapter 5.

Finally, you must have as a precontest goal to possess effective onstage presentation and a great personal appearance.

CYCLE DIETING

In this section, I am presenting the exact words of a great champion, Boyer Coe, on how he cycles his diet from off-season to precontest phases. Boyer is one of the greatest IFBB champions, having won the World Professional Bodybuilding Championships, World Grand Prix Championships, and more than 10 other major titles.

"In the off-season I mainly endeavor to follow a nutritionally balanced diet which will allow me to build a maximum degree of muscle mass without adding substantially to my body fat levels," Boyer Coe revealed. "I believe that, to gain muscle mass at an optimum rate of speed, you must maintain a high degree of health. And to be truly healthy, you *must* follow a nutritionally balanced diet supplemented with adequate vitamins and minerals to prevent nutritional deficiencies.

"There are a variety of theories on off-season diet, some in which bodybuilders consume up to 400 grams of protein per day. I used to eat steak after steak— between 300 and 400 grams of protein each day—for years. But I never made the type of gains then that I do now, and the large amount of fat in the beef was so difficult to digest that it overly burdened my digestive system.

"I believe that a bodybuilder's diet should be relatively low in fats year-round, since fats are more than twice as concentrated a source of energy as either protein or carbohydrates. In the off-season when total caloric consumption can be higher than prior to a competition, however, it is permissible to consume a few more grams of fats.

"I feel that the best sources of protein year-round are egg whites and white meats, such as poultry breasts and fish. To reduce fat consumption, all poultry should be broiled with the fatty skin removed before cooking. And no foods should ever be fried, since they inevitably soak up the cooking oil, adding substantially to the total number of calories in the food.

"If you are having difficulty gaining muscular body weight, you might consider consuming low-fat milk products. However, some individuals cannot drink milk or use some forms of milk products without having their stomachs become painfully bloated. This is because their digestive systems do not secrete lactase, the enzyme needed to digest lactose, the form of sugar in milk.

"This inability to digest milk is called 'galactose intolerance.' It becomes more common as any individual grows older, and it's more common among blacks and Orientals than among Caucasians. Individuals who suffer from galactose intolerance can usually consume hard cheeses however, since lactose is removed from most cheeses as they are processed.

"Overall, I don't feel that any bodybuilder will need to consume more than 200 grams of animal-source protein per day. Should you be experiencing difficulty gaining weight, break your protein intake into five or six smaller and evenly spaced meals per day, rather than the traditional three huge repasts that so many people normally consume. The human body can digest and utilize only 25–30 grams of protein per meal, so smaller and more frequent feedings make good sense when it comes to increasing protein assimilation and improving muscle-growth rates.

"When eating a greater number of smaller meals each day, two or three of these meals can come from a protein drink. The best way to mix such a drink is to use a blender to thoroughly blend two tablespoons of protein powder in 8–10 ounces of milk or juice. You can also blend in some type of soft fruit, such as a banana, as flavoring.

"Biologically, the best form of protein powder comes from milk and egg sources. Meat-based protein powders are next in biological quality, but many of them taste rather bad. Generally speaking, you should avoid vegetable-source protein powders, such as those made from yeast and soya beans, since they are low in some of the essential amino acids that your body can't manufacture on its own.

"Other than protein foods, the remainder of your off-season food intake should come

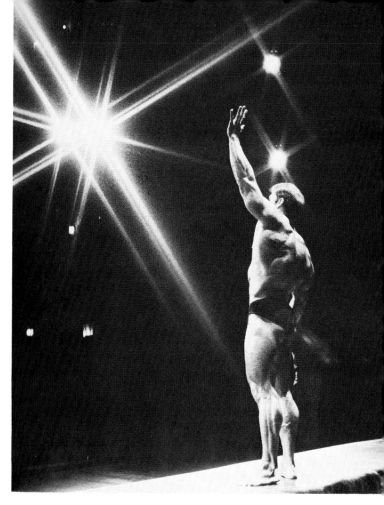

Boyer Coe acknowledges the cheers at the 1981 New York Grand Prix.

from good-quality carbohydrate foods. Some types of carbohydrates are more complex and they break down relatively slowly in the body, yielding a sustained flow of energy. I personally prefer to include plenty of these complex carbohydrate foods in my diet. They include baked potatoes, rice and other grains, and most vegetables.

"Simple carbohydrate foods tend to break down very quickly once they are eaten, resulting in a quick rise in blood-sugar levels and hence in short-term energy levels. But you can just as quickly have an energy crash an hour or two later, particularly if you are borderline hypoglycemic. Most fruits fall into this category, as does honey and other forms of natural sugar.

"Year-round you should avoid refined carbohydrates—such as white sugar and white flour—in your diet. Other than merely providing your body with a quick source of calories, these foods yield few other useful nutrients, such as vitamins and minerals. As such, refined carbohydrates provide your body with what can be called 'empty calories.'

"I know that there's always a temptation to eat junk food from time to time in your diet. But generally you should avoid junking out, even in the off-season. A good rule to follow is to eat for function rather than for taste.

"Through experimentation, you can soon determine your caloric maintenance level. Your off-season diet should include a total of no more than 100–200 calories per day over that level. And you'd be better off keeping only *slightly* above your caloric maintenance level. In the off-season you should never allow yourself to gain enough body fat so that your abdominals become smoothed over enough that you can't see the major separations between the muscles.

"My precontest diet is almost devoid of fats, since they are so high in calories. Still, it's difficult to totally avoid fats and a small amount of fat is necessary for optimum health, particularly of the nerves. Even such low-fat meats as fish and skinned chicken breasts have a degree of fat in them. Therefore, I have found that it's difficult to reduce fat intake to much under 40–50 grams per day.

"My diet prior to a contest still contains approximately 200 grams of protein and a minimum of 200 grams of carbohydrates. Figuring in about 50 grams of fats, this would amount to a daily caloric consumption of 2,000 calories (well below my caloric maintenance level prior to competition when I'm training hard in the gym and also doing at least an hour a day of aerobic exercises.)

"I will adjust my carbohydrate intake upward or downward according to how quickly I am losing body fat and how close I am to my competitive peak. Essentially, for each 3,500-calorie deficiency that I can create below my maintenance level by working out more and/or eating less calories, I will lose one pound of body fat.

"The trick to peaking exactly on time with a precontest diet is to play with the total number of calories consumed according to how your body looks in the mirror at various checkpoints prior to your competition. If I'm personally looking too smooth at a particular checkpoint, I cut back on my calories a little, and I will also increase my aerobic training. And if I'm peaking too quickly I will eat more calories, primarily in the form of complex carbohydrate foods.

"When you're on a strict precontest diet, it's essential that you supplement it with extra vitamins and minerals in capsule or tablet form to prevent developing nutritional deficiencies. With experimentation, you'll learn which individual vitamins and minerals you need, as well as in what potencies, during a precontest cycle.

"With time and careful observation, you will be able to gradually develop a perfect off-season eating program and an optimum precontest diet. And once you have done this, you will have won more than 50% of the battle when it comes to building a contest-winning physique!"

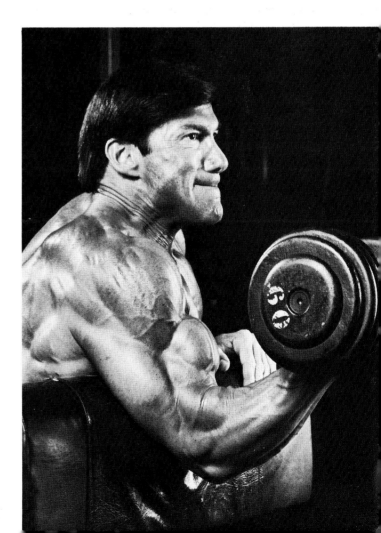

CYCLE TRAINING

In this section, I would like another great IFBB champion to explain, in his own words, how he trains cyclically to develop maximum muscle mass with tremendous cuts. This champion is Roy Callender, who has won the Mr. Canada, Amateur and Pro IFBB Mr. Universes, and the IFBB Diamond Cup Professional Championships titles, as well as placed in the top five at the 1981 Mr. Olympia.

"I don't believe that there is a bodybuilding champion anywhere today who doesn't train in cycles," Roy Callender stated. "Cycle training is the only way to build a maximum degree of muscle mass combined with great cuts at contest time, and all without burning out and overtraining or incurring an injury.

"During my off-season cycle, I try to improve my weak points, as well as generally add to my muscle mass. There is a direct relationship between the amount of weight you use for reps in strict form in an exercise and the relative mass of your muscles. Very simply, the heavier the weights you use, the larger will be your muscles.

"Since the use of heavy weights results in more massive muscles, it's best to work primarily with basic exercises on which you can use very heavy weights during an off-season cycle. I personally use two or three basic exercises per muscle group—plus perhaps one or two isolation movements—in the off-season. Less experienced bodybuilders should stick to doing only one or two basic movements for each muscle group.

"I feel that total recuperation between workouts is a requirement for the promotion of maximum muscle growth. Therefore, it's essential that you train each major muscle group only twice per week. At lower levels of bodybuilding, this will involve following a four-day split routine, hitting half of the body on Mondays and Thursdays and the other half on Tuesdays and Fridays. Calves and abdominals can be trained on all four workout days.

"At higher levels—and I am at this higher level—you should split your body into three parts and work them on a six-day split routine. This means you will do one third of your body on Mondays and Thursdays, the second third on Tuesdays and Fridays, and the final third on Wednesdays and Saturdays. On this six-day, off-season split routine, you can train your calves and abdominals 4–6 days per week, depending on how much work they need. I personally do my calves, a weak point, daily and my abdominals four or five days per week.

"Another recuperation factor involves the total number of sets that you do for each muscle group. I firmly believe that you must do a relatively low number of sets for each body part during the off-season in order to recuperate between workouts and really *grow*. Many novice bodybuilders make the mistake of being too enthusiastic in the off-season and performing so many total sets that they can't fully recuperate. You can't expect to make good gains in muscle mass while following precontest-type routines!

"As a general guideline, I feel that beginning-level bodybuilders should do only 6–8 total sets for large muscle groups like the thighs, back and chest, and 3–5 total sets for smaller bodyparts. Intermediates should do 8–10 for larger muscle groups and 6–8 for smaller ones, while advanced men can do 12–15 and 8–10 total sets, respectively, for each body part and still fully recuperate between workouts.

"In order to use very heavy weights in my basic exercises—and still be able to put in a good enough warm-up to prevent injuries—I pyramid my poundages and reps. This means that I begin with 12 reps at a light weight, slap on a few plates and 10 reps with the increased poundage, add more weight for eight reps, more weight for six reps, more weight for four reps, and even more weight for a final set of one or two reps. This pyramid system will allow you to add weight to every exercise very quickly. I don't think that it can be beat for helping to add muscular body weight to your body during the off-season.

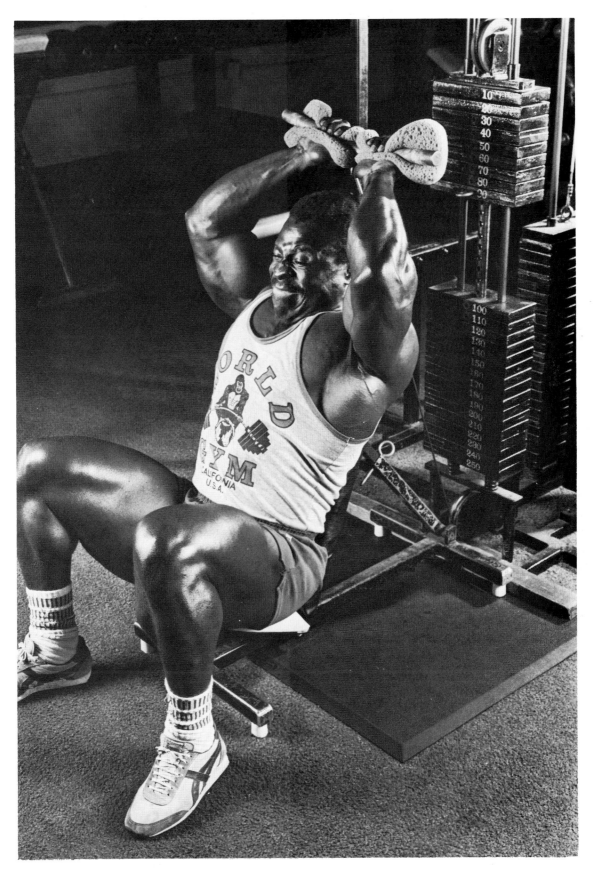

Roy Callender.

"Since you're using heavy weights during an off-season cycle, you'll need to take relatively longer rest breaks between sets. On exercises for large muscle groups, you can rest 1½–2 minutes between sets. Don't go past two minutes very often, however, since doing so allows your body to begin cooling down, whereupon it becomes susceptible to injury. On smaller muscle groups—even when using very heavy poundages—hold your rest intervals down to about 60–90 seconds.

"As a final off-season training tip, try to avoid injury as you increase your training poundages on each exercise during an off-season cycle. This involves staying well warmed-up, wearing a full warm-up suit, weightlifting belt and body wraps, and—above all else—using impeccable biomechanics (body form) on all exercises. These rules should allow you to use max poundages without risking injury."

Turning to precontest training, Roy Callender stated, "I like to think of my transition into a precontest training cycle and the actual cycle itself as one long and gradually building crescendo which reaches its peak just prior to a competition. It is then moderated for the final three or four days leading up to competition to allow the body sufficient time to recuperate and the muscles enough time to fill out completely before stepping onstage to compete.

"During my precontest crescendo, I use more and more isolation exercises. I gradually add to the total number of sets I do for each body part; I switch to training each major muscle group three times per week rather than two; I train with much shorter rest intervals between sets, and I do a number of other things to intensify my training.

"Inevitably, this faster training and the workout intensification principles I follow—to say nothing of the reduced number of calories I am eating, which results in lower energy levels—lead to the use of considerably lighter training weights than what I can handle in the off-season. But by keeping the weights as heavy as

possible nonetheless, I am able to build great muscular density.

"In addition to quality training and using a greater number of sets prior to competition, my favorite intensification techniques include the use of supersets, continuous tension, peak contraction, double-split system training, staggered sets, burns, preexhaustion, descending sets training, and isotension contraction. (Author's Note: All of these Weider Intensification Training Principles will be discussed and explained in Chapter 3.)

"I don't use all of these principles in one workout, but instead use various combinations of them for each body part. Through long use of the Weider Instinctive Training Principle (Author's Note: Please see Chapter 2 for a full discussion of this principle), I have discovered which principles work best on each individual body part, and I apply them accordingly in my precontest training.

"The only Weider Training Principle that I use consistently on every body part is the Weider Iso-Tension Contraction Training Principle, which goes a long way toward bringing out the maximum degree of muscle striations in every part of my body. I use it both while I am practicing my posing and in between sets as I am training each individual body part.

"Correctly orchestrated, my long training crescendo and a well-modulated precontest diet allow me to go into competition in peak condition and markedly improved over my physical condition at my previous contest. And this has helped me to be a winner as a pro bodybuilder!"

A FINAL WORD

All of the great champions use the Weider Cycle Training Principle—as well as all of the other Weider Training Principles—to maximum advantage in their workouts. But while training all of the great champions of our sport since 1936, I have noticed that each one of them interprets and applies the various Weider Training Principles differently. And each great champion trains quite differently than all of his comrades in iron.

The reason for these differences in training and dietary methods lies in the unique physical and mental makeups of each individual bodybuilder. Just as everyone has uniquely different muscle shape and body proportions, every champ has differing body chemistry and other factors that make his body respond uniquely to every type of training and dietary stimulus.

Each bodybuilder also has a unique mental makeup and temperament toward bodybuilding training. All of the great champs are incredibly positive about gaining additional muscle mass and further improving their physiques. But each also has a unique temperament that interacts with his mental and physical makeup to dictate the way he trains to improve his physique.

There are excitable bodybuilders who thrive on supersets and other types of high-intensity, fast-paced training. There are also more phlegmatic types who prefer to train slowly and methodically. There are dependent bodybuilders who can't get in a decent workout without the use of a training partner. And there are rugged individualists who prefer to train alone and in maximum privacy. In short, you will find every type of training temperament among champion bodybuilders (as I have learned over the years) but each champ has discovered what style of training works well for him and has stuck with it until he succeeded.

The secret of how to discover what works best for you lies in the next chapter on the Weider Instinctive Training Principle. Read it carefully, and you will have a maximum chance of becoming a champion. The Weider Instinctive Training Principle is truly bodybuilding's master training principle!

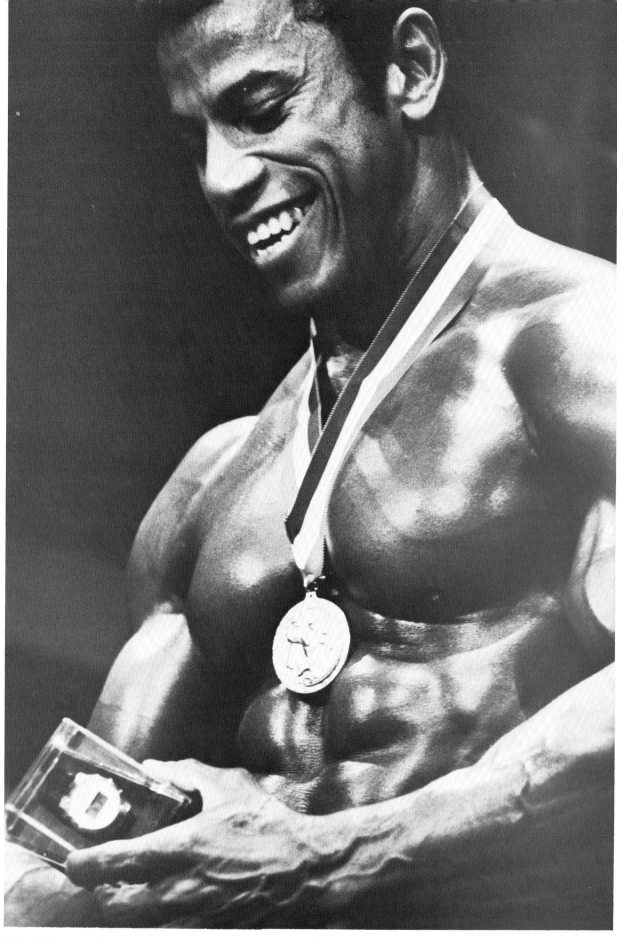

Chris Dickerson enjoys the reward of having championship instincts.

2

The Weider Instinctive Training Principle

"The Weider Instinctive Training Principle is the master training principle," said **Roy Callender** (Pro Mr. Universe). "Without first having mastered instinctive training ability, you won't be able to evaluate the effect of various other principles on your own unique body. To a great degree, you will live or die as a competitive bodybuilder according to how thoroughly you have mastered instinctive training ability and how well you put this knowledge into practice in developing your own unique training philosophy."

Roy Callender has accurately presented the value of the Weider Instinctive Training Principle. It is, indeed, the master principle in bodybuilding training. It also is an advanced training principle that can require several years to completely master.

I firmly believe that beginning bodybuilders should stick consistently to a basic training program. Trying to copy the training philosophies of IFBB pro bodybuilders too early invariably leads to a severely overtrained body, and hence to failure in our great sport. Initially, you need to learn how to do the exercises prop-

erly, develop a degree of physical power, and accustom your body to regular high-intensity training.

It's only later that the instinctive training principle comes into play. You can only go so far as a bodybuilder when you stick to someone else's system of training. A true champion needs to determine whether he should train every day or follow a double-split routine, what time of the day to work out, how forced reps affect his physical development, and so on. To become a great champion, you *must* understand your body and what works best for you. And every successful bodybuilder has learned to do this.

Although there are general physiological principles that all bodybuilders share as they build larger and stronger muscles, individual bodies do not react consistently to each principle. Unfortunately, I discovered early on during my involvement with bodybuilding that every one of my pupils reacted differently to a particular training program or technique. As a result, while I have been able to formulate a number of training principles to give you guidelines as you learn how to train, I am unable to predict how your body will react to each training stimulus.

A casual examination of several training articles in *Muscle & Fitness* magazine will quickly convince you of the variety of training philosophies followed by the IFBB bodybuilding superstars. Mike Mentzer thrives on short, high-intensity workouts featuring forced reps and retro-gravity reps. But, what works well for Mike Mentzer may not work at all for Chris Dickerson, and what builds a great physique for Chris won't necessarily work equally well for you.

As I wrote in *Bodybuilding: The Weider Approach:* "The essence of serious bodybuilding is the **Experiment.** Bodybuilding is a continually ongoing group of experiments, in which you try technique after technique in your bodylab, to determine what will work best to build muscle on your unique body. . . . As you experiment with various bodybuilding techniques, exercises and routines, replace what isn't working . . . with the exercises, body part routines, and techniques that you have discovered to work best for you. . . . Only **you** can tell what works and doesn't work in your body. No one can climb into your body and do this for you."

Ultimately, you alone must bear responsibility for making your own bodybuilding decisions and then live with the consequences of those decisions. I can only advise you on the probable results of the entire spectrum of bodybuilding techniques and practices. In the end, you must give each technique, exercise, and routine a trial and evaluation.

Every successful bodybuilder has learned to interpret the sometimes subtle messages his body is sending to him 24 hours a day. Knowing how to tune in to these biofeedback signals and interpreting them correctly is an example of mastery of the Weider Instinctive Training Principle. And possessing good instinctive training ability is invaluable to a serious bodybuilder, because it saves him a great deal of time and energy that might have ordinarily

been wasted in hit-and-miss experiments with the gamut of training techniques, routines, and bodybuilding exercises.

As Bill Reynolds and Ken Sprague note in their excellent training manual, *The Gold's Gym Book of Bodybuilding* (Contemporary, 1983): "The only way to develop an accurate training instinct is to monitor the biofeedback signals that your body gives you. These signals can be as obvious as a great muscle pump from a particular set or as a good psychological response to a new training technique.

"Muscle pump is probably the biofeedback signal that most bodybuilders monitor. Around Gold's Gym you constantly hear Lou Ferrigno or someone else saying, 'Wow, I really got a good pump in my biceps with the routine I'm on!' And a good pump (a tight, blood-congested feeling in a muscle) is a reliable signal that you've trained a particular muscle group optimally."

There are numerous types of biofeedback that will be obvious to you and will give you very clear messages once you tune in to them. A good example of this is muscle soreness following a stiff workout. As Lou Ferrigno has said, "You want your muscles to be a little stiff and sore to the touch, but having very sore muscles a day after training means you've pushed too hard in a workout. Press your fingers into a muscle to test how sore it is. If you feel sharp pain, your muscles are too sore.

"The secret to bodybuilding in general, and to instinctive training in particular, is a willingness to learn from experience. Sure, it's good to go for a full pump in each working muscle group, but pushing past this point is deleterious to the muscles. If you go too far in a workout, you'll lose your pump, a sure sign that you've done too much. Do just enough to achieve a maximum pump in each muscle group, and then move on to work your next body part.

"Working for a deep growth burn in the muscles is another positive biofeedback signal that your body will send you. Going for this burn every workout guarantees you a maximum growth stimulus from a work-

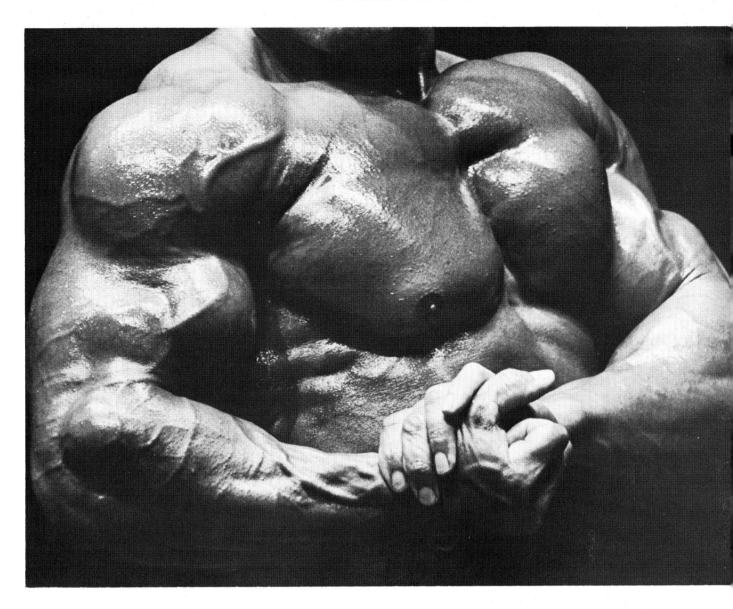

out. Try to feel a maximum growth burn on only the final set or two of each exercise, however. Going too deeply into a growth burn can turn off your mind and body to training. For some bodybuilders, it's just too painful to go for a deep burn on every set!"

Another good biofeedback signal is an increase in the exercise poundage you do on a particular movement. There is a direct linear relationship between the amount of weight you handle in a particular movement and the mass of those muscles that are activated by that exercise. Simply put, the stronger your muscles are, the larger they will be.

Ordinarily, your training poundages will improve rather slowly. Over a longer period of time, however, they will be markedly evident. For this reason, as well as a few others, maintaining an accurate training diary is very helpful when attempting to master the Weider Instinctive Training Principle. You can leaf back through your diary and visually note progress patterns and advances in your training weights. These can later be correlated with the types of training techniques you were using at various times, thereby revealing which work best for you.

I have compiled a very nice *Muscle & Fitness Training Diary* (Contemporary,

1982), which you can use to record accurate notes on your training. Or, you can use a looseleaf notebook to record such observations.

As you maintain your training log, you should periodically refer back to your notes. This will provide you a clear indication of which training techniques, exercises, and routines give you the best results. Without precise records in your training and nutritional log, it's difficult at first to make these decisions. With such detailed diary notes, you can more quickly master the Weider Instinctive Training Principle.

At the lower levels of your bodybuilding involvement, records of your body weight and body measurements can give you valuable clues to whether you are making good progress. As you become more advanced, however, these measurements will be of less value. Body weight and measurements do not reveal the relative quality of your muscular development, while photos will do so quite efficiently.

Again, quoting Reynolds and Sprague: "There are tactile and visual factors that can also improve your training instinct. You can test your muscle density (hardness) simply by feeling each muscle group from time to time. Greater muscle density indicates that your training and dietary techniques are successful. It's also easy to see improvements in your physique in various poses in front of a mirror."

The following is a list of several other biofeedback signals that you should continually monitor as you progress as a bodybuilder:

1. The "feel" of an exercise (your perception of particular muscles being strongly stressed by the weight you are using).
2. Presence or lack of joint pains.
3. Nervousness, jumpiness, irritability.
4. Chronic fatigue.
5. An inability to sleep soundly.
6. Hunger.
7. Feeling of physical power.

You should also consider subconscious sources of biofeedback.

Frank Zane (Mr. Olympia 1977–78–79): "Successful bodybuilding depends on expansion of awareness into particular areas. A great deal of information is being fed to you unconciously. You receive clues from the subconcious mind all of the time, and a bodybuilder who shuts off his unconscious mind to live only in the conscious side of his life misses more than half of the input he *could* receive. The unconscious mind is the source of all creativity. If you disregard this in your mental approach to bodybuilding, you will not develop a unique physique. Remain open for ways to improve your physique. Don't feel that you know everything there is to know about bodybuilding and get locked up in your own ego."

There are several ways in which you can open your mind to unconscious feedback signals. Initially, you need only resolve to maintain an open mind, which will in turn open up your conscious mind to stimuli it would never notice otherwise. Later, you can use hypnosis and various meditation techniques to further reveal the subconscious biofeedback signals that you would normally fail to recognize.

Implicit in the use of the Weider Instinctive Training Principle in evaluating various training techniques, exercises and routines is a thorough knowledge of bodybuilding training and nutrition. You should read every book and magazine on bodybuilding and related sports you can collect in an effort to further advance your knowledge of the sport.

I also firmly believe that you should carefully study science and technical books which might include information that has a bearing on your approach to bodybuilding. Some of the subjects that you should study are anatomy, kinesiology, biomechanics, exercise physiology, biochemistry, and psychology.

In addition to an instinctive approach to training, you can also use the Weider Instinctive Training Principle in developing a diet plan suited to your unique body.

Reynolds and Sprague: "Nutritional instinct is a little easier to develop than

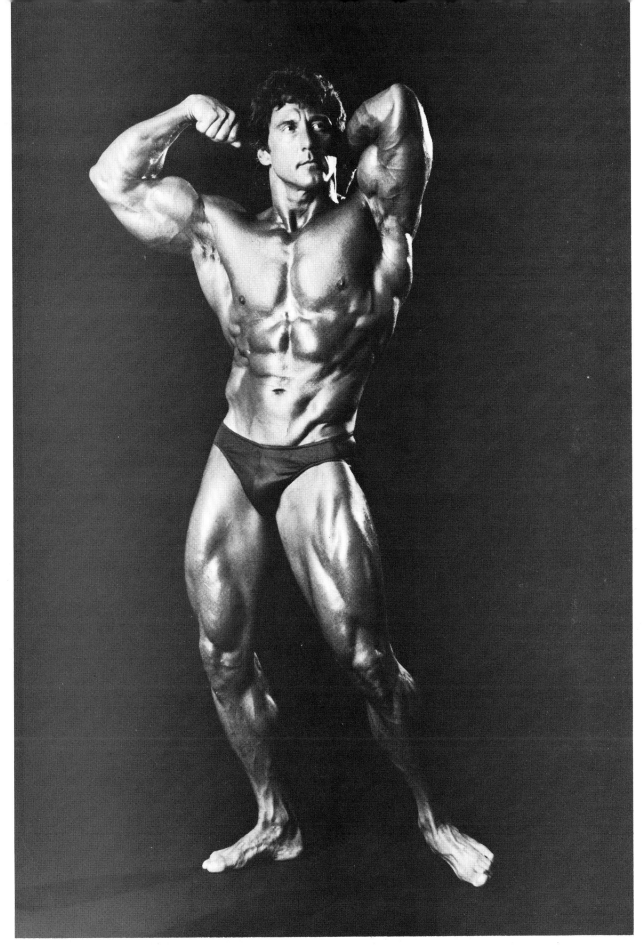

Frank Zane.

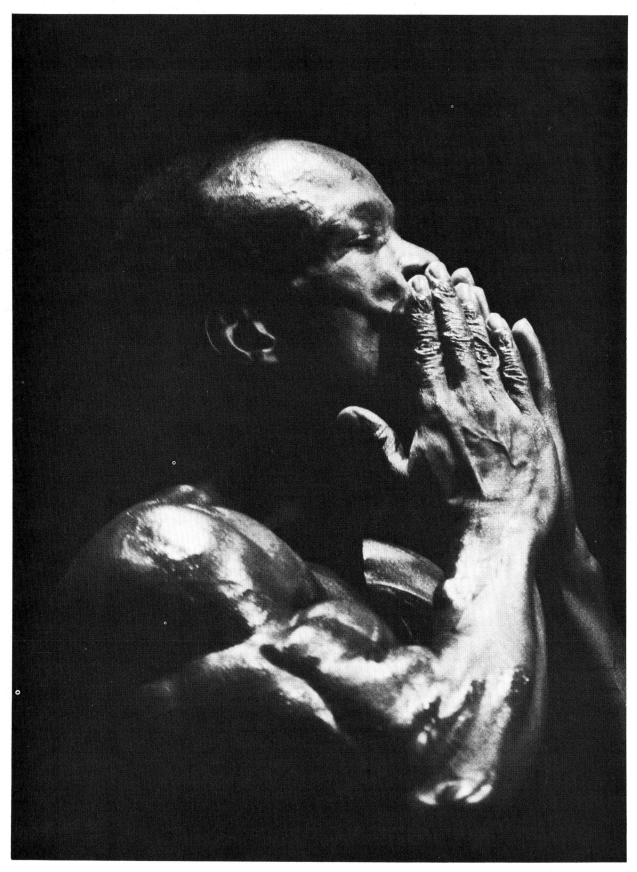

The joy of Albert Beckles.

training instinct. What foods make you fatter? Are there certain foods that bloat your body with water? Which foods have you eaten that cut you up quickly? Is a low-calorie diet or a low-carbohydrate diet best for cutting up your body? Do certain supplements give you greater training energy? Simply answering these questions through a series of dietary experiments will quickly give you a good nutritional instinct.

"Within a year or two of monitoring your body's biofeedback signals you'll develop a feel for what does and doesn't work in your unique bodylab. At that point you will have achieved true training instinct."

This may be somewhat difficult to believe, but once you have developed optimum training instinct, you can actually determine how valuable a new technique, exercise, or routine is to you within a day or two.

Albert Beckles (Professional World Champion): "When I inject some new technique into my routine, I can feel how it works on my muscles almost immediately. If it feels a certain way, I know it's going to help improve my physique. But if it feels another way, I know it's worthless and immediately reject it. It may take a year or two to develop this type of judgment, but it *will* come for you. And once you have it, you can take better advantage of every opportunity to become a champion. Instinctive training ability is the most valuable weapon in a bodybuilder's arsenal."

Once mastered, the instinctive principle allows you to be in harmony with the natural up and down energy cycles through which your body goes. No one feels highly energetic very frequently, but when you *are* bursting with energy you should take advantage of it by training long, hard, and heavy. But, pushing this hard when you are on an energy downswing will result in a progress-slowing injury or an overtrained condition.

If your instinctive training ability has been finely honed, you will be able to easily identify your up and down days, matching the intensity of your workouts to sync with your energy levels. This way, you will always train as intensely as possible, but still far enough within your abilities that you can avoid injuries and the chance of overtraining.

In conclusion, I can't stress strongly enough how valuable the Weider Instinctive Training Principle can be to a serious competitive bodybuilder. You can make or break yourself by how well or poorly you master the Instinctive Training Principle. Indeed, the Weider Instinctive Training Principle is the master principle in bodybuilding training and diet.

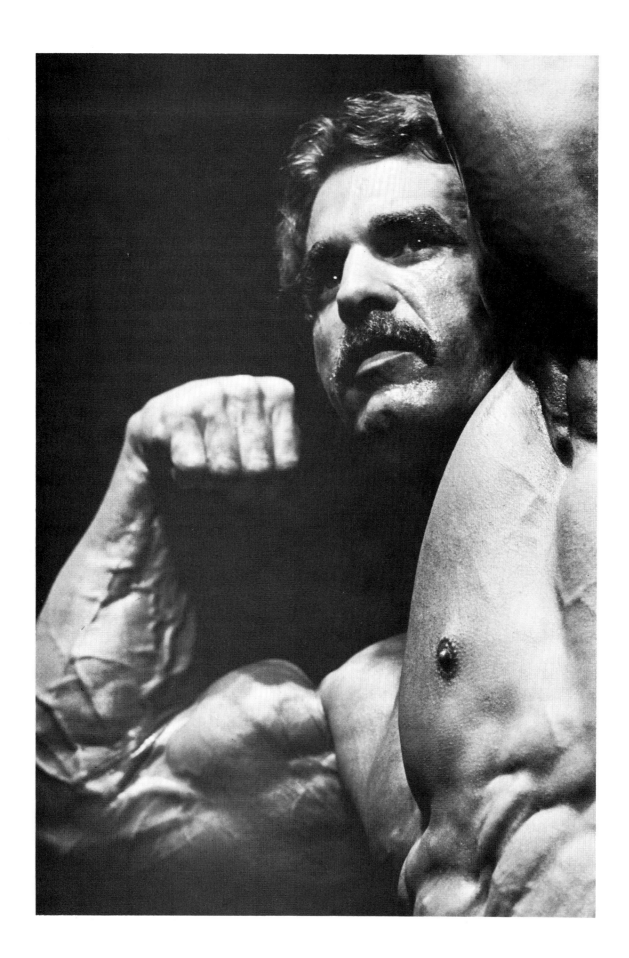

3

Weider Training Intensification Techniques

Most of the Weider training principles discussed in this chapter were previously discussed in my earlier book, *Bodybuilding: The Weider Approach* (Chicago: Contemporary Books, Inc., 1981—available in a softcover edition for $8.95). A few of the Weider Training Intensification Principles covered in this chapter, however, have not been previously discussed.

Whenever you encounter a discussion of some previously presented training principle in this chapter, you will note that I have attacked its discussion from a slightly different angle. In most cases my discussion will be much longer in this book than in the previous one but still I could devote an entire chapter to discussing each principle. Due to space limitations, however, my discussion of the Weider Training Intensification Principles must be kept somewhat brief.

When it has been possible to do so in this book, I have used the exact words of a wide variety of IFBB superstar bodybuilders to further clarify and validate most of the training principles discussed. To a man, all of the top bodybuilders heartily endorse and faithfully follow the Weider system of training.

QUALITY TRAINING

The Weider Quality Training Principle is a vital tool in the arsenal of any serious bodybuilder during a precontest training cycle. Quality training consists of progressively reducing the average rest interval between sets from approximately 60–90 seconds during the off-season down to as little as 15–20 seconds at the end of a precontest cycle.

The Weider Quality Training Principle works hand-in-glove with a tight precontest diet to bring out the maximum degree of muscularity and muscle density in a competing bodybuilder's physique. Inevitably, however, a precontest diet results in lower energy levels. And combined with the drastically shortened rest intervals between sets, this results in quite a drop in exercise poundages.

Tim Belknap (Mr. America): "Like every other modern champion bodybuilder, I use the Weider Quality Training Principle for

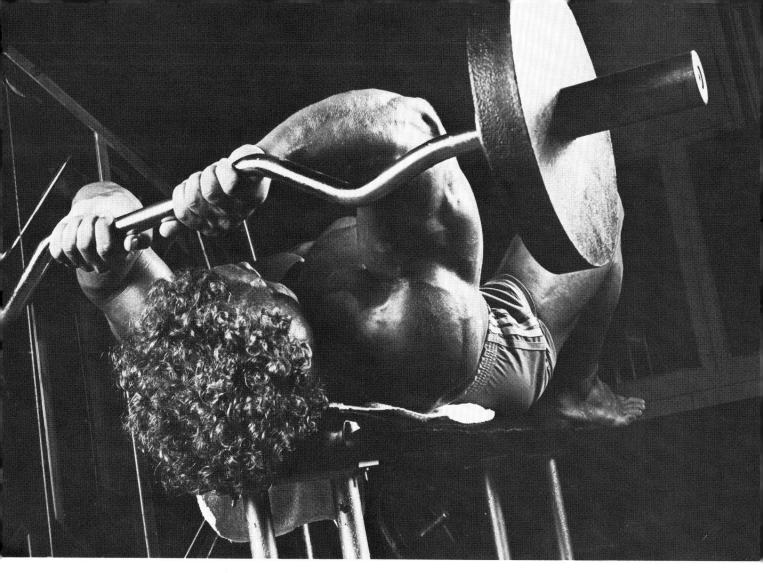

Tim Belknap pumping his triceps.

8—10 weeks prior to a competition. I also follow a low-calorie diet, sometimes eating as little as 800—900 calories per day. Naturally quality training and such a tight diet combine to drastically reduce my workout weights. In the off-season I use 500+ pounds for reps in the Bench Press, but usually I can't handle much over 350 pounds in the same movement prior to a competition. Still, I endeavor to keep my exercise weights as high as possible. By combining quality training with my precontest diet, I can step onstage at a competition with huge muscle mass, but at the same time I can appear ripped to the bone. And, that's a difficult combination to beat!"

Robby Robinson (Mr. America, Mr. World, Mr. Universe, and winner of several IFBB professional bodybuilding titles):

"The *only* way to achieve the type of muscle mass and deep cuts necessary to win titles today is to use quality training during a precontest cycle. In the off-season I train with very heavy weights and rest for 60—90 seconds between sets. But prior to a contest, I shorten my average rest interval to approximately 20 seconds. I use lighter weights, of course, but the intensity is still there because I also use continuous tension and peak contraction reps on each exercise. You have to train like a rabid dog when following the Weider Quality Training Principle, but it'll get you into great shape."

SUPERSETS, TRISETS, GIANT SETS

"One of the best ways to effectively reduce the average rest interval between sets when quality training," states **Ken Waller** (Mr. America, Mr. World, Mr. Universe, and a Mr. Olympia class winner), "is to use supersets, trisets, and giant sets in your workouts. Since you rest minimally between the exercises in these groups of two, three, or more movements, you can easily reduce the length of your average rest interval between sets."

The most basic type of superset consists of a grouping of two exercises for antagonistic muscle groups (e.g., biceps + triceps, quadriceps + hamstrings, or pectorals + lats) with as little rest as possible between the exercises. This superset is followed by a rest interval of 30–60 seconds (depending on whether you are in a precontest or an off-season training cycle) and another run through the superset.

Here are several examples of this most basic form of superset:

- Biceps + Triceps = Barbell Curls + Lying Triceps Extensions
- Quadriceps + Hamstrings = Leg Extension + Leg Curls
- Pecs + Lats = Bench Presses + Chins
- Biceps + Triceps = Incline Dumbbell Curls + Pulley Pushdowns
- Pecs + Lats = Flyes + Lat Machine Pulldowns

Pat Neve (Mr. USA, Mr. America class winner): "I've won the Best Arms trophy in five national-level bodybuilding competitions primarily because I superset my biceps and triceps exercises to increase the intensity of my arm workouts. Even a relatively inexperienced bodybuilder can successfully superset his biceps and triceps exercises. This should be the first area in which you experiment with supersets."

A second—and much more intense—form of superset involves grouping two exercises for the same body part and doing them with no rest between exercises. Here are several examples of this type of superset:

- Calves = Seated Calf Raise + Standing Calf Raise
- Thighs (quads) = Leg Extensions + Leg Presses

- Thighs (hamstrings) = Stiff-Leg Deadlifts + Leg Curls
- Lats = Seated Pulley Rowing + Lat Machine Pulldowns
- Traps = Upright Rowing + Barbell Shrugs
- Pecs = Bench Presses + Flyes
- Delts = Seated Press Behind Neck + Side Laterals
- Triceps = Lying Triceps Extensions + Pulley Pushdowns
- Biceps = Seated Dumbbell Curls + Standing Barbell Curls

Tom Platz (Mr. Universe): "When a body part has been stubborn in the past, I have had good success in nudging it into growth again by supersetting two exercises for it. This is a very intense type of training, and as a result it is ordinarily quite productive. To give you an example, I have had good success in developing my upper pectorals by supersetting Dumbbell Incline Presses with Incline Dumbbell Flyes."

Moving up one rung on a ladder of training intensity from supersets, we come to trisets, which are groupings of three exercises done with no rest between sets. I originally designed the Weider Trisets Training Principle for use with muscles with three or more areas that need work, such as the deltoids, and which require greater-than-normal training intensity.

The three areas of the deltoids that require work are the muscle group's three heads: the anterior (front), medial (side), and posterior (rear) heads. Here is a triset that works all three of these heads:

- Military Press (anterior head)
- Side Laterals (medial head)
- Bent Laterals (posterior head)

For some large and complex muscle groups, a triset can be used to intensify training strictly for that muscle group. As an example, the front thighs are a large muscle group, and here is a tough triset that you can use for your quadriceps muscles: **Leg Press** + **Leg Extension** + **Squats.**

Casey Viator (history's youngest Mr. America winner): "I've used a lot of trisets

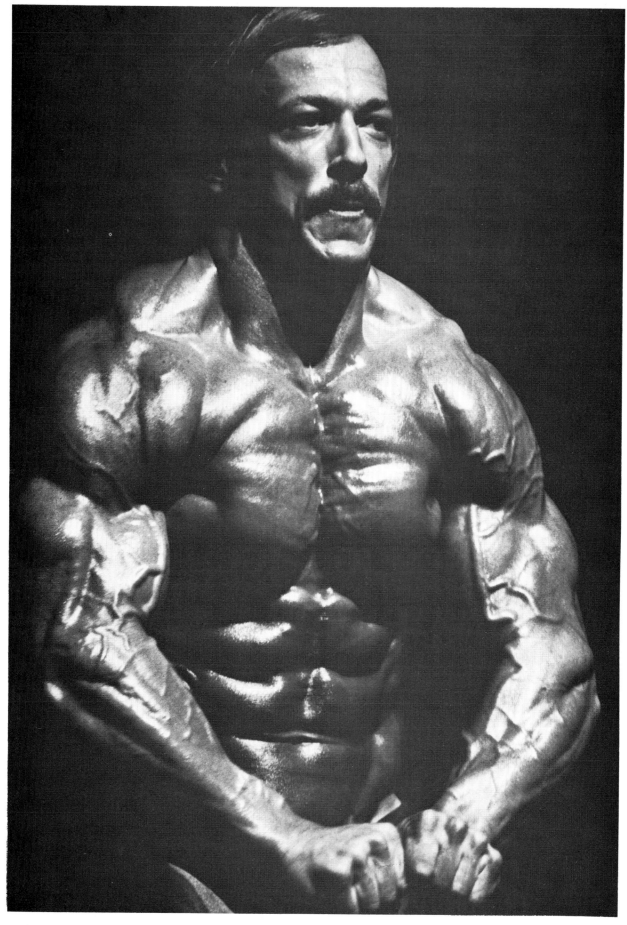

Casey Viator.

in my training. As an example, I've used a thigh triset of Leg Presses, Leg Extensions, and Squats. One or two such trisets is all I ever need to do for my quadriceps. Averaging 15–20 reps per set, I have used 750 pounds on Leg Presses, 320 pounds for Leg Extensions, and 525 pounds in the Squat during use of this triset. It's rugged training, but produces great results because of the great intensity of the triset."

Moving up the ladder of intensity from trisets we come to giant sets, or groupings of 4–6 exercises for either a single body part or two antagonistic muscle groups. The greater the number of exercises in a giant set, the greater the degree of intensity that it has. And, a giant set consisting of exercises exclusively for one muscle group is much more intense than one including movements for two body parts.

The following is an example of a four-exercise giant set for the pectorals: **Incline Dumbbell Presses + Cross-Bench Dumbbell Pullovers + Parallel Bar Dips + Cable Crossovers.**

And here is an example of a five-exercise giant set for the back muscles: **Seated Pulley Rowing + Dumbbell Shrugs + Chins Behind Neck + Hyperextensions + Front Lat Machine Pulldowns.**

Robby Robinson: "In my training, I frequently use a giant set for my pecs and lats. It consists of the following six exercises: **Bench Press** (pecs), **Front Chins** (lats), **Incline Dumbbell Press** (pecs), **Seated Pulley Rowing** (lats), **Parallel Bar Dips** (pecs), and **Lat Machine Pulldown Behind Neck** (lats).

"It was my experience that this giant set pec–lat routine did a great deal to improve my torso development. I would rest about 1½–2 minutes between giant sets in the off-season when I was using this routine, and allowed as little as 45–60 seconds between giant sets prior to a competition. Giant sets are so intense that they're not for every bodybuilder, but for experienced men like myself, they work very well in producing quality muscle tissue."

"Finally, here is an example of a six-exercise giant set for the chest structure: **Incline Machine Press** (upper pecs) + **Pec Deck Flyes** (inner pecs) + **Parallel Bar Dips** (lower and outer pecs) + **Cross-Bench Pullovers** (rib cage, general pecs) + **Incline Flyes** (upper pecs) + **Cable Crossovers** (general pectoral muscularity).

"Echoing Robby Robinson, I must be very experienced and in good physical condition to successfully use the Weider Giant Sets Training Principle. But giant setting a body part is very high-intensity exercise that works any large and complex muscle group to the maximum."

PREEXHAUSTION

By comparing the relative size and work output potential of the body's various muscle groups, you will immediately note that your torso muscle groups (the lats, traps, delts, and pecs) are quite a bit larger and stronger than your upper arm muscles (the triceps and biceps). As a result, your arm muscles generally weaken and fail before the torso muscle groups when you do basic exercises such as Bench Presses, Military Presses, Upright Rows, and Seat Pulley Rows for the torso muscle groups. And, because of this weakness in the arm muscles, your torso groups are often trained with less intensity than they should be.

By using the preexhaustion method, however, you can circumvent this weakness of your upper arm muscles and train your torso groups much more intensely than you can under normal circumstances. Preexhaustion involves using a superset (or, occasionally, a triset) of an isolation movement for a muscle group with a basic exercise for the same muscle complex.

In this kind of superset the first exercise fatigues the muscle being worked, but without also tiring the arm muscles. The isolation exercise, then, effectively makes the arm muscles momentarily weaker than the torso group being trained. Therefore, when a basic movement is immediately supersetted with the isolation exercise, you can work the torso muscles involved to the limit with the basic movement before the arms would fail.

It's essential when using this preexhaustion superset that you not rest at all between exercises. As you will learn in greater detail later in this chapter (the Weider Rest–Pause Training Principle), a fatigued muscle will recuperate very quickly when it's allowed to rest. As a result, too long of a rest interval between exercises in a preexhaustion superset negates the preexhaust effect.

The following are examples of preexhaustion supersets that you can try in your own training for a variety of body parts:

- Pectorals (upper) = Incline Flyes + Incline Presses
- Pectorals (lower) = Decline Flyes + Decline Presses
- Pectorals (general) = Flat-Bench Flyes + Bench Presses
- Deltoids = Side Laterals + Press Behind Neck
- Trapezius = Shrugs + Upright Rows
- Latissimus Dorsi = Pullovers + Chins

For large muscle groups (e.g., the thighs) you may profit more from trisetting a basic exercise, an isolation movement, and another basic exercise for that body part. As an example, one which Casey Viator mentioned earlier, your front thighs can profit from a superset of Leg Extensions and Squats, but the muscle group will benefit even more from a triset of Leg Presses, Leg Extensions, and Squats.

TRAINING TO FAILURE

The concept of "training to failure" on some or all of the sets that you perform in a workout has been related to the Weider system of training since its inception, because many Weider Training Principles allow a bodybuilder to actually push a fatigued muscle *past* its normal failure point. Still, the actual process of training to failure has not reached great popularity among high-level bodybuilders until just recently.

Regardless of the exercise employed, training to failure amounts to continuing a set until the muscles that move the weight are so fatigued that you cannot complete a full repetition of the movement in strict form. After you have put in five or six weeks breaking in your muscles to the heavy work of bodybuilding training, you should go to failure on at least one set per body part. And you should gradually add to the number of sets you take to failure, until most of your workout amounts to sets taken either to the point of failure or past that point.

Tom Platz sums up the concept of training to failure quite well: "Once I'm fully warmed up, I keep pushing on absolutely every set in my workout until I can't move the weight even an inch. And it's only when I have pushed a muscle momentarily to failure like this several times in a workout that I feel I've gotten the muscle growth stimulus I've been after. Only then do I *know* that my muscles will increase in mass and power from that workout."

CHEATING

Up to this point, you may have been told never to use extraneous body movement to "cheat" a weight up in an exercise. This is a good practice for beginning and intermediate bodybuilders to follow, because they invariably tend to cheat to make an exercise *easier* to do. An advanced bodybuilder, however, intelligently uses the Weider Cheating Training Principle to make an exercise *harder* on the muscles involved.

Properly exploited, the cheating principle is one of the easiest ways in which to push a tiring muscle group past the point of failure in an exercise set. And you needn't have a training partner standing by to assist you in using the Weider Cheating Training Principle to good advantage in your training.

To illustrate how to cheat correctly, let's assume that you are doing Barbell Curls with 100 pounds. Using this weight you are able to do six full reps in strict form before your seventh repetition stalls out less than halfway up. All that missing this seventh repetition means is that you can't, at that precise moment, do a Curl with 100 pounds, since your biceps muscles are too fatigued to do so. In all likelihood you would still be able to curl 95 pounds, or at worst, 90 pounds. So, you are faced with having to somehow instantly make your barbell 5–10 pounds lighter, and one way to do this is through cheating.

Using *only enough* extraneous body movement to swing the barbell past your sticking point, cheat on a rep of your barbell curls by swinging the bar up with torso movement. Be sure, however, that you complete the repetition in good form. And once you complete this repetition, lower the bar slowly back to the starting point to take full advantage of the negative or downward part of the exercise. (For more detailed information on negative reps, please see the section on the Retro-Gravity Principle later in this chapter.)

You will profit most from doing two or three cheating reps at the end of a set. Doing more than three is generally of little value because your muscles are fatiguing so rapidly that it becomes difficult to judge how much of a "cheat" you must use to get the weight up in an extra rep.

Chris Dickerson (all-time IFBB pro bodybuilding victories leader and 1982 Mr. Olympia): "While I personally prefer to use very strict form in most of my sets of an exercise—particularly in a precontest cycle—cheating can be very valuable in helping to increase muscle mass in the off-season. I suggest doing at least 5–6 reps in a movement quite strictly before loosening up your form for 2–3 cheating reps."

FORCED REPS

If you have a training partner available, you can conveniently do forced reps, a very efficient method of pushing your fatigued muscles well past the normal point of failure. When you use forced reps, your partner will pull up on the middle of your barbell or other apparatus just enough to remove the 5–10 pounds weight that your fatigued muscles couldn't handle on their own. And, a training partner can do this

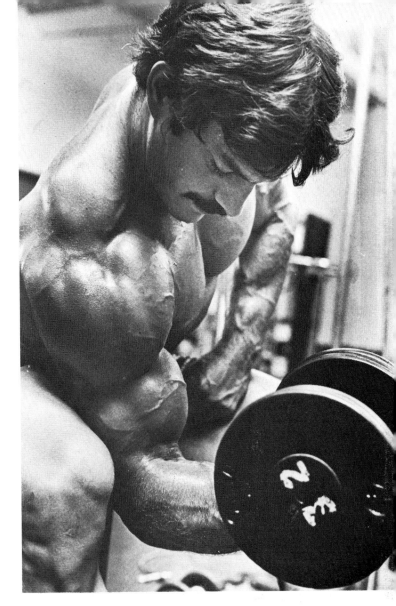

Mike Mentzer grunts out forced reps.

more efficiently than you can when using the cheating principle.

One of my best known pupils, **Mike Mentzer** (Mr. America, IFBB Mr. Universe, and runner-up in the 1979 Mr. Olympia competition), uses forced reps extensively in his training. Mike has even worked out a method by which he gives himself forced reps on one-arm exercises. In Dumbbell Concentration Curls, for example, he uses two or three fingers of his free hand to press up on the wrist of his working hand sufficiently to grunt out two or three forced reps.

Casey Viator (Mr. America, Mr. USA, and winner of two IFBB pro bodybuilding titles): "To build a maximum degree of muscle mass in the off-season, I make extensive use of the Weider Forced Reps Training Principle. If I don't consistently push my muscles well past their limit twice per week, I can't carry a maximum degree of muscle mass onstage at my next competition. And forced reps on basic exercises are my primary method of pushing my muscles this hard. I do two or three forced reps on virtually every exercise that I perform in the off-season. And, I'm so strong on the basic movements that I have to use two training partners to help me do my forced reps."

RETRO-GRAVITY REPS

By using the Weider Retro-Gravity Training Principle (often called "negative reps" or "negatives") you can push your muscles even further past the point of failure than you can through forced reps. Exercise physiologists have discovered that a bodybuilder or other strength athlete can develop more strength and muscle mass in the negative (lowering) phase of a movement than is possible in the positive (raising) phase if he goes about it correctly. Retro-gravity reps take advantage of this discovery.

To most easily utilize retro-gravity reps, you can simply emphasize the negative phase of a movement by lowering your barbell, dumbbell(s), or other apparatus more slowly than normally. Ordinarily, you should take 3–5 seconds to lower the weight, so during a negative emphasized repetition, take 10–15 seconds to lower the weight. You will quickly find that negatively emphasized reps fatigue your muscles very quickly, and you won't be able to do the same number of negative emphasized reps as you can when you perform your repetitions with a normal cadence.

In doing pure retro-gravity reps you must thoroughly warm up and then have one or two training partners to lift a weight 10%–20% heavier than you can normally handle in an exercise to the top point of the movement. Then, you slowly lower the weight down to the bottom point of the

exercise, strongly resisting the downward momentum of the weight. Lastly, your partner(s) lift the weight back up for other retro-gravity reps. You can get quite a bit out of doing one set of 4–6 retro-gravity reps each week.

Of course you will soon learn that it's difficult to secure training partners willing enough to sacrifice some of their workout time and energy to help you with regular retro-gravity reps. Therefore, you must learn how to give yourself negative reps from time to time.

If you train on machines such as a leg extension apparatus, you can easily give yourself retro-gravity reps. To accomplish this you simply use two legs to raise the weight to the finish point of the movement, remove one leg and lower the effectively doubled weight using the muscles of one thigh to resist it. By alternating legs this way, you can give yourself as many retro-gravity reps as you desire.

Using the foregoing method, you can give yourself negative reps for most of your body's major muscle groups. Some of the more obvious exercises on which you can use this method are Leg Extensions, Leg Curls, Leg Presses, Standing and Seated Calf Machine Toe Raises, Machine Bench Presses, Machine Shrugs, Machine Overhead Presses, and Seated Pulley Rowing.

A training partner can give you forced retro-gravity reps by pushing *down* on the barbell, dumbbell(s), or other apparatus that you are using to do an exercise. Once you are thoroughly warmed up, such forced negatives are an excellent way to intensify virtually any exercise. Try them on your Standing Barbell Curls and Lying Barbell Triceps Extensions for a couple of workouts, and you'll notice that your upper arm muscles become very sore, a sure sign that you have stressed them much more intensely than usual.

A final method of using retro-gravity reps has been outlined by **Ray Mentzer** (Mr. America, Mr. USA): "When my brother Mike and I train together we do maximum-intensity sets for each muscle group at least once per week. To illustrate our method, let's say that I'm doing Barbell Preacher Curls. With 180 pounds on the bar I can do 4–5 full, positive-and-negative reps to failure. Mike then helps me to do 2–3 forced reps, which almost annihilates my biceps. But I don't stop there. Mike then lifts the barbell to the top point of the movement for me so I can do 2–3 fully negative reps to push my biceps even further past the limit. Doing such maximum-intensity sets once per week has allowed me to develop an incredible degree of hypertrophy in my muscles."

BURNS

Another way to push your muscles past the point of failure, without the assistance of a training partner, is to use the Weider Burns Training Principle. Burns are quick, short reps at some point along the full range of motion of an exercise, but usually at the beginning or the end of the movement. Done at the end of a set—when the working muscles are already very fatigued—these reps build up huge quantities of fatigue toxins and evoke their characteristic burning sensation in muscles.

Usually burns are done over a two- or three-inch range of motion, and their cadence is quite rapid, only slightly slower than the cadence of skipping rope at a normal pace. The reps are somewhat bouncy in character, and you can initially practice them at the stretched position of Toe Raises on a standing calf machine.

On your Toe Raises, do a full set of 10–15 reps to failure. Then, bounce up and down for 10–20 quick partial reps of burns. Doing these burns will force your fatigued muscles to keep on working hard well past the point of normal failure.

Andreas Cahling (IFBB Mr. International and a top professional bodybuilder) is one of the leading exponents of the use of burns in hard bodybuilding training. Andreas recently stated, "When I am training at maximum intensity, I do burns on one or two sets of virtually every exercise I perform in my workouts. They are a convenient way of pushing a muscle group past the failure

threshold without requiring the use of a training partner. I simply do as many full reps as possible and then perform 10–15 burns at either the start or finish position of each movement. Without using either burns or forced reps, I can't have optimum muscle density onstage at a competition."

DESCENDING SETS

The Weider Descending Sets Training Principle is another way to keep pushing your muscles past the normal point of failure. In a way, they are somewhat like using forced reps, since in descending sets you utilize a lighter and lighter weight each few reps. But rather than having a training partner lift up on the weight, you have two partners actually strip plates off the barbell as your muscles grow tired. And on many exercises you can provide these changes in weight by grasping steadily lighter dumbbells during descending sets.

Let's use the Barbell Curl and two training partners to illustrate this training principle in action. Without using the collars on the barbell, load on a weight with which you can do approximately 6–7 strict repetitions with the Barbell Curl. Be sure that you load on a combination of five- and ten-pound plates so you can easily strip five or ten pounds off each side—or a total of either ten or twenty pounds—two (or perhaps three) times.

Grasp the barbell with the initial full load and stand erect with it, your partners standing ready at the ends of the bar. Do your 6–7 strict reps to failure, whereupon your partners immediately strip a total of 10–20 pounds, whatever seems most appropriate. With the reduced weight you should do as many reps as possible, say another 3–4. Again the weight is quickly reduced for 3–4 more reps. Usually two weight reductions will be sufficient, but with exercises for large muscle groups, you may need to reduce the weight three times in using descending sets optimally.

Bertil Fox (Mr. Britain, Mr. Europe, Mr. World, and Mr. Universe) is a great booster of the Weider Descending Sets Training

Principle. As Bertil recently explained, "I use descending sets for at least one basic exercise per muscle group. Let's take Seated Presses Behind Neck for the deltoids as an example. Over five or six warm-up sets I work up to 310–320 pounds for 7–8 reps. Then I load on a peak weight of 330–340 pounds in such a manner that I can have 40–50 pounds stripped off the bar for three descending sets.

"Next, I sit down on a bench that braces my back with my torso in a perfectly upright position. My training partners lift the barbell off the rack so I can position my grip correctly on the bar, then rest it across my traps behind my neck. From there I do 5–6 good, solid reps to the failure point, have the weight reduced for 4–6 more reps, have another reduction for 4–5 additional reps, and have a final weight reduction for 3–4 delt-blowing reps!"

Bertil Fox.

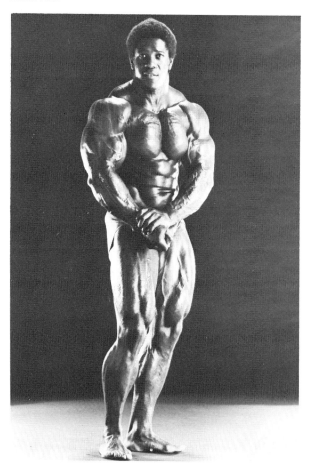

REST–PAUSE TRAINING

It is a physiological fact that fatigued muscles recuperate very quickly with a minimum rest interval following heavy exercise. Indeed, a fully fatigued muscle can recoup approximately 50%–60% of its endurance and strength when given a mere 10–15 seconds of rest.

It is equally certain physiologically that the buildup of fatigue toxins prevents the working muscles from doing a high enough number of reps in some exercises to develop a maximum degree of muscle mass and power. More than 30 years ago I made an inspired connection between these two physiological facts that produced the Weider Rest–Pause Training Principle, a superadvanced producer of the ultimate in muscle mass and density.

Let's use the Incline Barbell Press as an example of how to utilize rest–pause training. Warm up thoroughly on the movement, then load up the bar with a weight you can handle for a good 2–3 reps to the failure threshold. Do the 2–3 reps and place the bar back on the rack for a 10–15-second rest pause. Immediately pick it up again and force out 1–2 more reps.

You'll probably have to quickly strip 20–30 pounds from the bar then regrasp it, all within 10–15 seconds. Do 2–3 more reps and take your 10–15-second rest pause before forcing out a final 1–2 reps. This will totally saturate your muscles with growth stimuli, and it will build very massive and powerful muscles all over your body.

Shoot for a total of 8–12 reps when doing rest–pause training. And never try to do a rest–pause workout more than once per week for each muscle group, keeping in mind the fact that your upper arm muscles work quite hard when you do your torso movements. Therefore, you might profit best from one rest–pause arm workout each two weeks. Since the rest–pause system is such super-intense work, it shouldn't be overworked, or it will lead to an overtrained state.

Mike Mentzer is an enthusiastic booster

of rest–pause training. Mike has stated, "I have made some of my best gains using rest–pause training. But I've had to be very careful to use the rest–pause method infrequently on each body part. You make such quick gains in muscle mass and power on it that it's easy to get carried away with the system. It takes an iron hand on the reins to get maximum gains with rest–pause training without actually overtraining."

MUSCLE CONFUSION

Depending on a bodybuilder's basic temperament and physical makeup, he may find that his muscles quickly grow used to a particular routine and his mind becomes bored with it very quickly. Lou Ferrigno is typical of this type of athlete, while Arnold Schwarzenegger is typical of the stoic battler who can stick to the same routine for many years and still make good progress.

In Lou's case, his mind and body become accustomed to a particular exercise routine within a week or two. Then boredom sets in and his muscles are no longer challenged by the training program. At that point, Lou's muscles fail to improve, regardless of how hard he trains them on a particular bodybuilding program.

The Weider Muscle Confusion Training Principle is tailor-made for bodybuilders like Lou Ferrigno. When you are following this principle, you are encouraged to use a particular training schedule for each body part only once. Then, the next time you train that muscle group you should move on to a new routine for it. In effect, you follow a "nonroutine routine."

Use of the Weider Muscle Confusion Training Principle keeps your mind and muscles totally off-balance, and hence they are continually forced to adapt to new stresses. Since they never know what to expect next, the muscles must keep growing in mass and power to accommodate new stresses placed on them.

Lou Ferrigno (Mr. America, Mr. International, Mr. Universe, and screen and televi-

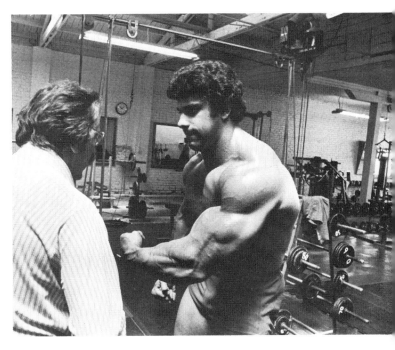

Joe Weider and Lou Ferrigno.

sion star): "To keep my individual muscle groups responding at a good speed, I never use the same training program twice. I constantly play with the order of exercises, the body angle with which each exercise is done, the actual exercises used, training poundages, sets, reps, training pace, everything. Using muscle confusion training like this keeps my mind fresh and interested in my workouts. Similarly, my muscles are unable to adapt to a specific routine, as they tend to do when I follow a set routine for a period of time. They must continually grow larger and stronger. And, *that* is what bodybuilding is all about!"

DOUBLE-SPLIT ROUTINES

As an advanced bodybuilder, you no doubt are already familiar with the various permutations of split routines that can be used in bodybuilding training. In the event that you are not, I will briefly review the Weider Split Routine Training Principle before discussing the Weider Double-Split Routine Training Principle.

After three or four months of training, you will have built your workout intensity and volume to the point where you won't have sufficient energy reserves to do justice to each muscle group when training only three days a week. Then, you must switch to a split routine and train only a part of your physique each training day.

Split Routines

The most simple split routine involves training four days per week, hitting each muscle group twice every week. Here is an example of such a four-day split routine:

Monday-Thursday	Tuesday-Friday
Chest	Back
Shoulders	Thighs
Upper Arms	Forearms
Calves-Abs	Calves-Abs

Note in the foregoing example how abdominals and calves are stressed in each workout, a total of four training sessions per week. Generally speaking, you can profitably train your abdominals six days each week. Calves can accept 4–6 workouts per week and still keep growing in mass and density.

Moving up to greater intensity, you can use a five-day split routine. On the five-day split you will again divide your body into halves, and you will train each half on alternate weekdays. Monday workouts will always be devoted to training the muscle groups that were worked only twice the previous week.

To clarify the information in the foregoing paragraph, below is an example of how a five-day split works over a three-week period. "A" and "B" have been arbitrarily assigned to represent the respective division of the body into equal groupings of body parts.

	Mon	Tue	Wed	Thu	Fri
Week 1	A	B	A	B	A
Week 2	B	A	B	A	B
Week 3	A	B	A	B	A

In terms of allowing sufficient recovery time for full recuperation between workouts, a five-day split allows less than the four-day split and more than any type of

six-day split routine. As on the four-day split routine, you can train abs and calves each workout if you like.

There are two types of six-day split routines, one in which each muscle group is trained twice per week and another in which major muscle groups are trained twice per week. The first type of six-day split is less intense than the second, and it's the type of split routine that a large number of champion bodybuilders use when gaining muscle mass and power during the off-season. And, the second type of split is frequently used when trying to harden up during a precontest cycle.

Here is an example of how the body can be divided up into three groups for the first type of six-day split routine:

Mon–Thu	Tue–Fri	Wed–Sat
Abdominals	Abdominals	Abdominals
Chest	Upper Back	Thighs
Shoulders	Biceps	Lower Back
Triceps	Forearms	Calves
Forearms	Calves	

The following is an example of the second type of six-day split routine, when each major muscle group is trained three days per week:

Mon–Wed–Fri	Tue–Thu–Sat
Abdominals	Abdominals
Chest	Thighs
Shoulders	Lower Back
Upper Back	Upper Arms
Forearms	Forearms
Calves	Calves

Prior to competition—when the volume of each workout has been greatly increased—it soon becomes difficult to complete an entire workout in one daily session. When this threshold has been reached, many bodybuilders switch to using the Weider Double-Split System Training Principle in which each day of a normal split routine is further subdivided into two workouts per day.

Double-Split Routines

Initially, you can use a double-split routine in which your major muscle groups are

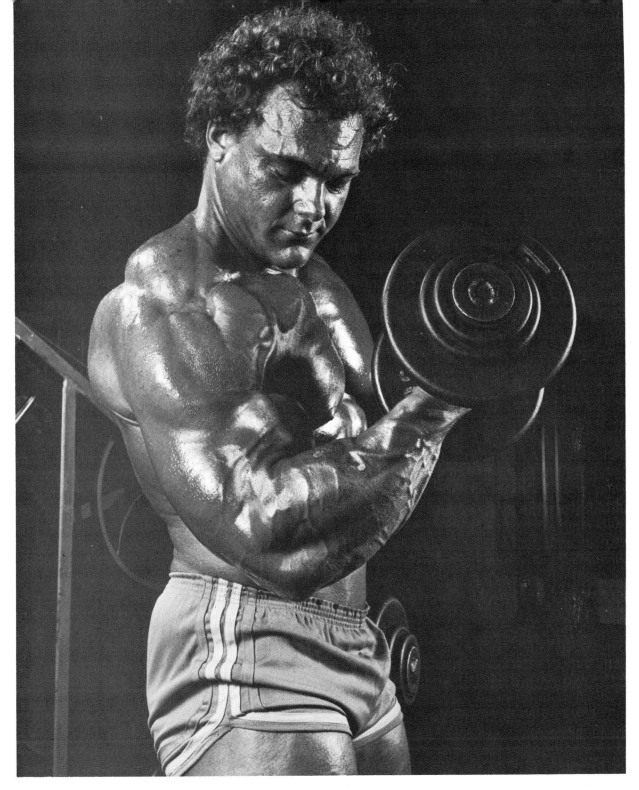

Tim Belknap.

worked in your morning session and your calves, abdominals, and forearms are blasted in an evening session. This type of double-split routine is ideal for use prior to a competition, when a much greater volume of abdominal training needs to be undertaken.

Very experienced bodybuilders can use a modified double-split routine in which they work out twice a day three days per week and only once each day on the other three training days. Here's an example of how you can split up your body for this type of modified double-split routine:

Mon-Wed-Fri (AM)

Abdominals (hard)
Chest
Back
Calves

Mon-Wed-Fri (PM)

Abdominals (easy)
Shoulders
Upper Arms
Forearms

Tue-Thu-Sat (AM or PM)

Abdominals (medium to hard)
Thighs
Forearms
Calves

Finally, in a full double-split you will actually train twice a day six days a week. Here is an example of how you can split up your body for such a full, double-split routine:

Mon-Wed-Fri (AM)

Abdominals
Chest
Shoulders

Mon-Wed-Fri (PM)

Calves
Upper Back
Biceps

Tue-Thu-Sat (AM)

Abdominals
Thighs
Forearms

Tue-Thu-Sat (PM)

Calves
Lower Back
Triceps

You won't be able to stay on a full, double-split routine very long since it's extremely strenuous. While you are on it, however, you will find that it helps greatly to achieve peak physical condition for a competition.

STAGGERED SETS

The Weider Staggered Sets Training Principle is ideal for use by bodybuilders who have many sets of relatively boring abdominal or calf training to do in their workouts. This is particularly true just prior to a competition when up to 25–30 sets of abdominal training is done each day in order to have very sharp abdominal delineation onstage.

To illustrate how to use the Weider Staggered Sets Training Principle, let's assume that you are training your chest and back muscles in a particular workout, and that you also have a total of 20 sets of abdominal training to do. Start your workout with two sets of chest training, followed by a set

of ab work, two more sets of chest, one set of abs, two sets of chest, and so on until you finish your workout by intersetting one set of abs between each two or three sets of chest and back training.

By using the staggered sets principle, you can easily do 20 sets of otherwise boring abdominal work almost without noticing it. And, you can do so without any deleterious effects on the rest of the body. Indeed, you will probably notice an overall positive effect on your physique, particularly on your abdominals.

Dennis Tinerino (winner of the Teenage Mr. America, Junior Mr. America, Natural Mr. America, and Mr. America titles, the only man to win all four "America" events): "I've successfully used staggered sets for both my abdominals and calves. I feel that intersetting calf and abdominal training between work for the rest of my body has been quite beneficial for my physique."

PEAK CONTRACTION

Anatomically speaking, muscles are made up of long, thin fibers of muscle. And these fibers are composed of single muscle cells strung together end to end. A huge number of muscle fibers must be bundled together to form any muscle group.

Physiologically, the mind sends nerve impulses to the muscle group that will be contracted to move a weight in an exercise. This nerve impulse causes a given number of individual muscle cells to contract, and a muscle cell either contracts fully or doesn't contract at all. This is called an "all or nothing" model by exercise physiologists.

The contraction of one muscle cell in a fiber causes the entire fiber to shorten in length, and the contraction of two cells in a fiber causes it to shorten even more. Overall, the number of muscle cells in a muscle fiber that actually shorten to contract a muscle group depends on the strength of the nerve impulses sent by the brain to the individual cells. The stronger this nerve impulse, the greater the number of cells caused to shorten. And the more cells you

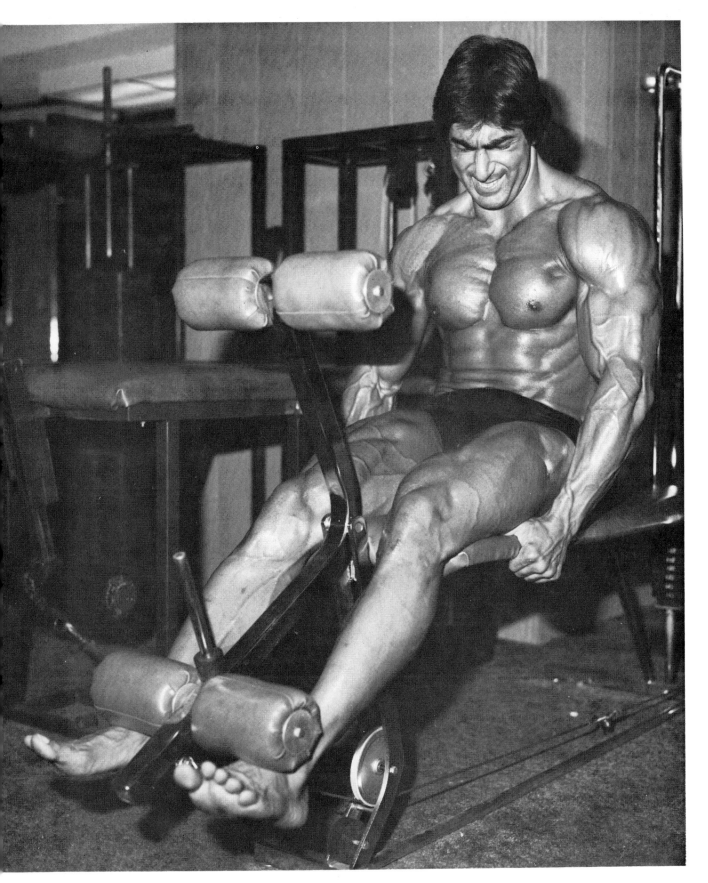

Dennis Tinerino.

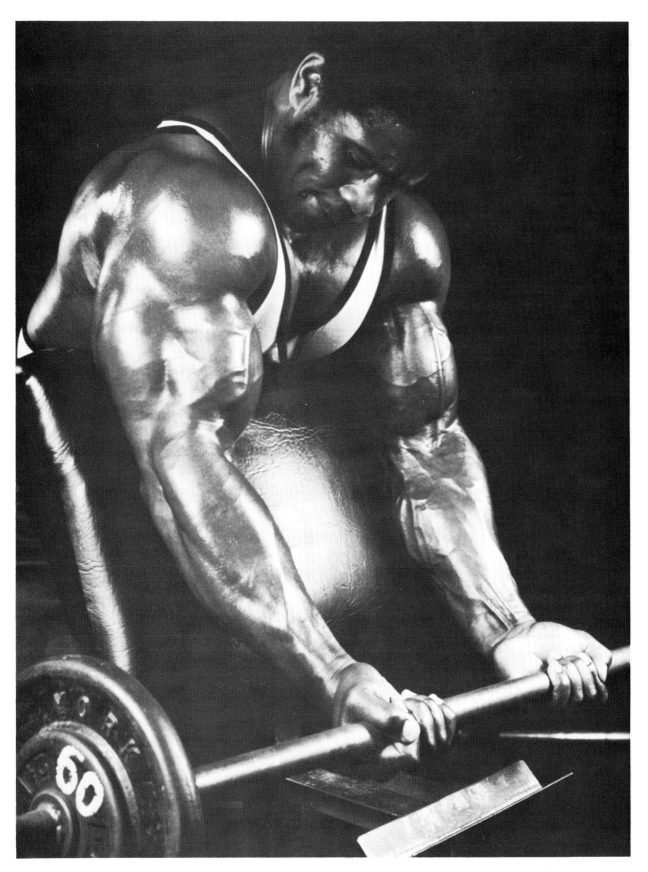

Peak contraction wrist curls by Bertil Fox.

can shorten like this, the stronger and more complete the contraction of a full muscle mass.

Furthermore, the more a joint is bent by a working muscle group, the greater the number of individual muscle cells necessarily contract to produce that effect. So, I theorized many years ago that a bodybuilder could develop a greater degree of muscle hypertrophy if he could place a heavy load on the muscle when it was fully contracted, something that often isn't possible when using most bodybuilding exercises.

After considerable experimentation on my own body and those of a large number of "human guinea pigs," I conclusively proved my theory. Thus was born the Weider Peak Contraction Training Principle, which has been responsible for much of the huge, high-quality muscle mass displayed by competitive bodybuilders in recent years.

In using this principle, you will utilize exercises in which you have a full weight load on the working muscles when they are completely contracted, as is the case in most latissimus dorsi (Chins, Rows, Pulldowns, etc.) and calf (all types of Toe Raises) exercises. A few other movements in which you can have a peak contraction effect include Dumbbell/Cable Side Laterals, Dumbbell/Cable Bent Laterals, Front Raises, Leg Extensions, Leg Curls, Hyperextensions, Barbell/Dumbbell/Cable Concentration Curls, Dumbbell Kickbacks, Pec Deck Flyes, Shrugs, Upright Rows, and Wrist Curls done with the forearms running down a decline bench.

Ordinarily, most bodybuilding movements done on machines provide a peak contraction effect. This is particularly true of machines—such as the pec deck—which operate with a circular or oval cam (or cams). Such "rotary resistance" is one of the few features I like on Nautilus machines, incidentally, because it allows for both a peak contraction and for continuous tension (please see the next section for a detailed discussion of Continuous Tension).

At the top of each peak contraction movement, you should try to hold the weight for several seconds with your fully contracted muscles, building as much tension as possible into the working muscle groups. Holding the weight for a slow count of three at the top of the Leg Extension movement, for example, allows you to contract your quadriceps much harder, thereby adding mass, quality, and deep cuts to your front thighs.

Pete Grymkowski (Mr. World, owner of Gold's Gym): "Experience has shown me that I have to do plenty of peak contraction movements in my bodybuilding routines. Without peak contraction, I feel that I would have at least 10% less muscle mass, density, and muscularity. I recommend this training technique to all of the bodybuilders who train at Golds, and the ones who use it always seem to have an edge over the bodybuilders who don't."

CONTINUOUS TENSION

For a muscle to receive full benefit from an exercise, the weight used should continually be felt along the fullest possible range of motion. Unfortunately, many exercises do not allow for stress to be placed on a working muscle at all times, and when it is, many bodybuilders use such loose exercise style that they waste much of the stress that they place on a muscle.

As a result of the foregoing factors, I codified the Weider Slow, Continuous Tension Training Principle in an effort to provide a bodybuilder with the resistance he should place on each muscle. In using this principle, you will first build tension into the working muscle by contracting the antagonistic muscle group, then holding that contraction for the duration of the set you are doing. As an example, when you are working your biceps, you will have your triceps tensed as you do your Curls. And while your triceps are in this contracted state, you automatically have your biceps working hard over the full range of the curling motion.

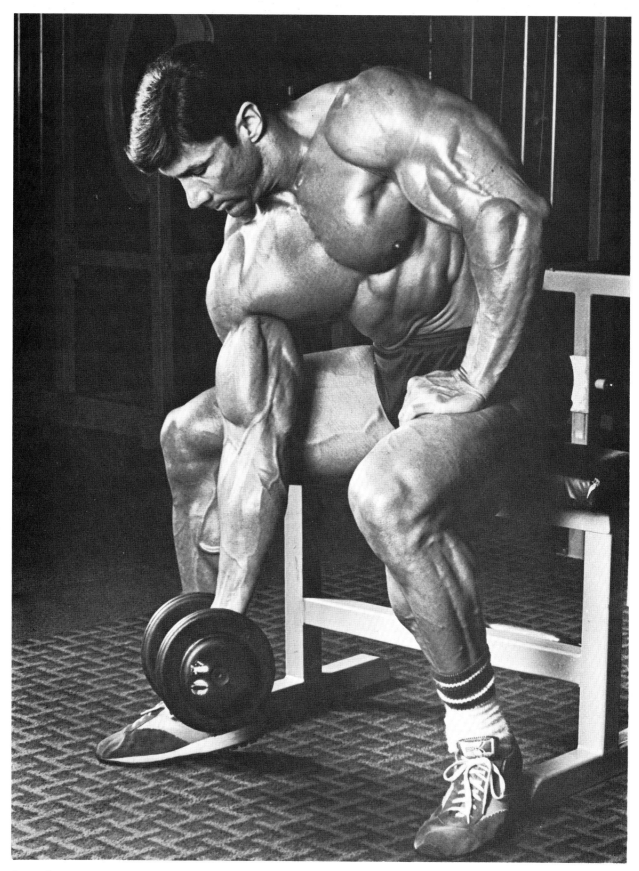

Boyer Coe curling with continuous tension.

In addition to contracting antagonistic muscle groups, you must also move the weight you are using slowly and over the full range of motion in each exercise. Doing so will add to your chance of feeling heavy resistance over every inch of the range of motion of any exercise you're doing.

Adding together this slow and full type of movement and the contraction of antagonistic muscle groups to add tension to working muscles, you will be profitably using the Weider Slow, Continuous Tension Training Principle. And, when you do this, you will be getting the most out of each movement you do in terms of building a massive and highly detailed physique.

Prior to a competition, most bodybuilders like to combine both continuous tension and peak contraction movements in their workouts. And this combination—abetted by quality training and a tight precontest diet—is greatly responsible for developing the type of highly striated physique displayed by Frank Zane, winner of three Mr. Olympia titles.

Boyer Coe (holder of more than 10 World Bodybuilding Championships): "I faithfully use continuous tension in my training, particularly for the last five or six weeks prior to a competition, and it has gradually helped to give me a maximum degree of muscle mass and density, which in turn gave me the World Grand Prix Championships title in 1981. Overall, I recommend that you use an eclectic approach to your training—use every possible training principle, exercise, and routine over a period of time. This way you'll be guaranteed of maximizing your physical potential. Then, if you have good potential, you will win many bodybuilding titles, and you will perhaps one day even become a professional bodybuilder."

ISO-TENSION CONTRACTION

One of my more recent innovations is the Weider Iso-Tension Contraction Training Principle, which has also helped bodybuilders to achieve the type of ripped-to-shreds muscularity necessary to win today's high-level bodybuilding titles. In utilizing this training principle, you will do repetition flexes of each muscle group, tensing the muscle hard in a variety of positions and holding each rep flex for 8–10 seconds before taking a rest interval of about 20–30 seconds between flexes.

I first became aware of the value of iso-tension contraction when I noticed that bodybuilders who put in a great deal of posing practice invariably had the hardest looking physiques onstage. Since these men trained and dieted virtually the same as other bodybuilders, I felt that the large amount of muscle flexing that they did in their posing practice made them look harder.

Next, I theorized that tensing the muscles hard—either individually, or in groups, as is the case when practicing posing—would both help a bodybuilder to better control each muscle group as he posed onstage, and would actually assist in hardening up the muscles. After exhaustive investigation of my hypothesis on my own body and those of my "guinea pigs," I was able to prove this theory to my satisfaction. Therefore, I codified the Weider Iso-Tension Contraction Training Principle, so bodybuilders everywhere could understand and use it to improve their physiques.

To initially practice iso-tension contraction, let's use your biceps muscles. Stand in front of your posing mirror clad in your posing trunks, and run quickly through your routine to decide in which three or four basic positions you hold your arms to contract your biceps muscles for the posing routine you use. No doubt some of these positions will include holding your arms in a double-biceps pose, holding each arm at the side of your torso as for a side-chest shot, and holding your arms out in front of your body as in a most-muscular pose.

Given three or four positions in which you contract your biceps, begin with the first. Tense your biceps as hard as you can in this position, and hold the flex for about 8–10 seconds, breathing as shallowly as

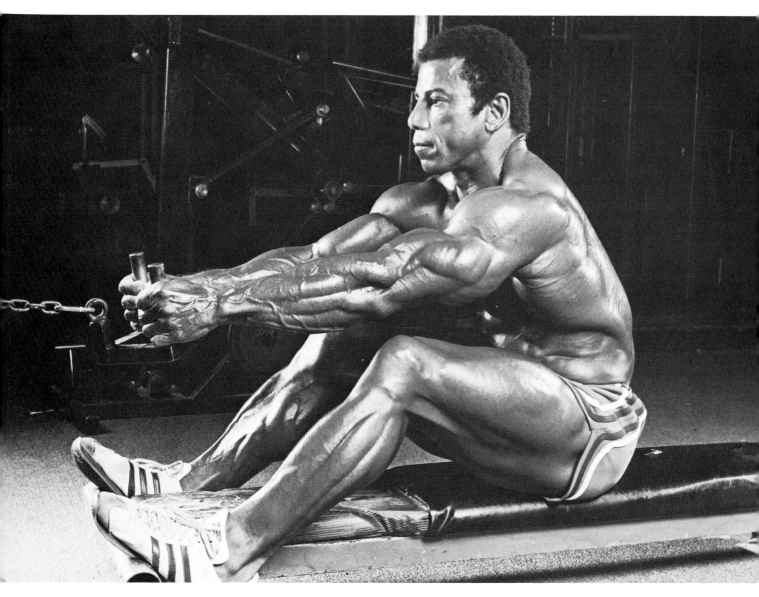

Chris Dickerson at full flex while rowing.

possible in order not to interfere with the tensing of your biceps. Relax your arm muscles for 20–30 seconds, breathing normally, then repeat flexing your arms in the initial position.

At first, you will probably make your biceps muscles quite sore by simply holding each position at full flex for two or three such "reps," or a total of perhaps 8–10 rep flexes. As you become more experienced with this technique, however, you will be able to build up to about 10 rep flexes in each position, or something in the neighborhood of 30–40 flexes lasting 8–10

seconds per flex for each muscle group. And this will greatly aid in hardening up your physique.

While I recommend iso-tension contraction work for use at home away from the gym, you can also use it between sets as you train each muscle group.

Rick Wayne (Pro Mr. America, Mr. World, and formerly Editor-In-Chief of, and now a respected writer for, *Muscle & Fitness* magazine): "You will greatly improve a muscle group if you flex and pose it at a variety of angles between sets of exercises for that muscle. As an example, you can really harden up your pectorals if you tense them very hard for about 10 seconds per flex between each two or three sets of your training for that muscle group. Look in the mirror so you can vividly see each strand and groove of muscle brought out as you practice posing and flexing a particular muscle group. I used this method quite effectively when I was competing, and my muscularity won me a number of national and international titles and high placings."

Frank Zane (Mr. America, Mr. North America, Mr. Universe, Mr. World, and three times Mr. Olympia): "I practice iso-tension contraction as part of my posing practice, and particularly on the Round II compulsory poses. Onstage at the prejudging for a competition, I have found that I often must hold a compulsory pose for 30–40 seconds without shaking like a leaf while comparisons are made. And the only way to hold one this long—plus to look hard and muscular in it—is to actually practice holding these poses for 30–60 seconds at home prior to the show. And by going very slowly through the compulsory poses and the rest of the poses I normally do in my free-posing routine—holding each pose for 30–40 seconds—I have been able to gradually harden and striate my physique for the best chance of winning a Mr.

Olympia title. My formula has worked now three times, and I'm sure that it will help me to win another Olympia before I retire."

Chris Dickerson (Mr. Olympia Pro World Champion): "I have practiced the Weider Iso-Tension Contraction Training Principle since Joe Weider taught it to me in 1980. I think that doing these hard repetition flexes of each muscle group has greatly improved my overall muscularity. I particularly feel that it has helped me to maximize my upper arm development."

CONCLUSION

Reread this chapter several times, if need be, to understand how you should use each of the Weider Training Intensification Principles. Then actually practice each training principle until you fully master it. And, finally, work with each principle long enough to be able to use the Weider Instinctive Training Principle to determine if it works well for your individual mental temperament and body makeup.

In the balance of this book, I will repeatedly refer to the Weider Training Intensification Principles discussed in this chapter, so you will need to at least thoroughly understand each one, even if you don't use it in your own workouts.

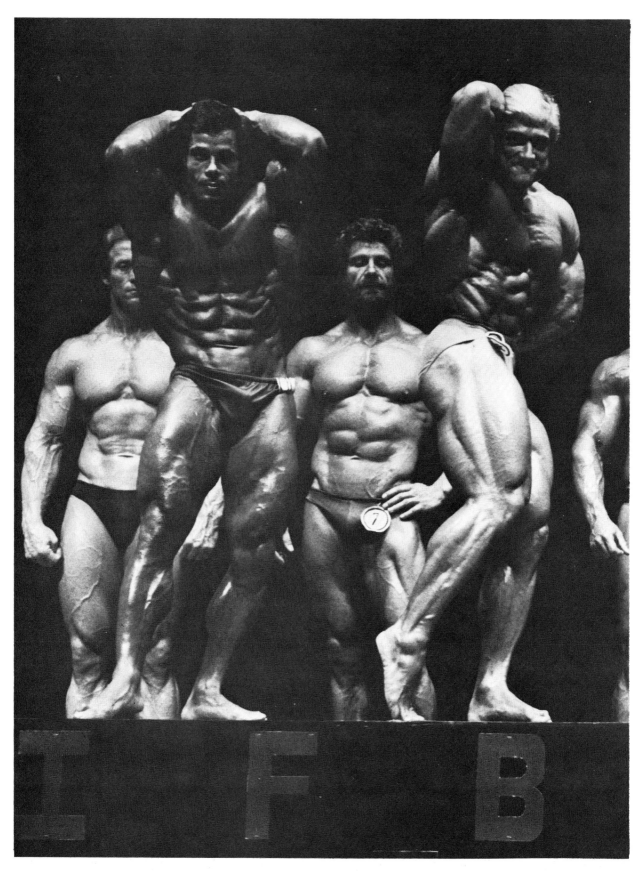

Franco Columbu and Tom Platz at the 1981 Olympia.

4

Contest Preparation

Physique contests are what keep most bodybuilders in the gym training hard.

For younger novice bodybuilders, the lure of a contest trophy is what gets them into the gym in the first place. And often each new trophy that is won is displayed along with the others on a sort of altar at which the bodybuilder pays homage to his previous efforts and renews his enthusiasm for the sport before going off to train each day.

Even for great champions, contests serve as an incentive for harder and more consistent training. As the incredibly developed Boyer Coe has noted, "The trophies don't mean that much to me anymore, but I love to compete against the sport's best athletes. I enter every upcoming IFBB professional contest, because using these competitions as goals keeps my enthusiasm at a peak level. As a result, I consistently train with maximum intensity and have been able to continue improving year after year!"

Unfortunately, for young bodybuilders contest preparation has long been a hit-and-miss, learn-as-you-go proposition.

Therefore, I hope that in this chapter I can pull together enough data on contest preparation to allow you to more quickly develop a personal contest preparation formula.

In its essence, contest preparation boils down to making your physique into a finished product, then presenting it in the best possible light. This involves developing a good degree of muscle mass, even proportions, and good symmetry in the off-season, then dieting and training in such a manner that you become as muscular as possible without losing too much of your hard-earned muscle mass.

I've seen top men look semi-pitiful a week before a competition, then be in true Olympian shape on the day of a show. Ken Waller was a great one for this, and I often joked, "Ken Waller is in top shape for only six hours per contest cycle, but he's always at his best for a big contest, and he consistently wins!"

WHAT DO JUDGES LOOK FOR?

Above all else, you must have a great body. Good body proportional balance is

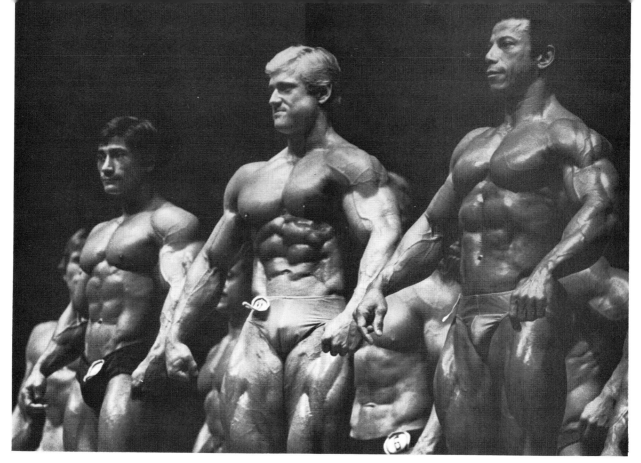

Danny Padilla, Tom Platz, and Chris Dickerson were finalists in the 1981 Olympia.

probably the foremost quality that judges seek (provided, of course, that a contestant has a reasonable amount of muscle mass). In this respect, you will often see a very good small man defeat an overbulked or ill-proportioned giant. One example of this occurred in 1968 when a smaller, better proportioned and crisply defined Frank Zane defeated a much larger Arnold Schwarzenegger (but one with less physique quality) in the IFBB Mr. Universe contest. Of course, Arnold learned from that loss and refined his proportions while developing superb muscle quality to go with his phenomenal mass. He ended up winning a record seven Mr. Olympia titles (1970-1975, 1980).

As the judges look for good proportional balance between muscle groups, they are probably assessing body symmetry as well. Symmetry is the shape and relative silhouette of the body. A bodybuilder with good symmetry will have broad shoulders, a narrow waist—hip structure, and flaring lats, which results in a great V-shaped torso.

Ideally, he will also have relatively small joints, which will make the surrounding large muscle volumes look even more impressively full. As an example, Sergio Oliva (a three-time Mr. Olympia) has very small knee and ankle joints, which make his calves look much larger than they are. But Oliva unfortunately does not have a high-peaked biceps, which is a definite minus in terms of body symmetry.

There is also such a factor as "bilateral symmetry," or an equality of shape, size, vascularity, and other physical factors on each side of the body. Only a few bodybuilders have very good bilateral symmetry, so they disguise this fact through skillful posing. If, for example, one biceps has a high peak and the other is somewhat more flat looking, a bodybuilder won't do a straight front double biceps pose. Instead, he will twist his body a little to display the peaked biceps dead on and the flatter biceps at somewhat of an angle, so it appears that it might look the same as the good biceps.

A third quality the judges look for, and

the one that you can most enhance in your precontest preparations, is muscularity (or the absence of fat over your muscles). Your body could have the symmetry of Michelangelo's statue of David and the muscle mass of a Farnese Hercules, but if it's not cut up you won't win even local titles.

This diamond-hard muscularity is not overly difficult to attain, although it does require a disciplined diet and hard training. And yet potential champions enter national contests year after year with the same five or six pounds of superfluous fat filming over the deep cuts they could so easily have.

A fourth quality that will help you to win is muscle mass, which is developed through heavy training on basic exercises during the off-season. Bodybuilders seem to be getting bigger and bigger every year, and when you can combine good muscle mass with equal body proportions, aesthetic body symmetry and great cuts, you'll have a winning physique.

The final category that can influence judges is that of onstage presentation. It's easy to pick up points here by obtaining a good tan (where applicable), being well-groomed, posing to display your physique to its maximum advantage, and choosing the right pair of posing trunks. After reading this chapter, you should be able to utilize these presentation techniques to best advantage, adding about 10 percent to your chance of winning a contest.

PRECONTEST TRAINING

For most physique champions, precontest training involves a progressive intensification of workouts (see Chapter 3 for a more thorough discussion of Weider intensification training principles). Olympian-level bodybuilders who compete only once a year will gradually intensify their training over a 3–4-month period, holding peak intensity for four to six weeks. Less experienced bodybuilders, however, will usually intensify their training over 6–8-week cycles, holding peak training intensity for only two or three weeks.

Although a handful of top bodybuilders do not change their training at all prior to a contest, most follow one or more of these intensification methods:

1. Reduce rest intervals between sets to a minimum (which is using the Weider Quality Training Principle).

2. Do additional sets for each body part.

3. Use the Weider Continuous Tension and Peak Contraction Training Principles.

4. Use supersets, trisets and giant sets rather than straight sets for a body part in a workout.

5. Use the Weider Descending Sets Training Principle.

6. Use the Weider Staggered Sets Training Principle.

7. Train certain body parts more frequently.

8. Train more than once a day (which is using the Weider Double-Split System Training Principle).

9. Use the Weider Iso-Tension Contraction Training Principle.

10. Add running, bicycling, or some other form of cardiorespiratory training to the overall workout plan.

Let's allow the superstar bodybuilders themselves to explain how these 10 variables help them to increase precontest training intensity and result in better onstage muscularity.

Reducing Rest Intervals

Chris Dickerson (Mr. Olympia, Grand Prix Champion): "In the off-season, I rest 60–90 seconds between sets, because I am using heavier weights on basic exercises and am eating more in order to build muscle mass. Then prior to a contest I diet strictly and train in certain ways to burn off all of my body fat and reveal in bold relief the more massive and the better developed muscles under my skin. One of the training methods that helps most to sharpen up my muscularity is quality training. In this method, I gradually reduce my rest intervals to 20–30 seconds, which makes it seem to me like I'm training virtually nonstop. Of course, when I am training

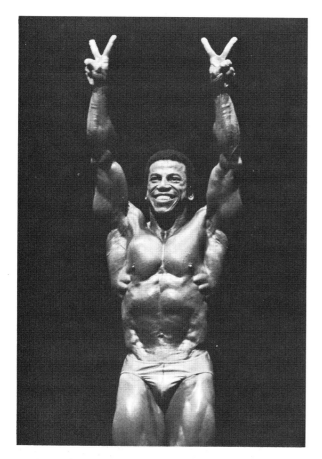

Chris Dickerson's victory sign.

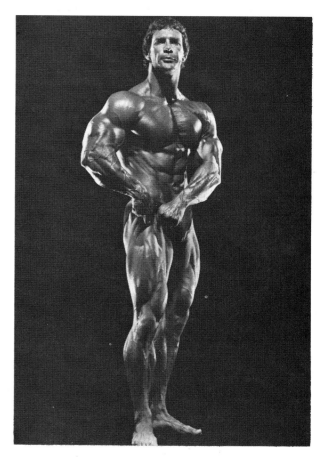

Scott Wilson.

with so little rest between sets and following a restricted calorie diet, my training poundages suffer. I'm simply unable to use as heavy weights as during the off-season, but I still force myself to use maximum weights in strict form. If I don't push really hard like this, I won't achieve maximum muscular density."

Scott Wilson (Pro Mr. America, Mr. International): "I progressively shorten my rest intervals before a contest from about 60–70 seconds between sets eight weeks before competing to 20–30 seconds between sets for the final three or four weeks. One way I achieve an average of 20–30 seconds rest between sets is to switch from straight sets for all body parts to doing supersets and occasionally even trisets for some muscle groups. Combined with a tight precontest diet, these shorter rest intervals result in a definite drop in my exercise poundages, but by keeping up my effort

level, I can build muscle density using these lighter weights. The key to effectively using quality training is to keep the weights as relatively heavy as possible all the time, regardless of how light they become."

Adding Sets

Casey Viator (Mr. USA, history's youngest Mr. America winner, and twice an IFBB Pro Grand Prix Champion): "Adding sets to a workout for each body part is a technique that I—and many other top bodybuilders I know—use to zero in on contest condition. Contrary to what has been written about me in the past by non-Weider authors, I prefer to do 20–25 total sets per muscle group in the off-season and 30–35 sets per body part prior to a competition. Sometimes adding so many sets to a workout is courting overtraining, but with the enthusi-

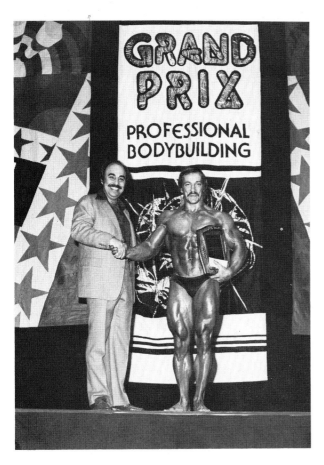

Suitably humble, Casey Viator.

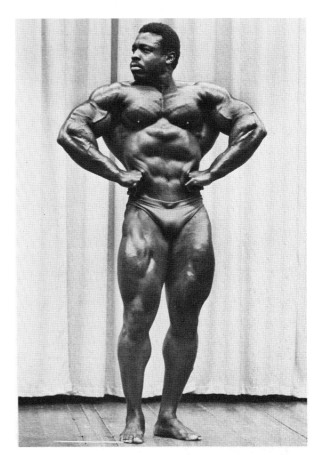

Roy Callender.

asm I develop for my training prior to a high-level contest, my workouts seem to automatically accelerate in pace and grow longer. And I simply can't achieve the degree of muscular detail necessary to win an IFBB pro competition without adding appreciably to the number of sets I do for each body part prior to a competition."

Roy Callender (Mr. Canada, Amateur and Professional Mr. Universe, Diamond Cup Professional Champion): "I used to find it very easy to build muscle mass, but very difficult to reach the type of cut-up condition needed to win the most prestigious titles. After only two years of bodybuilding training, I had developed a world-class physique, with nearly 20-inch upper arms. But I was as smooth as a baby's behind. It was only when I switched to doing more total sets for each muscle group prior to a competition that I finally was able to get really muscular. Before a contest, I will

train from six to eight hours a day, doing up to 60–70 total sets for each muscle group. I wouldn't recommend this technique to too many bodybuilders, but it has certainly worked wonders in allowing me to combine maximum muscle mass with crisp muscular definition."

Continuous Tension and Peak Contraction

Robby Robinson (Mr. America, Mr. World, Mr. Universe and winner of numerous IFBB pro bodybuilding titles): "To bring out the maximum degree of muscle striations at a contest, I have to feel the weight in every exercise over each millimeter of the full range of motion of that exercise. In a Barbell Curl, for example, I'll move the barbell very slowly over its full range of motion, and with great tension built into my biceps and the antagonistic muscle group, the triceps. Using this method, I can make a 70-pound barbell feel like it weighs 140 pounds."

Mike Mentzer (Mr. America, Mr. North America, Mr. Universe and an IFBB Pro Grand Prix Winner): "It's only when a muscle is fully flexed that the maximum number of fibers in that muscle are contracted. And, to build a muscle group to the greatest possible mass and degree of quality, you must have a heavy weight on the muscle when it is fully flexed like this. That's the reason for peak contraction, and I frequently use this technique in my own training, particularly prior to a competition."

Supersets, Trisets, Giant Sets

Steve Michalik (Mr. America): "To cut down on the average rest interval between sets when I am quality training prior to a competition—plus to increase the overall intensity of my precontest training—I will use supersets, trisets and giant sets for up to six to eight weeks prior to competing. I mainly use supersets for my upper arms, alternating biceps and triceps exercises. I like to use trisets for three-faceted muscle groups such as the deltoids, and I prefer to use giant sets for large multifaceted muscle groups such as my back. Supersets, trisets and giant sets are extremely strenuous to perform, but they give me great results."

Tony Pearson (Mr. America, Mr. World, Mr. Universe): "I'll sometimes superset two exercises for the same muscle group when I'm in my precontest cycle, because this greatly intensifies my training for that particular muscle group. As an example of this, you could do a set of 6–8 reps in a full-range Barbell Preacher Curl, step back from the preacher bench and immediately do 6–8 reps in a Standing Barbell Curl, all without even letting go of the barbell between exercises. You just won't believe the growth burn you'll feel in your biceps from this type of superset!"

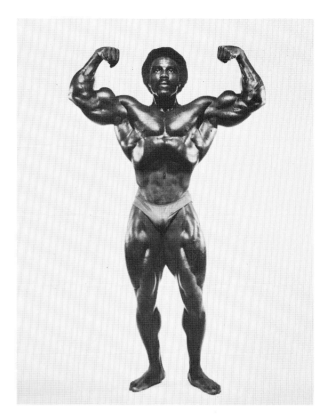

Robby Robinson, the Black Prince.

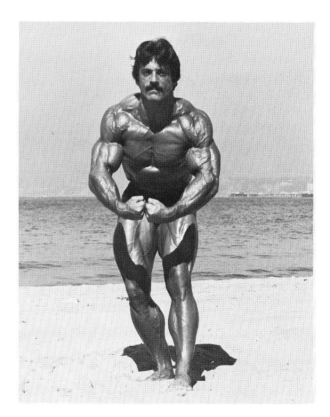

Mike Mentzer.

Descending Sets

Arnold Schwarzenegger (Mr. World, Mr. International, Mr. Universe and seven times Mr. Olympia): "I would often use the stripping method, or descending sets principle, in my training close to a competition, particularly for my biceps. As an example, I would have two training partners stand at the ends of a barbell that was loaded with plates, but did not have the collars in place. Then I would pick up the barbell and do about 5–6 strict reps of Barbell Curls. Without setting the bar down, I'd have my training partners strip 10–15 pounds of plates off each side, whereupon I'd do another 5–6 strict reps with the lighter weight, not having rested even five seconds between the first set and the descending set. Then I'd immediately have my partners strip off 10–15 more pounds from each side so I could do a final super-intense 5–6 strict reps of Barbell Curls."

Bertil Fox (Mr. Britain, Mr. Europe, Mr. World, Mr. Universe): "I use the Weider Descending Sets Training Principle on at least one basic exercise per body part during my precontest cycle. As an example, I'll work up through four or five sets on the Bench Press to fully warm up my pecs, delts and triceps. My final 'warm-up' set will be with 450–475 pounds for six reps, depending on my relative energy levels on a particular day. Then I'll load up my barbell with 505–525 pounds, again depending on how I feel on a particular day, in such a manner that I can have two training buddies each strip off a 45-pound plate, or a total drop of 90 pounds, on each descending set. Then I do 5–6 reps with the top weight, 5–6 reps with my second descending set, and so on for a total of four descending sets on the Bench Press. And, man, are my pecs blown away after *that* type of descending sets training."

Staggered Sets

Jusup Wilkosz (Mr. Germany, Mr. Europe, Amateur and Professional Mr. Universe): "Before a contest, when I have a lot

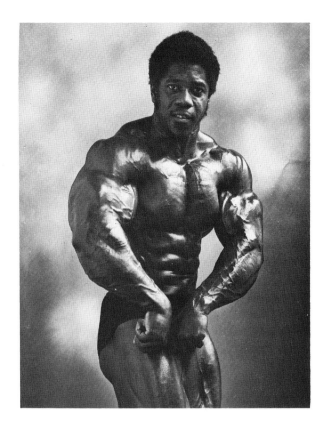

Bertil Fox.

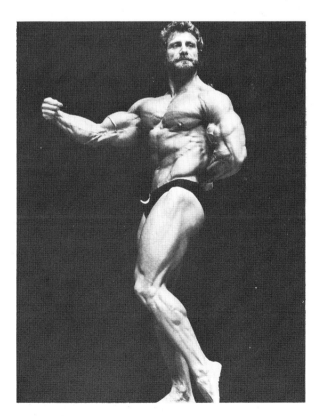

Jusup Wilkosz.

of abdominal training to do, it's difficult for me to perform 20–25 sets of abdominal work in one grouping. Frankly, I'd find doing 20–25 straight sets of abdominal training to be terribly boring. Therefore, when I have a lot of abdominal training in my program, I'll use the Weider Staggered Sets Training Principle. In this principle, I'll do a couple of heavy sets of chest work, a quick set of light abdominal training, a couple more sets of chest work, another quick set of ab training, and so on until I've intersetted all 20–25 sets of abdominal work between my exercises for other muscle groups. And by the end of my workout, through using the Weider Staggered Sets Training Principle, I will have hardly noticed that I've done all of these sets of abdominal exercises!"

Training Body Parts More Frequently

Tom Platz (Mr. Universe): "During my off-season training cycle, I find that I am able to build muscle mass most easily if I train each major muscle group twice a week. But to harden up prior to a competition, I must train each major body part three times a week for about 10 weeks prior to my contest. I feel that this method of training less frequently and more heavily in the off-season to build muscle mass and more frequently and lighter prior to a show to harden up will work quite well for any bodybuilder."

Dennis Tinerino (Teenage Mr. America, Natural Mr. America, Mr. America, Mr. World, Amateur and Professional Mr. Universe): "Not only do I train each major muscle group three times a week instead of two prior to a contest, but I'll also occasionally train a few body parts, such as my abdominals, calves and forearms, either twice a day, or daily in cases when I wasn't already training them every day. Working my abdominals on a twice-daily basis is particularly effective in sharpening them up just prior to a major competition."

Double-Split System Training

Johnny Fuller (Mr. Britain, Mr. International, Mr. Universe): "Close to an important competition such as the Mr. Olympia, I am up to doing so many total sets for each body part that I simply can't do my entire workout with any degree of energy left toward the end of it by training only once a day. Therefore, I will follow a Weider Double Split System of training, working out twice a day. This way I can do half of my training in the morning when I'm well-rested and can devote full energy throughout the workout. Then, after resting during the day, I can come back and do the second half of my workout with equal energy. The net result is that I can add to the overall intensity of my training. When I'm really going berserk close to a show, I might even work out three times a day!"

Pete Grymkowski (Junior Mr. USA, Junior Mr. America, IFBB Mr. World, owner of Gold's Gym): "Prior to a competition, I'd usually adopt a partial double-split routine in which I'd do two workouts a day three days each week and only one on the other three training days. This worked really well for me, because I could do calves, chest and back on Monday, Wednesday and Friday mornings, then come back and blast abs, thighs and forearms on Monday, Wednesday and Friday evenings. On Tuesday, Thursday and Saturday afternoons I'd do calves, abs, delts and arms. The net effect is somewhat like using a full double-split, but this partial double-split prior to competition allows me a little more time to recuperate and grow between workouts."

Iso-Tension Contraction

Boyer Coe (winner of more than 10 World Bodybuilding Championships): "By doing rep flexes of each muscle group, holding each flex at maximum tension for 8–10 seconds, I am able to really harden up my physique before a competition. I'll do 10–20 reps of flexes for each muscle group daily for three or four weeks prior to a competition. The Weider Iso-Tension Contraction Training Principle works extremely well in helping me to harden up for competitions."

Frank Zane (Mr. America, Mr. World, Mr. Universe and three times Mr. Olympia): "I'll work hard every day for several weeks holding each of my poses for up to 60 seconds at a time. This gives me both better control of my muscles when I'm posing—particularly during my compulsory round—and greater muscle hardness."

Aerobics

Andreas Cahling (Mr. International): "I will ride my bicycle for at least five days a week for four to six weeks prior to a competition. I ride about 40 miles up and down a bike path along the Pacific Ocean Beach from Santa Monica southward to Palos Verdes, and prior to a major competition I see a lot of other champion bodybuilders out riding on the same bike path. This aerobic training really helps me to cut up to the max for an important competition."

Ray Mentzer (Mr. USA, Mr. America): "I will run 6–10 miles at a time several times a week prior to a competition to help burn off extra fat and achieve maximum muscular definition. I'll usually do my running relatively late at night. I'll also frequently ride a stationary bicycle for an hour at a time during the early evening while watching television, and I'll go for long walks when I'm having difficulty sleeping. Every little bit of aerobic activity helps to make me more cut."

Danny Padilla (Mr. America, Mr. USA, Mr. Universe): "For about six weeks before a competition, I will alternate days of bicycling 1½–2 hours with days of running 45–60 minutes. And to keep from getting too bored while I'm doing my aerobic workouts, I'll wear earphones with a radio in them so I can listen to my favorite music. I've personally discovered that aerobic training is absolutely essential if I plan to be in peak condition onstage at a competition."

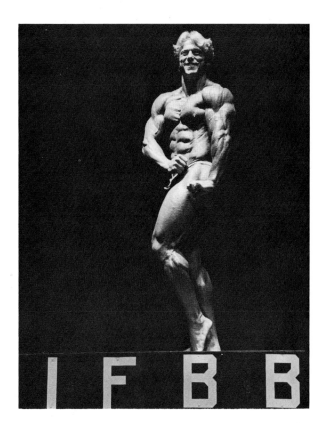

Andreas Cahling.

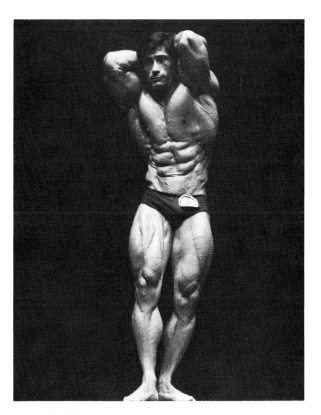

Danny Padilla.

PRECONTEST DIET

The two main types of precontest body-building diets are low-carbohydrate and low-fat/low-calorie diets. There are still adherents to the classic low-carb diet, but a majority of bodybuilders today rely on a low-fat/low-calorie dietary regimen to get cut up for a competition.

You can change the appearance of your body greatly in a short period of time through following a tight precontest diet. The only problem is that different bodies have different biochemical makeups and react differently to each diet. Therefore, you must experiment with each type of diet and use the Weider Instinctive Training Principle to evaluate the relative results of each diet.

Regardless of the type of precontest diet you follow, you should restrict carbohydrate intake for four days prior to competition and then carb-load either the night before competing or the morning of the contest, depending on how your body reacts to carbohydrate loading. Each gram of carbohydrate in your body holds four grams of water, blurring sharp contest definition; hence the elimination of carbs.

Carbohydrate deprivation will flush out all excess water from your body, but it will also temporarily flatten your muscles and make your vascularity virtually disappear. This is because liver and muscle glycogen (sugar) is depleted. But by consuming 80–100 grams of low-bulk carbohydrates, such as dried fruit, you will fill the liver and muscles with glycogen, which in turn fills out your muscles and makes your vascularity as prominent as garden hoses, all without smoothing out your physique.

You must experiment with how much and what type of carbohydrate to take in—as well as the timing of such carb intake—using the Weider Instinctive Training Principle to decide which combinations are most effective in enhancing your appearance. However, in my experience with training a wide variety of champion bodybuilders, consuming more than 100 grams of carbs will usually result in water spilling in under the skin, blurring normally sharp muscularity.

Once you have determined which diet

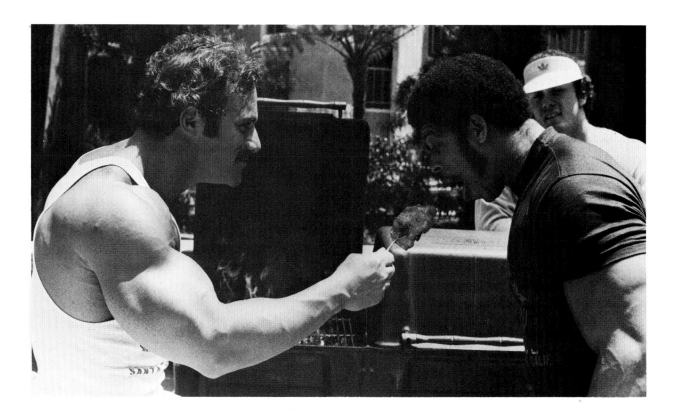

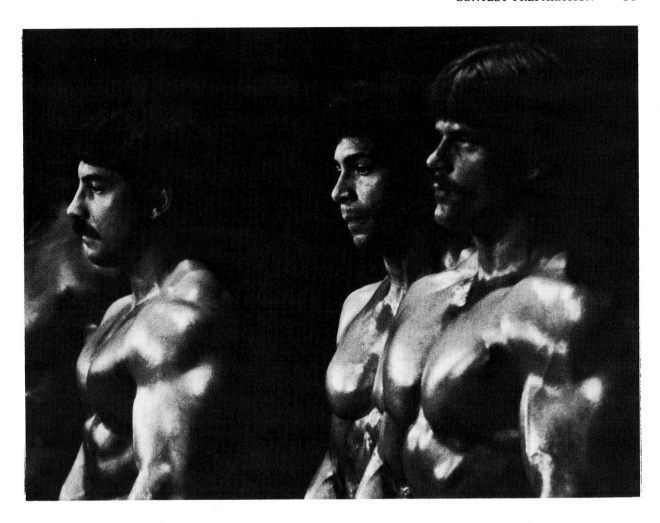

will work best for you, it's vital that you experiment with combining its timing with that of your bodybuilding and aerobic workouts to learn to peak perfectly on the day of a show. Peaking is an art form, and it will take several attempts at peaking—taking detailed written and photographic notes of how each training and dietary factor affects your peak timing—before you master the ability to peak on a specific day for a competition.

Eventually you will become so adept at timing a peak that you will hit it dead center every time. If you seem a little too heavy at a particular checkpoint leading up to your competition, you'll be able to diet a little more strictly and do additional aerobic training to accelerate your peak. And conversely, if you are peaking too quickly, you can retard the peak by eating a bit more and perhaps decreasing your aerobic

training. Only experience, good notes and several peaking attempts will give you this type of precise timing.

PERSONAL APPEARANCE

Personal appearance is a contest preparation factor about which you can do quite a bit prior to a show. Be well-groomed and have a good tan (unless you already have dark skin). Cut, comb and style your hair, and shave just before the contest (unless you wear a mustache or beard, of course).

Tom Platz recently summed up the subject of personal appearance for physique contestants: "Bodybuilding competitions are essentially judged from the neck down, but if you entered a contest with a super physique and grooming that looked as though you just fell off a boxcar, chances are good that you'd lose. Skin tone is important. I've seen men enter contests covered from head to toe with acne, caused either by a bad diet or excessive usage of steroids. I always stress that bodybuilders should follow a healthy diet, even if they don't need it to cut up for a competition. A bad diet usually leads to bad skin."

A natural tan is always best, although there are several chemical agents that you can use to enhance your skin color. A natural tan has the added benefit of flushing water from the skin, due to the sun's heat, and this makes your skin appear thinner.

Begin your tanning process at least 6–8 weeks prior to competing, so that you can gradually lie out more and more without suffering a skin-bloating sunburn. As you lie in the sun, rub a vegetable oil (e.g., almond or avocado oil) into your skin to keep it supple and moisturized.

I've had conflicting reports on the results of using tanning booths during the winter and at other times when the sun isn't cooperative enough to give you a good natural tan. Some bodybuilders, such as Andreas Cahling, have gotten good results from using tanning booths, while others haven't. You'll just need to experiment a little with such tanning booths to see what works best for you.

Numerous chemical skin creams have been used in the past to add to skin color, but usually they have resulted in a very yellowish tan. It looks almost as though a bodybuilder has been held by the head and dipped in a vat of nicotine! However, there's a new skin make-up on the market now that gives a deep brown color to the skin, easily takes on body oil, and then rinses off completely in a shower once a contest has been completed. It is called Indian Earth, and it's available at most women's cosmetic counters in larger department stores.

Indian Earth is a powder that must be rubbed very hard into the skin all over your body, preferably in two or three coatings. Later, when you apply oil over the makeup, the Indian Earth will appear a little streaky for a minute or two, but once the oil seeps into your skin, the makeup regains a very smooth appearance all over your body. Indian Earth makes your skin appear a mahogany brown, and with the oil over it, the makeup reflects light quite well. As far as I am concerned, Indian Earth is the state of the art in artificial tanning preparations.

Removing excess body hair is another factor that will improve your appearance at a contest. The number of novice bodybuilders who question this practice never ceases to amaze me, yet sooner or later they are chopping off body hair just like everyone else. The reason for this should be obvious. A thick mat of hair, such as on your chest, obscures the muscles you've slaved away to develop, and I've never seen anyone with much body hair ever win a big title.

There are three basic ways to remove body hair. You should experiment with each and then decide which is best for you. Some bodybuilders use cream hair removers. All you need to do in this case is smear the goop on, let it sit for a few minutes and wipe it and all of the hair away. Unfortunately, such depilatories irritate the skin of many users. I'd suggest trying just a dab of the cream on a small area of your body to see if it irritates the skin.

The two other methods of removing body hair involve the use of a safety razor or an electric razor. A safety razor is best used in a bathtub or shower, and once you have your body hair hacked back in that manner you can keep it down with an electric razor.

Experience has shown me that it's wise to shave down several weeks before a contest, then maintain your shave with the electric razor. This procedure allows you to get a better overall tan, and it also gives you plenty of time for any razor burns or rashes to heal before you step onstage.

Choice of posing trunks is very critical, and yet it is a very individual matter, and it's difficult for someone to help you choose a pair. What looks good on Danny Padilla or Frank Zane won't necessarily knock 'em

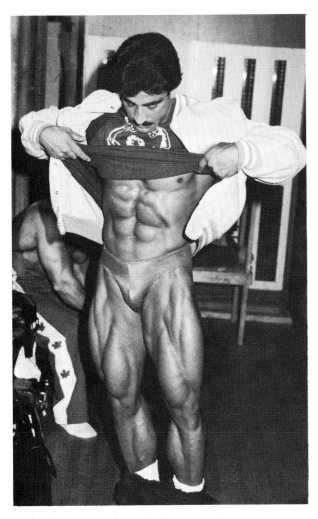

Samir Bannout "dressing" for the 1981 Olympia.

dead when you wear it. Therefore, I would like to give you the following six rules to use when choosing posing trunks:

1. Choose a pair of trunks cut to best display your physique. If you have a long waist, perhaps a high-cut waistline on your trunks will shorten it. Should you have great abdominals, you can get a low-cut waistline on your trunks. And if you have super-muscular upper thighs, you'll need to buy a pair of trunks that are cut high on the thigh to reveal this muscularity.

2. Stick to trunks of a solid color. Patterned trunks are very distracting and can draw attention away from your physique.

3. Be certain that the trunks fit snugly and do not bag or bunch up.

4. Choose a color that harmonizes with your skin and hair coloring. Blacks can look good in red, blue and purple. Blonds and redheads can usually wear dark green quite suitably. And brown looks good on almost everyone.

5. Choose relatively dark colors, since very light colors, particularly white, make the hips appear wide, detracting from your V-shape.

6. When in doubt, almost everyone looks good in basic black, so choose black or navy blue.

Better men's stores carry fairly wide selections of beachwear that make potential posing trunks. Or, you might have your wife, girlfriend, sister or mother custom fit and sew you a pair of posing trunks if you can't find any that you like in clothing stores. Additionally, numerous gyms and individual bodybuilders sell posing trunks in a wide variety of styles and colors through mail order ads in *Muscle & Fitness* magazine.

I recommend taking more than one pair of posing trunks to a competition. It's very easy for your trunks to be spotted or stained by oil during the prejudging, so a backup pair comes in handy for the evening public show. Or, you may merely like to wear a different color at night than you did in the morning or early afternoon prejudging. You might also like to own a variety of colors of posing trunks in the same size and with the same cut, so you can show a little variety on the beach and still develop an even tan line as you are lying in the sun.

LAST-MINUTE TRICKS OF THE TRADE

Muscle is largely composed of water, but if you have somehow also ended up with water under your skin a day or two before your show, you can often bring out more cuts than you ever knew you had simply by cutting back on your fluid intake for 24–36 hours. You might also experiment with taking a mild herbal diuretic the night before competing.

Under no circumstances do I recommend using a harsh chemical diuretic, such as the

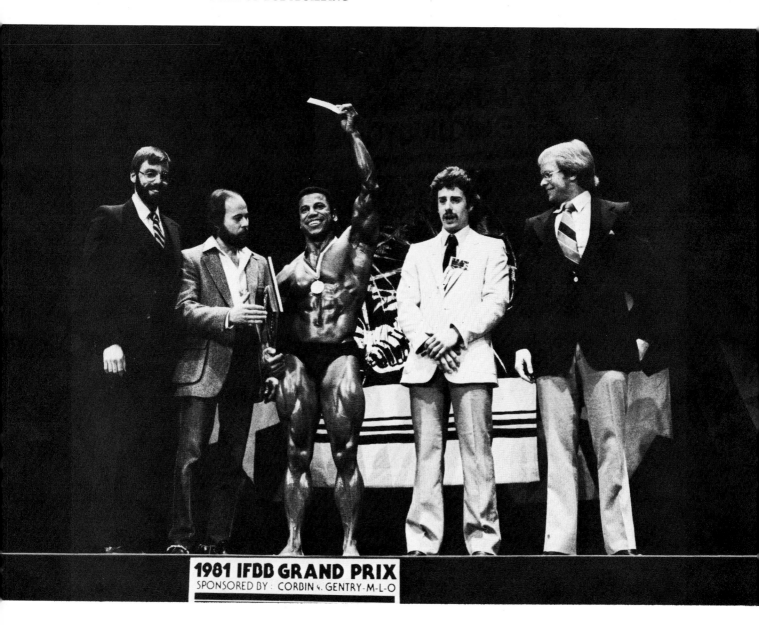

1981 IFBB GRAND PRIX
SPONSORED BY: CORBIN 4 GENTRY-M-L-O

Lasix that so many bodybuilders use. These harsh diuretics rob your bloodstream of electrolytes, which can lead to heart arrhythmia (irregular heartbeat) and possibly heart attacks. Heinz Sallmayer, the Austrian athlete who won the 1980 Lightweight Mr. Universe title, died of such a diuretic-induced heart attack in early 1982. Chemical diuretics can also cause massive muscle cramps and numerous other physical maladies. You're better off avoiding them!

Many bodybuilders take laxatives the evening before a competition, and they can often dramatically improve your appearance from one day to the next. Not only do they flush out the intestinal tract and result in a flatter-looking stomach, but they also draw excess water from beneath the skin, particularly in the abdominal area.

The proper use of body oil is also crucial to enhancing a bodybuilder's appearance onstage. At all costs, avoid the use of petroleum-based mineral oils, which simply lie on the skin and harshly reflect the posing light. With mineral oil on it, your body looks as though it's been wrapped in clear-plastic food wrapping.

It's best to use vegetable oils, and the most popular seems to be almond oil. Vegetable oils soak into the skin and then gradually emerge as you perspire to give your body a "glow," rather than the sheen that mineral oils impart to your skin. Smaller amounts of oil result in great three-dimensional muscle highlights under a posing light, while large amounts of oil tend to visually flatten out your musculature.

Your body oil should be applied evenly, so it's a good practice to bring your training partner along to the contest as your "oiler." If you've made several dry runs at oiling up in the gym prior to your competition, he should be able to apply just the right amount of oil to your physique to maximally highlight your muscularity.

Next, you should strategically pump up your body a few minutes before going onstage. Don't pump up too early, however, because then your pump will deflate before you're onstage, and it'll be difficult to re-pump.

Pumping up involves doing high-rep exercises with light weights for certain body parts. Or if you're blessed with the perfect muscular proportions of a Danny Padilla, you can merely run through your posing routine two or three times to warm up and give your physique a light overall pump.

The final last-minute technique that you can use, even though the seeds of this technique must be sown months before a show, is to project a confident and winning look onstage as you are being judged, or while running through your individual routine. Tom Platz discusses in detail how to achieve this winning look through positive mental visualization in Chapter 5.

SUMMARY

This has been an important chapter, so let's review the high points of achieving winning contest condition:

1. Intensify your training.

2. Follow an appropriate precontest diet.

3. Acquire a good tan (when appropriate) and pay attention to your personal appearance.

4. Learn to pose effectively.

5. Choose appropriate posing attire.

6. If you must, either cut back on fluids, take a mild herbal diuretic, or use a laxative.

7. Shave your body hair.

8. Use a light coating of vegetable oil to highlight your hard-earned muscularity.

9. Pump up your weak body parts before going onstage.

10. Project a confident and winning look onstage.

If you follow these 10 rules intelligently, and if you have trained long and hard enough to have developed a good physique, you *will* be a winner!

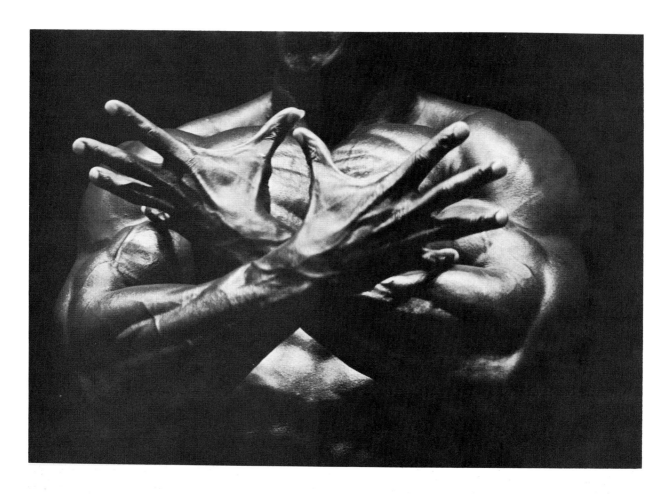

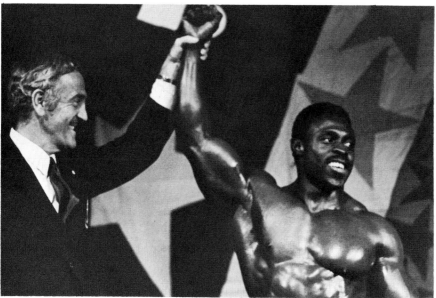

Ben Weider raises Roy Callender's arm in victory.

5

The Real Secrets of Bodybuilding Success

Most novice bodybuilders, and even a few more-experienced men, feel that the reason they aren't succeeding like the superstars is because the champs have well-guarded secrets to success that they don't share with others.

There very definitely are what we could call secrets to bodybuilding success, but they are just as definitely *open* secrets. By the time you finish reading this chapter, you'll probably say to yourself, "Well, that's logical enough, but I already *knew* all of that stuff." Undoubtedly this will be true, but hopefully this chapter will jog you into some type of positive action, because these "secrets" genuinely are major keys to your ultimate bodybuilding success.

KNOW YOURSELF!

Getting to know your body and how it reacts to such external stimuli as exercise, diet, and rest is undoubtedly the biggest "secret" in bodybuilding. In his usual fashion, Frank Zane (three times Mr. Olympia) has capsulized this concept very eloquently. "I treat my body as a living labor-atory," he said. "In this laboratory I conduct experiments and objectively evaluate the results of each of these experiments. As in the case of industrial research, I often come up with new ways of doing things better and more efficiently in my workouts, diet, and mental preparations."

That's it in a nutshell—you simply *must* constantly experiment on your body to discover what works and what doesn't. And this is where many potentially great body-builders blow it. You may, for example, have read Lou Ferrigno's arm routine in *Muscle & Fitness* magazine. Many bodybuilders will simply follow the routine as written for a couple of months, but unless they are very lucky they'll make only a minimum of gains.

The correct way to go about it is to try Ferrigno's exact routine and note the results. If you're making acceptable gains with it, great! Keep with it! But if you're not making noticeable gains after two or three weeks, change a few things around. Try using an EZ-curl bar instead of a straight bar for Preacher Curls. Move the reps up or down. Try more or less rest between sets, more or less weight, more or less sets of each exercise, or a different order of movements.

Each time you make a change, carefully note the progress you are making. Perhaps you'll eventually find that none of these combinations proves effective. Then you'll need to go on to something else. But occasionally you will run across something that really works. And then you will have taken a giant step to the top in bodybuilding.

As Chris Dickerson (the all-time pro bodybuilding victories leader) has noted, "I am constantly learning new things, new techniques that give me gains. I could give you the training schedule that I use today for my thighs or back, but a month from now it would be out of date. By then I would have learned how to do things better. I'm over 40, but I still learn something new and valuable every few days."

You can also experiment with diet. I recall the case of a famous bodybuilder who had been on a virtual zero-carbohydrate diet for several months without being able to cut up. He simply couldn't reduce the slight roll of fat he was carrying around his waist. He finally came to me for advice, and I decided to experiment a little by adding to his diet a bit of carbohydrate from low-calorie fruit and green vegetables. The champ was amazed that this slight dietary change resulted in an immediate drop in his body-fat levels, and within a few weeks he was sliced to ribbons and winning every title in sight.

The most fertile field for experimentation is in contest preparation. Without a doubt, all of the best bodybuilders have a tremendous knowledge of their bodies and how they react during the last few weeks and days prior to a competition. Boyer Coe will pinch the skin on the side of his waist and say, "Two more days of eating 1,800 calories a day and I'll peak. My contest is five days away, so I'll need to consume more calories for the next two days." And, Boyer is always very ripped up for important championships.

Knowledge like this is not gained overnight. You must peak for contest after contest, working out and dieting harder each time, and noting the results until you finally have arrived at an ideal formula for peaking perfectly. Even when you have this formula down pat, it can always do with more and more refinement. Eventually you may discover the perfect combination, but you could become Mr. America or Mr. Universe and still be experimenting with all the variables of bodybuilding diet and training. The essential ingredient here is the *experiment,* so keep at it.

DIET

If I had a dollar for every bodybuilder who has admitted to me over the years that he couldn't make good gains until he finally got his diet trip together, I could probably spend two years lying on a beach in Hawaii!

I discussed nutrition in great depth in *Bodybuilding: The Weider Approach,* so here I would merely like to mention that a huge number of champion bodybuilders credit the right diet for more than 50% of the reason for their success. Many hard gainers place that figure even higher. The great Larry Scott, for example, put it at 75%–80%.

THE HEAD TRIP

As you will discover later in this chapter, virtually all bodybuilders believe that a proper mental attitude toward diet and training is of paramount importance. And no contemporary bodybuilder has a better mental approach to his sport than Tom Platz. Even the greatly revered Arnold Schwarzenegger admits that, "Tom Platz has taken the mental aspects of bodybuilding much further than I'd dreamed of when I was winning seven Mr. Olympia titles." Therefore, I interviewed Tom to determine the secrets of his mental approach to bodybuilding.

"If you can learn to correctly harness the full potential of your mind," he stated, "it can become an unbelievably powerful force in shaping your physique, as well as in

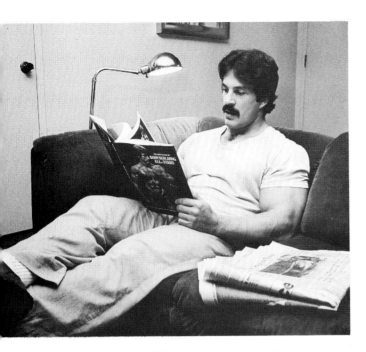

Reach for a bodybuilding book or magazine for inspiration—Mike Mentzer has a vast collection at his disposal.

every other aspect of your life. If the educated human mind has been able to create the baffling array of space-aged technology that we see about us every day, it is certain that you can use your own mind to build the ultimate physique.

"You need only to follow a few easy steps to full mastery of your mental powers in order to begin creating the ultimate physique. You must initially program your mind—much as an artificial brain, the computer, is programmed—to aid yourself in reaching your bodybuilding goals. Then you must constantly update your mind-computer program to keep improving as a bodybuilder.

"Crucially, you must also develop a positive mental attitude toward bodybuilding. The essence of any successful athlete's mental attitude is *positive thinking*.

"Unless my mind triggers off the will to improve my physique, I won't be able to make improvements. Essentially, the mind is the master potentiator in bodybuilding. I've actually trained optimally and dieted very strictly for more than two months prior to a competition—although I had not had my head into the peaking process—and

ended up miserably, failing to reach contest condition. I was so far from peak shape that it looked like I'd been eating jelly doughnuts every day. Yet, I'd actually been on fewer than 1,500 calories per day of chicken breasts, fish, salad, water, and food supplements!

"When I permit something to happen mentally, it quickly happens physically as well. Just as I can't get ripped up on my contest cycle unless I *think* about getting ripped, I also can't gain muscle mass in the off-season unless I permit it to happen mentally.

"At the 1981 Mr. Olympia, I competed weighing 218 pounds of ripped-up muscle, and for 1982 I decided I wanted to come in at 225, just as cut and with even more improved proportions than the year before. So, as soon as I returned to Santa Monica following the 1981 Olympia, I began to think about becoming fairly cut up at a massive 235 pounds, then training down to a supermuscular 225.

"Once I was thinking this way, I began to pack on muscle mass very quickly, until by the middle of the summer before the 1982 Olympia I could look in the mirror and see precisely the degree of muscle mass and muscularity that I had visualized for myself at the point when I would begin my precontest cycle. Oddly enough, although I had not weighed myself in nine months, I stepped on the scales and weighed 235½ *pounds!* My mind had erred by only a half pound in body weight, even though I hadn't remotely monitored my actual weight during my gaining cycle. This remarkable fact further validates the power of a bodybuilder's mind.

"I then immediately programmed myself to slowly train down to a ripped-to-shreds 225 pounds for the Olympia, and I weighed exactly that onstage at the 1982 Olympia. And this happened because I permitted it to happen mentally first. If you expect success, you will receive success. If you are totally convinced that you will succeed—beyond the shadow of a doubt—you will *always* succeed.

"Every negative situation can become

positive if you seek to make it so. Look for the positive and expect it to occur. Then, even a bad workout will be good. Otherwise, how else would you be able to tell when you've had a good workout? You need that reference point, so be happy with a terrible workout now and then.

"If you hate to see a particular photo of yourself, analyze it to discover what makes you look so bad in it. Then change the pose. Always program your mind to learn from your mistakes. Look for the silver lining in every dark cloud, and you will always find that silver.

"On the other side of the coin, when you have doubt and if you expect failure, you will very definitely fail. Hundreds of bodybuilders, and thousands of other athletes, actually fail to succeed because they fear success in their sport. To them, there are overwhelming responsibilities that go with success in a sport (e.g., having to maintain a high level of physical condition after winning a contest, because people expect you to remain looking good; or, living with the expectations of your friends that you will win again and again). This fear of success guarantees failure, so clear your mind of both fear and doubt.

"You have nothing to fear if you become a winning bodybuilder, because you actually compete only against yourself at the higher levels of the sport. Indeed, there are many very attractive perquisites that come with being a winner. Just as one example, I have been able to make a very good living solely from professional bodybuilding—sort of like making your hobby pay off in a big way—ever since I won the IFBB Mr. Universe title in 1978. And more intrinsically, the self-satisfaction I receive each year from constantly improving is more than enough to keep me bodybuilding.

"I take a supremely positive approach toward my entire life, not only to bodybuilding. As a successful bodybuilder, I am fascinated with applying my winning mental attitude and abundant energies to some other facet of my life. So, following Arnold Schwarzenegger's fine example, I am an athlete in the morning and a businessman

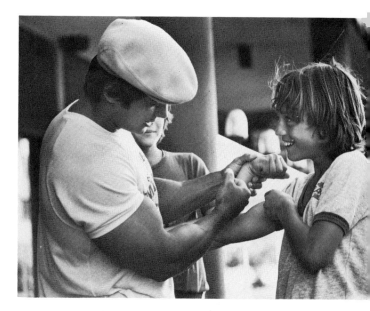

A positive approach to bodybuilding, and to life, is to share. The most important thing you can do is provide an example for others.

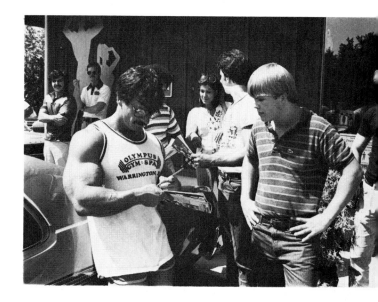

in the afternoon. And, business is great!

"Arnold is a perfect example of the value of a positive approach to life. Arnold came over from Germany in 1968 to train under Joe Weider, and at the time he was unable to speak more than a few words of English. But he knew that America was a land of opportunity for an intelligent and enterprising individual. He *expected* success both as a bodybuilder and businessman and never allowed doubt or fear to enter his mind. He's now a millionaire many times over, is the world's greatest body-builder, and has become an international film star. You can succeed as handsomely as did Arnold, if you want it badly enough.

"To me, learning that you have the ability to become a superman simply by eliminating fear and doubt and replacing it with positive mental programming is almost equivalent to meeting God. That's why in my seminars I try as hard as I can to help young bodybuilders to find this intangible mental ability within themselves and realize that with it they can do literally *anything!*

"The technique of visualization is the method by which you positively program your mind to aid yourself in reaching your bodybuilding goals. It involves a practical application of what psychologists call "self-actualization." Usually, self-actualization is a relatively unguided and unconsciously applied process, but through visualization you can and will consciously and with cold calculation be able to program your subconscious mind exactly the way you would like it to be programmed.

"To give you an example of self-actualization in action, think back about someone you've known who had wanted to become a doctor, lawyer, piano virtuoso, or whatever. Those who have successfully reached their goals in such areas are the ones who had total desire to reach them, desire so strong that they actually *lived* the occupation of their choice in their daydreams and fantasies. When desire is this strong, the subconscious mind is programmed to make decisions that ease the route to the desired goal. It becomes easy, for example, to sit down for six hours and practice a Brahms concerto time after time.

"Individuals find it easy to self-actualize their deepest desires because their subconscious minds actually make difficult decisions easy for them. And in normal self-actualization, one needn't do anything more than simply creatively daydream about becoming a certain type of person or holding a particular job.

"In visualization, we consciously and realistically seek to program our subconscious mind to help us make bodybuilding decisions an easy task. And when this is properly done, it's no longer an ordeal to diet or an unpleasant task to get into the gym and train. The entire bodybuilding process becomes a pleasant experience. I can assure you of this, because my own bodybuilding preparations each day are the best part of my life by a wide margin.

"To properly visualize your bodybuilding success, you should be relaxed and free from distractions for at least 15–20 minutes. At first, I think you can best practice visualization while lying in bed preparing to sleep. Then you will be relaxed and there is minimum potential for disruption of your thought processes. I also feel at first that it's a good idea to practice visualization in the dark, so bedtime is again an ideal time to do it.

"As you lie in bed, begin to imagine yourself as you would like to become one day, either in a year or ultimately. Gradually make this image more and more sharp, until it is almost as though you are projecting a film against the insides of your eyelids. Vividly visualize every lump of muscle, every Grand Canyon cut and every garden hose vein on your body. Vividly imagine what it would feel like to be inside that new body, what it would be like to walk onstage at a contest in it and hear the roar of the audience as it shouts its approval of your appearance.

"Night after night you should practice this, for at least 15 minutes. And as you practice every night, you will gradually become more adept at focusing this image and refining it until it is totally realistic. It's really a very enjoyable experience, very much like the creative type of daydreaming I mentioned earlier. What I am getting at is that you should soon be able to make the image of your ultimate self so realistic that in your visualization process you actually *become* that superstar bodybuilder.

"Regularity is a key in effective visualization. Keep at it night after night for at least 15–20 minutes at a time, and within a few months your subconscious mind will be strongly programmed for success. Ultimately, visualization should become as much of an ingrained habit as brushing your teeth or combing your hair.

"I personally visualize two things each day—how I will look at my next Olympia and how my entire super-productive workout will go that day. I can make my visualization of my next Mr. Olympia contest so realistic that I can actually smell the oil on my body. I can feel my massive and tight muscles contracting and relaxing as I pose. Not only can I see myself in action, but I can feel my skin pulled as tightly as freezer wrap over my huge muscles. I can *feel* ready to do battle with the sport's titans, and through dieting and hard training *I know I will be ready.* Mentally, you can make things like this happen if your visualized image is vivid enough.

"I must caution you, however, to be objective and realistic as you visualize yourself. If you happen to be only four feet tall, you aren't going to play in the National Basketball Association, are you? Take into consideration the strengths and weaknesses of your physique, as well as what you can realistically expect at contest time from your optimum training and dietary preparations. Set your target high, but not so high that you cannot realistically ever expect to hit it.

"Every morning before I go to the gym I also mentally picture every set and every rep of my workout, feeling the super pump I will get from it. I do this *every morning,* either just before breakfast or while eating breakfast. I used to also visualize my training poundages for each set, but I don't do that any more. Now my emphasis is more on how the working muscle *feels* than on the actual weight being used. Sometimes I don't even count the plates I put on the bar. I firmly believe that a bodybuilder has to be a 'feeler,' not a 'lifter.'

"While I recommend that you practice visualization before falling asleep, I have personally become so adept at this practice that I can do it throughout the day. Often a good song will come on the radio and trigger such a reaction. My own posing music ("Ride Like The Wind," by Chris-

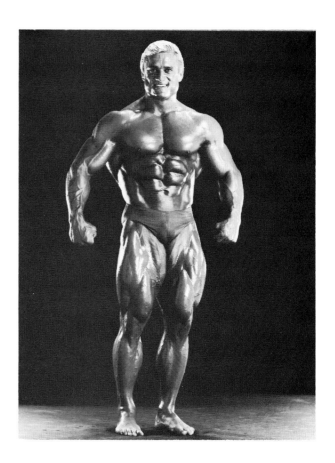

topher Cross) invariably sets me to visualizing how I will look at my next Olympia.

"More often than not, my visualization process is so automatic that it's triggered off by something in my environment at least once or twice a day. However, if it hasn't been triggered by the time I am ready for bed, I will consciously visualize myself in Olympia shape while lying in bed, just as I have recommended that you do.

"There are a lot of other little tricks I use to put myself in the correct frame of mind to win a competition. In the weeks leading up to my Mr. Universe win, I had a big sign that said 'Tom Platz—Mr. Universe' hung over my posing mirror, so I'd see it every time I practiced my posing or walked into that room. I don't want to mess up my apartment with a sign again, however, so I now do other things. In my training and nutrition log I'll sometimes sign an autograph 'Tom Platz—Mr. Olympia,' just to get used to signing it and to foster the belief that I *am* Mr. Olympia.

"It would be a very accurate characterization to say that I will have won a title hundreds of times in my mind before I actually accept the trophy and check. The actual winning of a contest is a mere formality if you have properly prepared yourself mentally for it.

"The final mental aspect of bodybuilding that everyone should master is the ability to concentrate during a workout. You must have a strong link between your mind and your working muscles on every repetition of every exercise. And this is what I mean by concentration in a workout.

"I believe that my ability to concentrate on a given muscle is better now than it's ever been. I can walk into Gold's or the World Gym in any kind of mood, sort of snap my fingers, and *presto!* I'm right into working a particular muscle optimally.

"In past years I'd have to push at it, and I'd get in a good workout here and there. But I usually couldn't tell how I'd gotten it. I'd attribute a good workout to something I'd eaten the night before, but never to my mental state or ability to concentrate. Once I'd begun to become conscious of my mental attitude, however, it became apparent that eating a piece of wholewheat toast wasn't the crucial factor. It was mental attitude and concentration that gave me optimum workouts.

"An upcoming bodybuilder will have to work hard to develop good concentration, this strong link between mind and muscle. Constantly experiment, trying different exercises and workouts. Consciously imagine your working muscles extending and contracting under a heavy load. And if you don't know what muscles are being worked by a particular exercise, read enough bodybuilding books and magazine articles to find out. Then look up the muscles on an anatomy chart so you know which ones you should be feeling as you do an exercise. You'd be amazed at how many bodybuilders do an exercise with no clear idea of what it's supposed to be building.

"Everyone can sense when he's having a good workout. Sometimes it just happens, but you're unsure of why it happened. Ana-lyze everything in your training diary, including your state of mind, after you've had a good workout. Then try to duplicate the conditions and see if you have another good one. When you have been able to concentrate totally on a working muscle group for an entire set, shoot for a second full-concentration set.

"Developing the mental abilities of a champion bodybuilder is like being a bricklayer building a house. Brick after brick, the house *slowly* takes shape. You can't expect to be able to fully concentrate after your first workout, nor after your hundredth. It takes at least two or three years before you have the type of concentration that allows you to shut out the world and concentrate totally on your working muscles during a set.

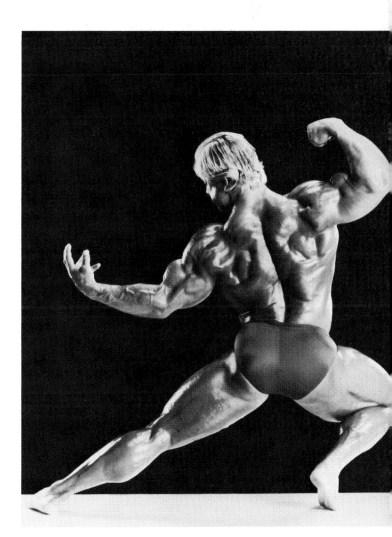

"When you can be doing a set of Preacher Curls and not notice that a jumbo jet has crashed into one side of the gym, you have developed full powers of concentration!

"In the final analysis, remember that the human mind is the most powerful force on earth, more powerful even than the hydrogen bomb. Properly programmed, your mind can carry you to bodybuilding superstardom. So, go for it mentally!"

CONSISTENT AND PERSISTENT EFFORT

"Never miss a workout, and always give 100% of your effort each training session," Bill Pearl advises. Pearl has been a great proponent of this bodybuilding secret. After only a couple of years of hard bodybuilding training, he won the Mr. America title. Many would have called it quits at this point, but Pearl persisted in his consistently hard training for 18 more years, reaching the zenith of his physical perfection when he won his fourth Mr. Universe title at the age of 41 in 1971.

The lesson here is as crystal clear as the old proverb, "Rome wasn't built in a day." Neither is a great physique. In my opinion, it will take you three to five years of consistently hard training to begin regularly winning contests. It will probably take you 8 to 10 years of hard training to win a Mr. America title, *if* you have the physical potential to do so. Therefore, one of the biggest secrets of bodybuilding success is to continue training consistently and intensely until you reach your bodybuilding goals.

SECRETS OF THE CHAMPS

In preparing this book, I quizzed a large number of the bodybuilding superstars I've trained about what they consider to be the "real secret" of bodybuilding success. On the following pages is a sampling of more than 35 of the best and most representative answers.

Lou Ferrigno (Mr. America, Mr. International, twice Mr. Universe): "It appears to me that many young bodybuilders think

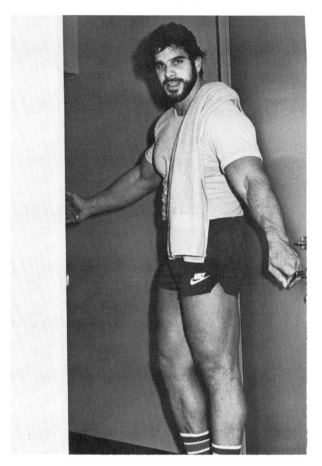

Lou Ferrigno.

the secret is having the right drugs. But drugs are a dead end. The best bodybuilders would still be the best without drugs, because they are mentally committed to bodybuilding and are willing to train hard and consistently, as well as follow a disciplined diet. Nobody will make it as a bodybuilder without having his mind totally in gear. Regardless of the sport, the head is the secret."

Boyer Coe (Mr. America, four times Mr. Universe, Pro World Champion, World Grand Prix Champion): "At the most basic level there are no real secrets, although it's only human nature for young bodybuilders to think there are. You must work hard and apply 100% effort 100% of the time. Hard work is something that 99% of the people in the world shy away from. If something proves to be the least bit difficult to achieve, they immediately give up. The man who doesn't give up, who goes on despite something being difficult to achieve, always comes out on top.

"Over and above all this, I am a firm believer in a positive mental approach to bodybuilding. I believe in the old proverb, 'Whatever can be conceived and believed can be achieved.' The body holds true to whatever course the mind sets as a future reality. Believing in yourself and being able to clearly visualize what you will soon become are the keys to bodybuilding success."

Chris Dickerson (Mr. America, Mr. Olympia, twice Mr. Universe, all-time IFBB pro bodybuilding victories leader): "This is a very complex question, because there are so many answers to it. Some of the most obvious factors to be considered are favorable genetics, desire, persistence, hard training on the right program, getting to know your body, the proper mental approach, and a nutritionally balanced diet. But there are thousands of bodybuilders who combine all of these factors and still don't win titles that they feel they deserve. At that level, seeking physical perfection by always working to bring up weak points is of paramount importance. And, with extensive contest experience, you'll gradually develop excellent onstage charisma."

Mike Mentzer (Mr. America, Mr. North America, Mr. Universe and Pro Grand Prix title winner): "Bodybuilding success starts with favorable genetics, which is a very elusive quality among all young men who begin bodybuilding. Add to that the intelligence necessary to understand and apply various scientific disciplines, such as anatomy, kinesiology, physiology, biochemistry, etc., and you have set the stage for future success. Then it is a matter of persistently training each muscle group with maximum intensity and minimum duration, following a good diet, and maintaining a positive mental approach to bodybuilding."

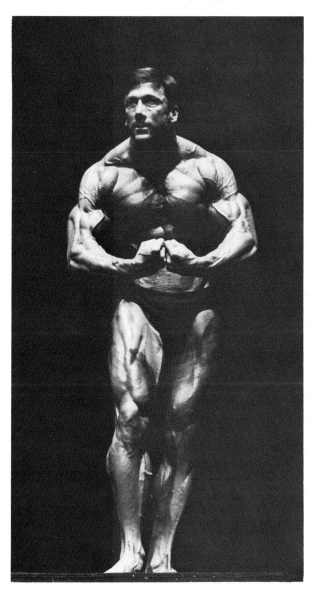

Boyer Coe.

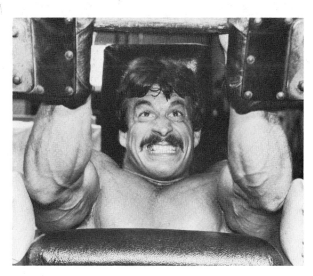

Mike Mentzer.

Shigeru Sugita (Mr. Japan, Mr. Universe, Mr. International class winner): "To me, bodybuilding is both an ennobling struggle for perfection and an art form. I receive great spiritual gratification from my struggle for physical perfection, and this is the reason why I have trained as hard as I have for such a long period of time. To achieve perfection, I always work my weaker body parts first in my program, using the Weider Muscle Priority Training Principle. Overall, I believe that any man who has enough desire to become a champion, and who is willing to make the required sacrifices, can actually become a champion if he is persistent enough."

Pat Neve (Mr. USA, former powerlifting World Record holder): "When I first started training, I thought there were secrets to success, just like everyone else. The longer I've trained, however, the more I've become convinced that there really are no secrets. Over the years I've used the Weider Instinctive Training Principle to gradually learn what sorts of things work well for me,

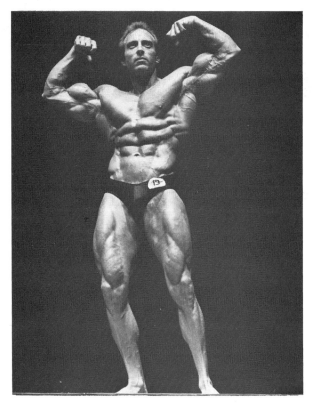

Pat Neve.

what diets to follow, what exercises are best, how to train. I would advise a beginner to seek out those particular combinations of foods and exercises that give him results. Then all he has to do is put in the time necessary to achieve his goals."

Dr. Franco Columbu (Mr. World, Mr. Universe, twice Mr. Olympia and a former powerlifting World Record holder): "First, you must have good genetic potential for the sport, and then you have to develop tremendous mental drive to carry you through many years of consistent hard training. You must get to know your body so you can give it the correct nutrition and training. Learn how to train hard and correctly, and don't waste time using exercises that don't work for you. Finally, if you want to become a superstar, you must work hard to develop personal charisma."

Bill Grant (Pro Mr. America, Pro Mr. World): "Success in bodybuilding comes as a result of total dedication and a great deal of consistent hard work. To be able to put such a large amount of hard work into your bodybuilding, you must have the right positive mental attitude. Follow this formula, and you will eventually reach the limits of your genetic potential. Whether or not that will make you a champion remains to be seen."

Scott Wilson (Pro Mr. America, Mr. International): "I feel that the secret is *determination*. Never lose sight of your goal. Place enough value on your goal for it to always be something you want to pursue. When it hurts to go on in a workout, try to accept the pain. Think of it as a sign of impending success. Sacrifice. Deny yourself the little pleasures of life to pursue your sport. Think like a winner!"

Arnold Schwarzenegger (Mr. Universe, Mr. International, seven times Mr. Olympia): "Bodybuilding is much like any other sport. To be successful, you must dedicate yourself 100% to your training, diet and mental approach. Be persistent and consistent in your training."

Tom Platz (Mr. Universe): "As anyone who has read my articles or attended my

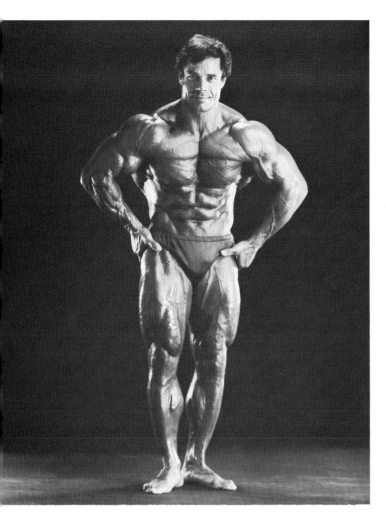

Dr. Franco Columbu.

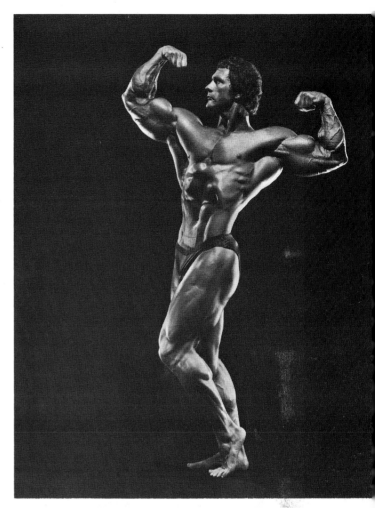

Scott Wilson.

seminars knows, I believe that the mind is a bodybuilder's greatest weapon. If you fully believe you will be successful and can visualize yourself being successful, you will succeed. Success ultimately breeds upon other success. Conversely, if you expect failure, that's exactly what you will get. Negative thoughts are a bodybuilder's greatest enemy."

Casey Viator (Mr. America, Mr. USA, winner of two pro Grand Prix titles): "I think that the secret of bodybuilding success—if there *are* any secrets—begins with having good potential for the sport. Then you must develop the ability to define your goal and then put everything you have into your workouts in order to reach that goal. You won't get any muscle from half-assed and inconsistent workouts. You *must*

work super-hard to win a high-level body-building title, and once you accept that fact, you're halfway to being a winner. Everything I do in my workouts is at 100% effort. I eat, sleep and *do* bodybuilding."

Roger Walker (Mr. Australia, Mr. Universe): "There's no doubt that I've been blessed genetically for building muscle mass. After less than three years of steady training, I was able to place in the top three at the Mr. Britain competition. But it's also true that I have trained exceedingly hard and consistently for a long period of time to reach the level of development I now possess. Over and above all of this, however, my positive mental approach and ability to visualize myself growing progressively better have been the keys to my achieving success as a bodybuilder."

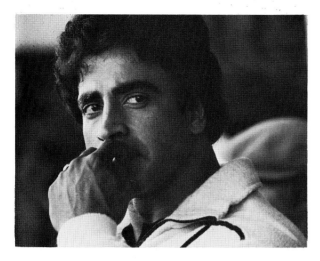

Samir Bannout.

Samir Bannout (Mr. World, Mr. Universe): "Above all else, I believe that I have been successful as a bodybuilder because I *love* the sport. I have definitely been gifted genetically to be a bodybuilder, but if I didn't sincerely love the sport, I could never have put in the long hours of intense training nor monitored my diet as strictly as I have to in order to win. Of course, I also supplement my great love for bodybuilding with a strong positive mental attitude toward my training and diet."

Bertil Fox (Mr. Britain, Mr. World, Mr. Universe): "I think that the key to bodybuilding success is in the mental attitude you have toward the things you do. People have many interests, but how intensely do they follow them? And how long do they keep them up? If you can maintain the same enthusiasm for your sport after ten years of daily workouts as you have now, then you will be a champion. When Bjorn Borg is on television and wins the Wimbledon title, many kids ask their parents for a tennis racquet. But after some weeks or months of practice, most of them lose interest and drop out. A few will continue and eventually have the chance to win professional tennis titles. So it is with bodybuilding. The man in tenth place at a competition has not been as dedicated as the man who won the title."

Don Ross (Pro Mr. America, IFBB professional bodybuilder): "It is no secret that bodybuilding success is the result of persistent training, maintenance of a good diet, hard work, accepting defeat as a yardstick for improvement, a vast amount of research into the science of bodybuilding, and a willingness to experiment with different training methods and diets."

Albert Beckles (Mr. Universe, Pro World Champion, Grand Prix Champion): "I've always figured that if I worked out harder and longer, lifted more weights, concentrated more, watched my diet more assiduously, was more consistent in my workouts, and persevered for a long enough period of time, I would stand a better chance of winning. And this formula has been quite successful for me."

Ray Mentzer (Mr. USA, Mr. America): "I think success comes from an accumulation of knowledge and the maturation of an objective mind. In bodybuilding you have to retain your childlike glee and creativity intact, so the dogmas of ordinary society don't drag you down. It's a matter of establishing a hierarchy of values and ethics, and then sticking to them. Your objective should be self-belief. If you lose the element of joy anywhere through the process, however, you ultimately won't succeed."

Ray Mentzer.

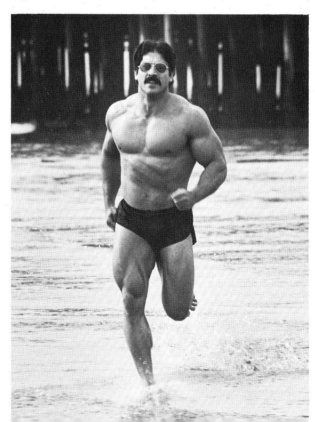

Tony Pearson (Mr. America, Mr. World, Mr. Universe): "Most of the champions I've talked to have labeled *perseverance* as the number one key to success. Most novices tend to get discouraged after their first or second attempt in competition, unless they are lucky enough to win. Bodybuilders who think they can instantly conquer the world are headed for doom."

Frank Zane (Mr. America, Mr. World, Mr. Universe, three times Mr. Olympia): "If there is a secret, it is first a willingness to study yourself objectively, so that you can identify your weak points and bring them up. Pay attention to detail, and train for proportion and symmetry rather than for pure muscle mass. Develop an effective mental approach toward your bodybuilding preparations. I would also advise beginners and intermediates to read science reference books to learn everything they can about how their bodies actually function."

Pete Grymkowski (Junior Mr. America, Mr. World, present owner of Gold's Gym): "A lot of young bodybuilders would think that the secret of my success has been heavy steroid usage, since so much has been written about myself and steroids. I freely admit that I have used steroids, but they have had little to do with my success. Right now I am able to look much better being totally off bodybuilding drugs than I ever did while using them. The secret for me has been a deep study of physiology, biochemistry and other scientific disciplines that affect bodybuilding, plus learning exactly what works for my body. If you don't know your own body inside and out, you'll never become a champion bodybuilder!"

Roy Callender (Mr. Canada, Amateur and Professional Mr. Universe, Pro Diamond Cup Champion): "To my mind, the Weider Instinctive Training Principle has been the real secret to my success. By using this principle while experimenting with a wide spectrum of training and nutritional philosophies, I have been able to gradually assemble a bodybuilding approach that is almost totally in harmony with my own unique body structure and physiology.

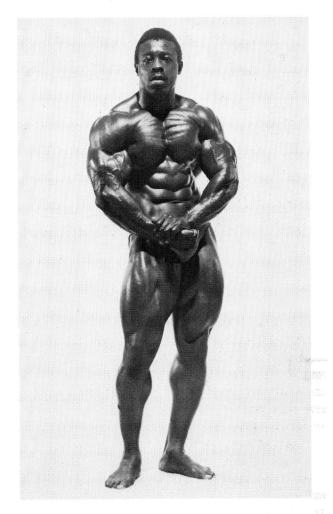

Roy Callender.

Know your body, be persistent, train consistently at 100% of your ability, maintain a healthy muscle-building diet, and you will ultimately succeed as a bodybuilder."

Dale Adrian (Mr. California, Mr. America): "To succeed in bodybuilding takes 100% effort all of the time. I think I've made it to where I am now because I train consistently hard, experiment with bodybuilding variables, follow a very good diet, and take inspiration from bodybuilding competitions. It is important to learn from your losses rather than becoming discouraged and dropping out of the sport. Find out why you lost, and then train to make your weak points very strong for your next contest."

Johnny Fuller (Mr. International, Mr. Universe): "I don't believe that there are any secrets in bodybuilding, or that there are really any shortcuts to success. I have been training with several bodybuilders who still look the same as they did five years ago, while I've improved tremendously during that period of time. So, what's the difference? I believe that I do have a few genetic advantages, but it's more a matter of being more dedicated, training consistently harder, having a better mental approach to my bodybuilding, and following a good bodybuilding diet. I wouldn't call these factors secrets. Would you?"

Richard Baldwin (Collegiate Mr. America, twice Class II Mr. America, twice IFBB Middleweight Mr. Universe runner-up): "I think my success has been a result of my attention to building a good combination of mass, proportions, symmetry, muscularity and posing presentation, so it becomes difficult for the judges to identify faults in my

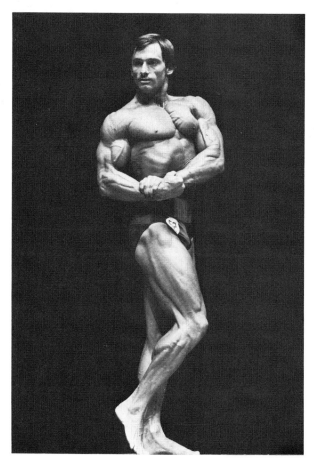

Richard Baldwin.

physique. Although other bodybuilders might be more massive, more muscular, better proportioned, more symmetrical, or may have more dynamic posing routines, I try to have better than average ratings in *all* of these categories. And this usually totals up to a higher score than is drawn by bodybuilders strong in only one or two categories. Consistency and perseverance are important factors in coming out on top. A loss in one contest can be beneficial if the weak point is identified and corrected before the next competition."

Mohamed Makkawy (Mr. International, Mr. Universe): "I think that all bodybuilders have certain hereditary potentials and limitations. As a result, a few can go only so far, despite the efforts they put into bodybuilding. I do not, however, know of any bodybuilder who has come close to his full potential, so don't let your potential worry you. Bodybuilding requires a great deal of desire, dedication and hard work. I believe I have won titles because I have certain hereditary advantages, desire and total dedication. Contest judges look for a combination of proportional balance, symmetry, muscle mass, muscularity, good personal appearance, athletic appeal, and onstage charisma. And, this is the combination toward which I strive at all times."

Chuck Sipes (Mr. America, Mr. World, Mr. Universe): "For me, the real secrets to success were determination and a willingness to sacrifice other pleasures in favor of bodybuilding. For me, training hard has always been enjoyable. I always planned ahead to win a title and devoted full effort for an entire year for one day of competition. Everything during that year was planned toward winning—nutrition, training, rest and recuperation, tanning, posing practice, and everything else."

Andreas Cahling (Mr. International): "The secrets are a healthy diet, a positive mental attitude, and consistent intense training. I have not missed a scheduled workout for more than five years. Even if circumstances beyond my control make it impossible for me to train for more than

15-20 minutes on a workout day, I still train for 15-20 minutes to keep up the rhythm of training. I have great mental concentration on my bodybuilding when I'm in the gym, but I feel strongly that bodybuilding should be confined to the gym and minimized in everyday life. I prefer not to dwell on bodybuilding in my normal conversations."

Robby Robinson (Mr. America, Mr. World, Mr. Universe, winner of many IFBB professional competitions): "In a word, *consistency* has been the key to my success as a bodybuilder. I never miss a workout and I never eat a bite of food that won't contribute to my success. I always eat totally for function rather than for taste. Bodybuilding also requires 100% effort in every single workout, great personal commitment and a good mental approach. There are no other 'secrets' that I know of."

Jusup Wilkosz (Mr. Germany, Mr. Europe, Amateur and Professional Mr. Universe): "In my case, the long preparatory period I spent as a competitive weightlifter greatly aided me in rapidly rising to the top as a bodybuilder. No doubt I have also been blessed genetically. Beyond these factors, it's been strictly a matter of hard work and more hard work, self-discipline and more self-discipline, persistence and more persistence."

Paul Love (Mr. California, Mr. Pacific Coast, Past 40 Mr. America): "I'm several years past 40 and still placed in the top five of my class at the last Mr. America class, competing against men 15-20 years younger. With every year that goes by, I learn new techniques that will improve my physique. If there is a secret to bodybuilding success, it can only be sticking with the sport long enough to become good at it. If you train hard for five years without missing a single workout and you always eat good food, you will be quite competitive in state- and regional-level competitions."

Danny Padilla (Mr. USA, Mr. America, Mr. Universe): "I've always believed in using the basic exercises to build muscle mass, and in paying strict attention to keeping my body proportions perfectly bal-

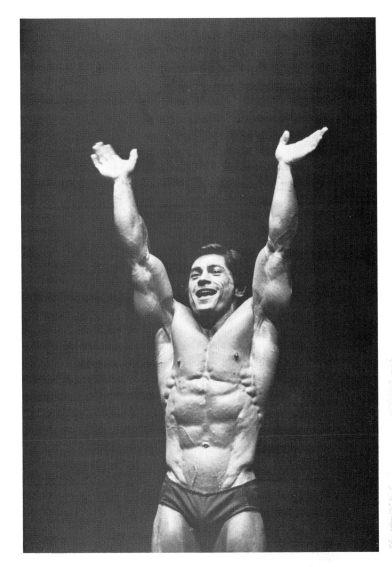

Danny Padilla.

anced. I've always had great drive and dedication, and have kept plugging along to reach the top. In recent years, my most exciting discovery has been finally developing a nutritional strategy that allows me to get ripped to the bone. Prior to a competition, I feel that nutrition is up to 75% of the battle."

Steve Davis (Mr. World): "The spark that put me over the top was using the Weider Instinctive Training Principle to discover what diets, exercises, routines and training methods are best for my unique body. I've always trained more for ideal shape, balanced body proportions, perfect symmetry and sharp muscularity than strictly to ac-

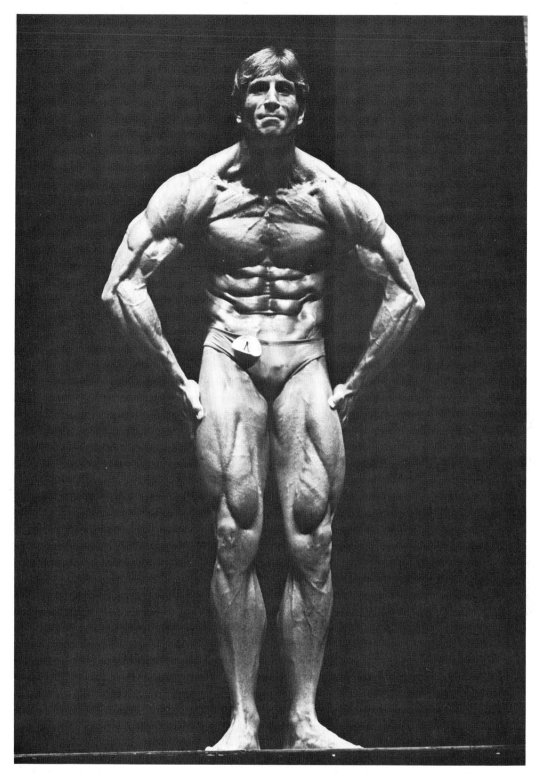

Steve Davis.

quire great muscle mass. Unbalanced mass won't get you anywhere as a competitive bodybuilder. I have also enjoyed the personal coaching of Joe Weider, 'The Master Blaster.' Joe's tremendous charisma has injected precious enthusiasm into my workouts."

Larry Scott (Mr. America, Mr. Universe, twice Mr. Olympia): "I wasn't born with optimum genetic potential to be a bodybuilder, so it took a great deal of persistence to reach the top. I constantly experimented with various exercises and training techniques, gradually discovering little

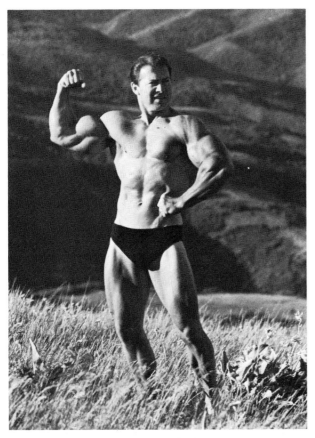

Larry Scott.

twists here and there to different exercises that helped me to more quickly add muscle mass to my body. I now teach these training tricks to all of my pupils at my new million-dollar racquetball and bodybuilding facility in Salt Lake City.

"Since I have always been a slow gainer, proper nutrition has also played a crucial role in my success formula. Ultimately, I discovered that I have to consume considerable milk and milk products—including a milk and egg protein supplement—each day in order to continue adding to my muscle mass."

Ron Teufel (Teenage Mr. America, Mr. USA, IFBB pro bodybuilder): "There's no substitute in bodybuilding for consistently training as hard as you can. I believe that there is a direct relationship between the amount of weight I use in an exercise and the size of the muscles that move the weight in that movement. Therefore, I train as heavily as I can, while maintaining strict exercise form during the off-season. And prior to a competition, I follow a low-calorie diet, while training as quickly and intensely as I can with moderate weights. In order to get ripped to shreds, you simply must use the Weider Quality Training Principle. My final secret to bodybuilding success is constantly keeping a positive mental attitude toward my diet and training. Because I can visualize success, I have often been successful in winning various competitions."

Dennis Tinerino (Mr. America, Mr. USA, Natural Mr. America, Mr. World, Amateur and Professional Mr. Universe): "I have come to believe firmly in doing four heavy workouts a week on primarily basic exercises during the off-season. This type of approach is perfect for full recuperation between training sessions. And without heavy exercise and full muscle recuperation between workouts, no one can develop a championship degree of muscle mass. You'll also need to follow a junk-free diet, be consistent and persistent in your workouts, and stay mentally committed to continued improvement as a bodybuilder. Following this philosophy, anyone with good genetics can build a great physique."

SUMMARY

The information presented in this chapter, particularly the comments of more than 35 Weider-trained bodybuilding superstars on the secrets of bodybuilding success, should give you plenty to think about. And I sincerely hope that this discussion of training secrets will help you to more quickly reach your goals as a competitive bodybuilder.

As the champions themselves have pointed out, there really aren't any deep, dark secrets in bodybuilding. There aren't any secret exercises, secret training routines, secret diets, or secret exotic combinations of bodybuilding drugs that will guarantee you quick success as a bodybuilder. All of the secrets in our sport are open secrets, and you simply must pay your dues in the gym for a considerable period of time to reach the top as a bodybuilder.

So, what are you waiting for? Get into the gym and pump some heavy iron!

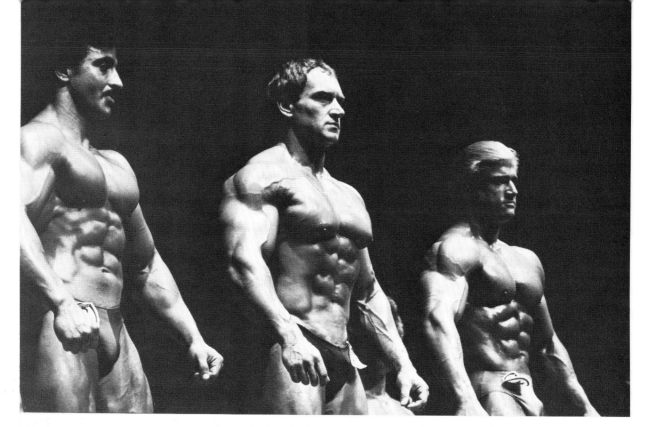

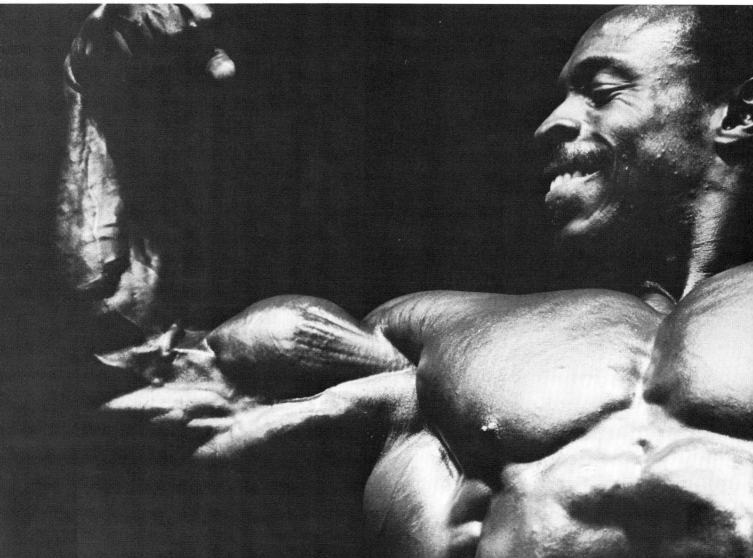

Part II:
Training Programs

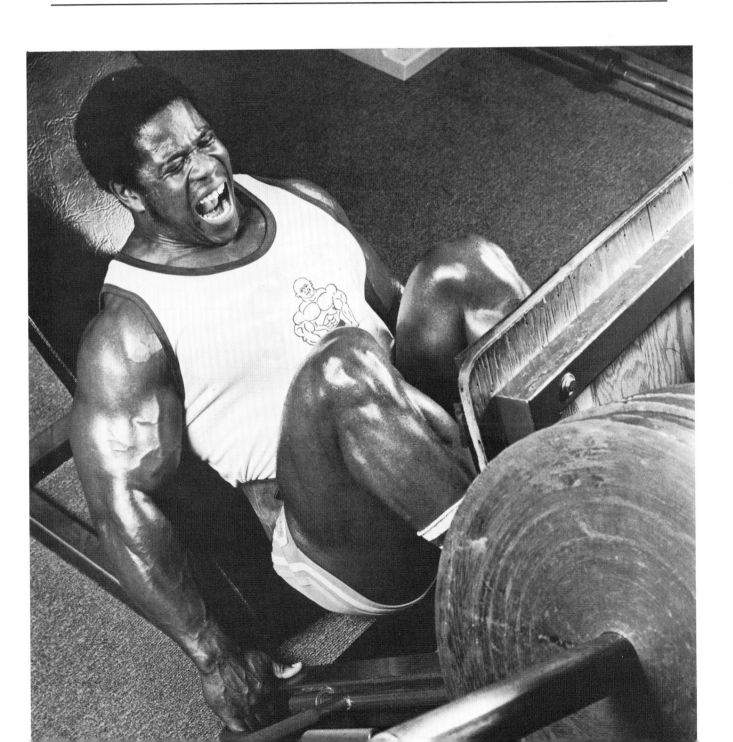

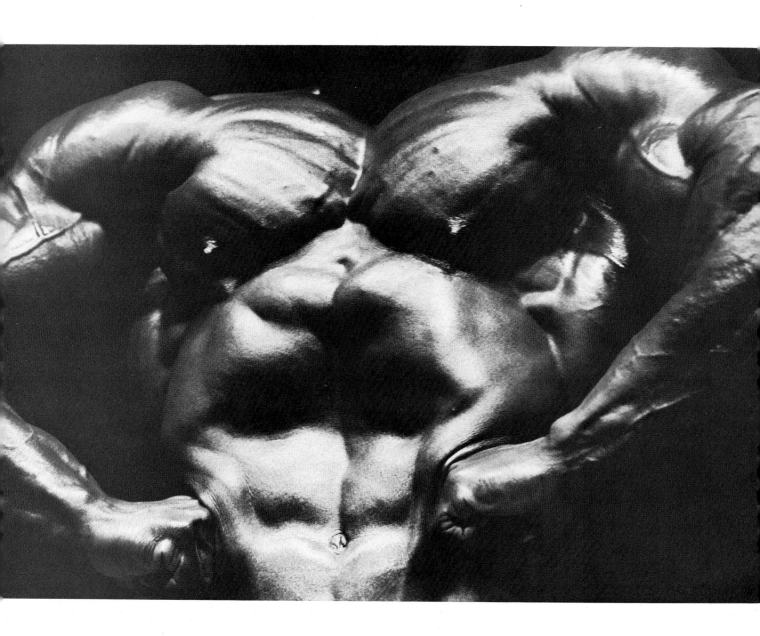

Amazing Abdominals

6

The abdominals are a key area to any serious bodybuilder, because a contest judge's eye normally settles on the middle of a bodybuilder's physique, the abs, first. Initial impressions count highly (if subconciously), and if the judge fails to see a fat-free, tightly muscled waistline, he may almost immediately dismiss you from the ranks of contenders.

Diet plays a vital role in the appearance of your abdominals onstage at a competition. Unless you are totally ripped to shreds, chances are good that your abdominals will be filmed over with a thick enough coating of fat to ruin your chances of taking the title. Therefore, it's essential that you diet down to the lowest possible level of body fat.

I caution you to remain within 6–8 pounds of your competition body weight at all times. The more you pork up during the off-season between competitions, the more difficult it will be to reduce your fat levels until your skin clings like plastic sandwich wrap to your abdominals.

Of course, you must also train quite intensely and regularly to build up the abdominal muscles. The abs *must* be developed, or your entire midsection will look weak. Fifteen or twenty years ago a bodybuilder could neglect his abs, diet down until his waist was small, and get by in a competition by doing a lot of vacuum shots. Today, however, sucking in the stomach is not enough; the judges and audience alike expect to see rugged ridges of muscle throughout the abdominal area.

The abdominal muscles *can* be built up, so every groove between the individual segments of abdominal muscle becomes deeper. And if you don't build up the thickness of your abdominal muscles, there will be little muscular development to add impact to your midsection once you have dieted down to contest condition. Overall, it takes proper diet and hard training working hand-in-hand to give you impressive abdominal development onstage at a major bodybuilding championship.

ABDOMINAL ANATOMY
AND KINESIOLOGY

In discussing abdominal anatomy, bodybuilders usually deal with four main areas:

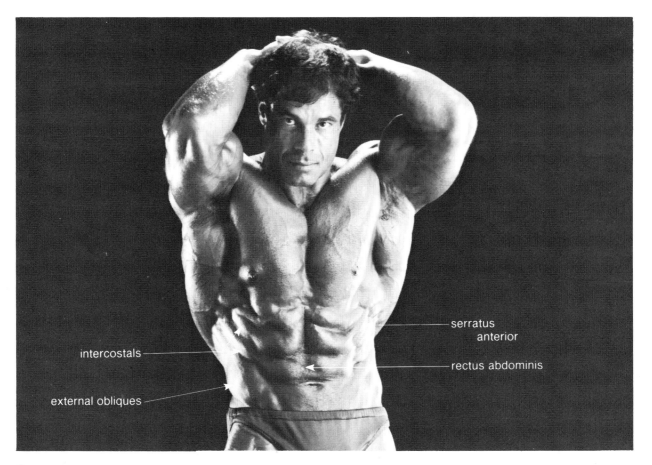

intercostals

external obliques

serratus anterior

rectus abdominis

The Abdominal Muscles.

the *rectus abdominis* (a large, flat, ridged muscle wall covering the front of the abdomen; this is often called the "front abs"); the *external obliques* (muscles at the sides of the waist; they are often called the "obliques"); the *intercostals* (bands of muscle angling downward like chevrons on the sides of the rib cage and upper abdomen); and the *serratus anterior* muscles (finger-like strands of muscle on the rib cage between the lats and front abs). Some bodybuilders feel that the serratus muscles are part of the chest complex and train them as such, but most bodybuilders treat them as part of the abdominal group.

Although most bodybuilders do thousands of Sit-Ups to "develop" their front abdominals, the rectus abdominis comes into play to flex the body only during the first third of the Sit-Up. Most of the body flexion in a Sit-Up is accomplished by the thigh muscles and such hip flexors as the *psoas* and *ilio-psoas.*

The primary function of the rectus abdominis muscles is to pull the upper torso toward the hips when the body is only slightly flexed at the waist. Their function is more one of scrunching the upper torso toward the hips than doing an actual Sit-Up movement. As a result, most modern bodybuilders rely heavily on variations of Crunches to develop the front abdominals.

The external oblique complex actually consists of three layers of muscle: the internal obliques, transverse obliques, and external obliques. The force vector of each of the muscles runs in a different direction from the other two. And, together, these muscles contract to *tilt* the torso from side to side, as well as to *twist* the torso from side to side.

Several variations of side-bending and

twisting resistance movements exist, but you should be quite careful about using very heavy weights for low reps in these exercises. The obliques respond and thicken very rapidly when stressed with heavy weights. And, if they grow too thick, the obliques can actually widen your waist and ruin the esthetics of your physique. Therefore, you should always use light weights for at least 50 reps to each side when doing oblique exercises.

The intercostals also come into play to a degree in flexing the torso and causing it to twist, so doing any type of Twisting Sit-Up or Twisting Crunch will stress that group. The primary function of the intercostals, however, is to depress the ribs, so you will stress these muscles most intensely when you do Twisting Crunches with all of your air expelled.

The serratus muscles depress the rib cage and also assist in bringing the upper arms from a position pointing directly up from the shoulders to one pointing directly down from the shoulders. The serratus muscles, as well as the intercostals, come strongly into play when you do Rope Crunches in your abdominal routine.

By studying the various functions of your abdominals as outlined in the foregoing kinesiology lesson, you should conclude that you must do a wide variety of movements to achieve complete abdominal development. And this conclusion is quite valid, as you will vividly see in the abdominal routines of the champs later in this chapter. Most of them will do 4–6 abdominal movements in order to stress their abdominal muscle complexes from a maximum number of angles.

THE CHAMPS' ABDOMINAL EXERCISES

In this section I will describe and illustrate nine major abdominal exercises that are used by all of the Weider-trained IFBB superstars. Counting variations on each movement, you can experiment with approximately 20 abdominal exercises from this chapter in your own waist-building routines. And, of course, you will use the Weider Instinctive Training Principle to evaluate the worth of each abdominal movement you try out.

Sit-Ups

Main Area of Emphasis–This basic movement stresses the front abdominal muscles, and particularly the upper third of the muscle group.

Method of Performance–Lie on your back on the floor or on an abdominal board. Hook your feet under a heavy piece of furniture, or under the foot strap or roller pads at the end of an abdominal board. Bend your legs slightly in order to take potential strain off your lower back (doing Sit-Ups with straight legs inevitably leads to lower back injuries). Place your hands behind your neck and interlace your fingers to maintain this arm position throughout the movement. From this basic starting position, use your abdominal strength to *curl* your shoulders, then your upper back, middle back, and lower back off the floor or abdominal board until you are sitting erect with your torso perpendicular to the floor. Try to conciously force your shoulders toward your hips as you sit upward in this movement. Reverse the movement to return

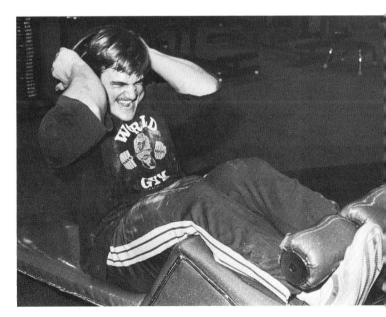

Sit-Ups with weight behind the head.

your torso to the starting position. Repeat for the desired number of repetitions.

Variations—If you are using an adjustable abdominal board, you can make this movement more intense by raising the foot end of the board in gradual increments. The higher the board, the greater the degree of stress placed on your front abdominal muscles. While lying either on the floor or on an abdominal board, you can hold a barbell plate or two behind your head to add resistance to the movement. And, the exercise can be done twisting alternately to each side on successive repetitions. Twisting like this brings the intercostals into play along with the rectus abdominis group.

Training Tips—The most common mistake in this exercise is throwing the head, shoulders and arms forward and upward to add momentum to the sitting-up movement. It's much better to do Sit-Ups slowly and deliberately in order to fully stress the abdominal muscles. Another error is to lift the entire torso off the floor or board at one time, rather than curling it off as described. Such a cheating movement robs your abdominals of much of the stress they should be receiving, and it also puts considerably more strain on the lower back.

Leg Raises

Main Area of Emphasis—Leg Raises stress the front abdominal muscles, and particularly the lower third of the rectus abdominis muscle wall.

Method of Performance—Lie on your back on the floor or on an abdominal board (on the abdominal board your head should be oriented in the direction your feet pointed when doing Sit-Ups). Grasp a heavy piece of furniture, or the feet strap or roller pads at the end of your abdominal board to steady your torso in position during the movement. Bend your legs slightly to take potential strain off your lower back, and keep them bent for the duration of your set. From this basic starting position, slowly move your feet in semicircles until they are directly above your hips. For a little additional stress, you can attempt to raise your hips from the floor or abdominal board. Slowly lower your feet back along the same arc to the starting point, and repeat the movement for the required number of repetitions.

Variations—If you are using an adjustable abdominal board, you can make this movement more intense by raising the head end of the board in gradual increments. The higher the angle of the board, the greater

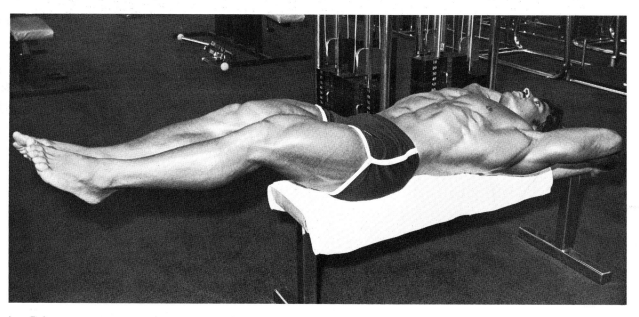

Leg Raise.

the degree of stress placed on your rectus abdominis muscles. While lying on the floor or on an abdominal board, you can do Leg Raises with iron boots on your feet (or with a dumbbell held between your feet) to add resistance to the movement. You can also do Bench Leg Raises with your hips at the end of a flat exercise bench to increase the range of motion of the exercise. On a bench like this, you can lower your feet quite a bit below the level that they reach when lying on the floor or an abdominal board, thereby making the movement more intense.

Training Tips—Do Leg Raises slowly and smoothly, avoiding the temptation to swing or jerk the legs upward. Some bodybuilders insist on doing Leg Raises with their hands under their buttocks, but this lessens the stress placed on the front abs. I am convinced that for best results in bodybuilding—regardless of the muscle group being trained—you should always endeavor to make an exercise *harder* rather than easier to do.

Crunches

Main Area of Emphasis—As mentioned earlier in this chapter, Crunches are the best exercise for directly stressing the rectus abdominis muscles at the front of the abdomen.

Method of Performance—In the most basic form of Crunch, you will lie on your back and drape your lower legs over a flat exercise bench so your thighs are perpendicular to the floor and your lower legs parallel to the floor. Place your hands behind your neck as you would to do a set of Sit-Ups. From this basic starting position, you must simultaneously do four things: (1) use your lower abdominals to raise your hips from the floor (there's a big temptation to use your hamstring muscles to do this, but you should avoid doing so); (2) force your shoulders toward your hips, effectively shortening your torso; (3) raise your head, shoulders, and arms from the floor with upper abdominal strength; and (4) exhale all of your air. When you execute

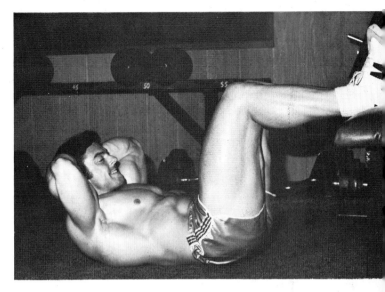

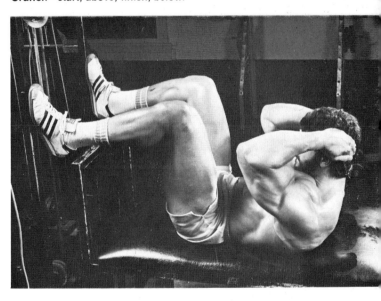

Crunch—start, above; finish, below.

these four actions, you will feel a very strong contraction along the whole of your front abdominal wall. Hold this contracted position for a second or two, then relax your abdominal muscles to return to the starting point of the movement. Repeat the movement until your front abdominals are fully fatigued.

Variations—There are several variations of this movement. In one, you leave the bench out of the exercise and do it by yourself in the middle of the floor, duplicating the leg position just described. In this variation, you can actually move your knees toward your elbows, which increases the intensity of the abdominal contraction. In a

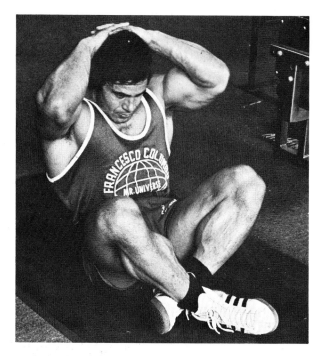

Free-form Crunch.

similar variation, you can lie with your hips about 1½–2 feet from a wall and place your feet flat on the wall at the same level as your knees, then do your Crunches in this position. The foregoing variation places your body in virtually the same position as the basic variation explained in the previous section. You can do L-Crunches with your buttocks wedged in the corner where the wall meets the floor and your legs running straight up the wall. This variation of Crunches is somewhat more intense than any of the foregoing versions. To stress your intercostals and obliques, you can twist alternately from side to side as you do all of the preceding variations of Crunches. The final variation, and the most recently evolved, is Inverted Crunches done wearing gravity boots and hanging inverted from a chinning bar. If you hold a heavy dumbbell against your chest and do Crunches in this position, the movement is very intense and produces great results.

Training Tips—I can't emphasize enough that the object in all variations of the Crunch is to *shorten your torso*. If you consciously think about shortening your torso on each repetition, you will provide your abdominal muscles with the highest intensity of stress.

Hanging Leg Raises

Main Area of Emphasis—Leg Raises done hanging from a chinning bar strongly stress the front abdominal muscles, and particularly stress the lower abdominals.

Method of Performance—Jump up and grasp a chinning bar with your hands set a comfortable distance apart. At the starting point of the movement your body should be hanging directly below the bar, and your legs should be held slightly bent to relieve potential lower back stress. From this starting point, slowly raise your feet forward and upward in semicircles until your thighs are above an imaginary line drawn through your hip joints and parallel to the floor. If you have the strength to do so, attempt to actually lift your hips upward toward your shoulders in order to contract your rectus abdominis muscles even harder. Slowly lower your feet back along the same arc to the starting point, and repeat the movement for an appropriate number of repetitions.

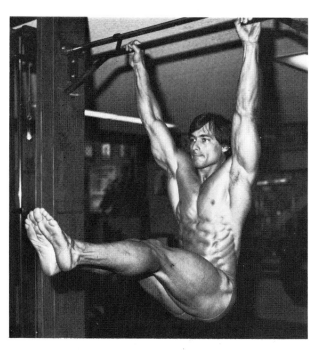

Hanging Leg Raise.

Variations—You can perform Frog Kick Leg Raises while hanging from the bar if your abdominal muscles aren't yet strong enough to do at least 10 repetitions of regular Hanging Leg Raises. In this movement, you bend your legs and pull your knees upward to touch your lower rib cage at the top of the movement. When doing Frog Kicks, you can twist alternately to each side if you wish to stress the intercostal muscles on the sides of your waist.

Training Tips—If you time each rep correctly, you can avoid swinging when you do Hanging Leg Raises. Or, if you have a problem with your torso swinging back and forth during the movement, I suggest that you have a training partner hold your hips in a steady position during the movement. After you have done a set or two of Hanging Leg Raises to thoroughly warm up your front abdominal muscles, you can profitably increase the intensity of the movement by either wearing iron boots (each of which weighs approximately five pounds) or holding a light dumbbell between your feet.

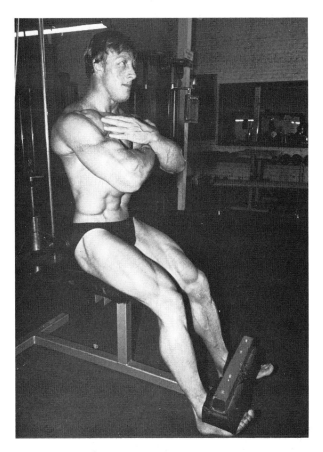
Roman Chair Sit-Ups.

Roman Chair Sit-Ups

Main Area of Emphasis—This movement stresses the whole rectus abdominis muscle wall, and particularly the upper third of the muscle group. If you do Twisting Roman Chair Sit-Ups, you can also stress the intercostals with this exercise.

Method of Performance—Sit on the seat of a Roman chair and push the insteps of your feet under the foot-stop bar near the floor in front of you. Cross your arms over your chest. Sit backward until your torso is only slightly above a position parallel to the floor. Sit forward until you begin to feel tension coming off of your abdominal muscles. Rock back and forth slowly between these two positions for the desired number of repetitions.

Variations—This movement can be done twisting your torso from one side to the other after each repetition. It can also be done while holding a weight on the chest,

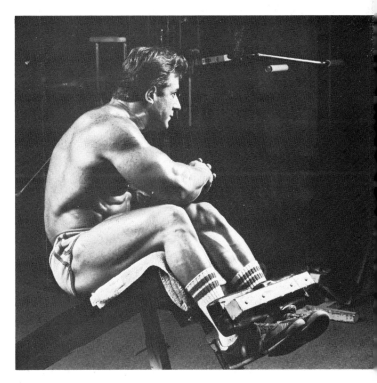
Twisting Roman Chair Sit-Ups.

although only a few bodybuilders seem to do weighted Roman Chair Sit-Ups.

Training Tips—A better way to add resistance to Roman Chair Sit-Ups involves placing a 4 x 4-inch block of wood under the foot end of the Roman chair to elevate that end and give you the equivalent of an Incline Sit-Up.

Rope Crunches

Main Area of Emphasis—This movement stresses the rectus abdominis, intercostal and serratus muscle groups quite hard. It also puts secondary emphasis on the latissimus dorsi muscles. Rope Crunches are a good finishing-off movement for both the abdominal muscles and the latissimus muscles.

Method of Performance—Attach a rope handle to the hook at the end of a cable running through an overhead pulley to the weight stack. Kneel down about 1–1½ feet back from where the pulley hangs down, holding the two ends of the rope handle in your hands. Kneeling erect, simultaneously bend forward to touch your forehead on the floor, do a partial pullover motion with your hands, and blow out all of your air. When you do this movement correctly, you will feel a strong contraction in all of your abdominal muscles. Hold this fully contracted position for a couple seconds, relax, and allow your body to assume the starting position. Repeat this movement until your abdominal muscles are fatigued.

Variations—Many bodybuilders twist alternately to each side to place greater stress on their intercostals and serratus for at least a couple of sets of this movement. You can also do Rope Crunches with one arm at a time for a very direct stimulation of your intercostal and serratus muscles.

Training Tips—You won't be able to use a very heavy weight in this movement, since you are not working large muscle groups with it. Rather than placing emphasis on the poundage you are handling for Rope Crunches, try to concentrate solely on the feel of the movement as you do it.

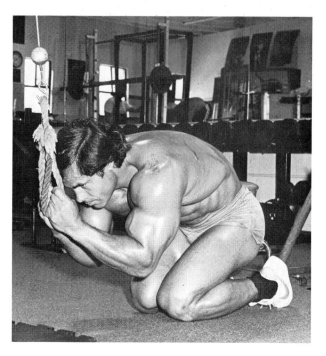

Rope Crunch.

Side Sit-Ups

Main Area of Emphasis—This movement strongly stresses all of the muscles at the sides of your waist—the obliques, intercostals, and serratus muscles.

Method of Performance—Lie on your right side with just your legs in contact with a high padded bench, such as across the top of a leg table. Have a training partner restrain your legs by draping his torso across them as you do the movement. Cross your arms on your chest. Allow your torso to sag from the waist directly to the side toward the floor as far as possible. From that position, use the muscles at the side of your waist to pull your torso upward as high as possible. Lower back to the bottom position of the movement, and repeat the movement for an appropriate number of repetitions to each side of the body.

Variations—The only real variation of this movement involves rolling your torso a bit forward and backward to stress a little of the front abdominals or lower back muscles.

Training Tips—You can add resistance to this movement by holding a light barbell plate across your chest.

Side Bends

Main Area of Emphasis—This movement stresses primarily the oblique and intercostal muscle groups at the sides of the waist.

Method of Performance—Stand erect with your feet set a little wider than the width of your shoulders on each side. Place a broom stick or an unloaded barbell bar across your neck and grasp the ends of it with your hands. Stiffen your legs and keep them stiffened throughout the set you are doing. From this basic starting position, bend at the waist as far to the right as possible. Immediately bend as far to the left as possible. Rhythmically move back and forth between these two positions for a full set of the required number of repetitions, counting each complete cycle of bending both to the left and right as one repetition.

Variations—This movement can be done while holding two light dumbbells in each hand or with a dumbbell held in one hand and the free hand placed behind the head. When you do this second variation, be certain to do an equal number of sets and reps with the dumbbell in each hand.

Training Tips—Again, remember to avoid using heavy weights and use low reps in this movement. You don't want to make your waist look any wider than it already is.

Twisting

Main Area of Emphasis—Although there is some doubt about it, many bodybuilders feel that variations of Twisting help to firm the sides of the waist and lower back.

Method of Performance—Assume the same starting position with a broomstick across your shoulders as for the start of a Side Bend set, but wrap your arms around the stick. Attempting to keep your hips and legs from deviating from this position, rap-

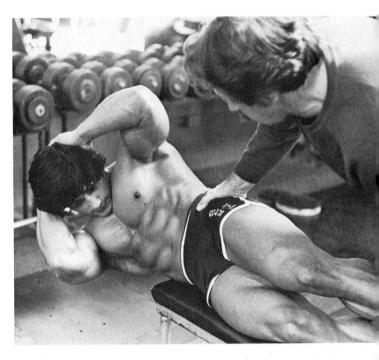

Side Sit-Ups.

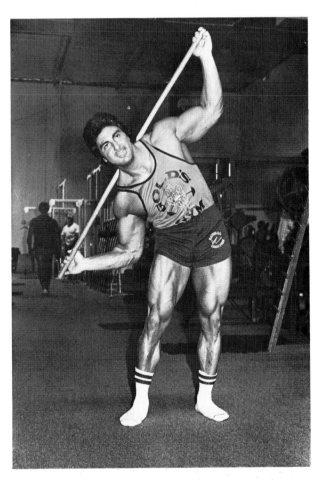

Side Bends.

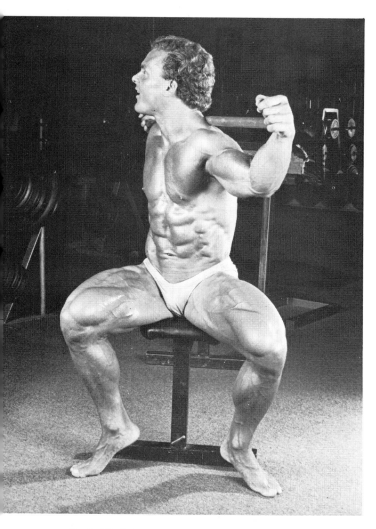

Seated Twisting.

idly and forcefully twist back and forth to the right and left. Count one cycle from right to left and back again to the right as a repetition.

Variations—To keep from moving the legs, some bodybuilders do this movement bent over at the waist with the torso parallel to the floor. Another way to restrain the hips and legs is to sit astride a flat exercise bench and wrap your legs around the upright legs of the bench. Or, you can sit on a roman chair with your toes wedged under the foot-stop bar to keep from moving your legs and hips as you do Twists.

Training Tips—You will notice if you do this movement at the beginning of your workout that it loosens up your lower back.

CHAMPIONSHIP ABDOMINAL ROUTINES

In this section I will present the abdominal training routines of 10 IFBB champions. In other chapters I have included 20 or more training routines for the body part discussed, but this isn't necessary with the abs, since most bodybuilders train them relatively the same.

Keep in mind as you read these routines that they are of very high intensity and suitable for use as written by only very advanced bodybuilders. You must adapt these routines to your own ability levels. If you are a beginner, you should do only one or two sets of each exercise and perform a total of only 6–8 sets. At the intermediate level of bodybuilding training, you can do 8–10 total sets of abdominal training, while at the advanced level you can do 12–15 total sets of ab work.

Lou Ferrigno

Exercise	Sets	Reps
1. Hanging Leg Raises	3–4	15–20
2. Roman Chair Sit-Ups	3–4	50
3. Bench Leg Raises	3–4	30–40
4. Crunches	3–4	30–40
5. Side Bends	3–4	50
6. Rope Crunches	3–4	25–30

Note: Exercises 1–6 are performed as a giant set.

Dennis Tinerino

Exercise	Sets	Reps
1. Roman Chair Sit-Ups	3–4	25–30
2. Hanging Leg Raises	3–4	15–20
3. Crunches	3–4	30–40
4. Bench Leg Raises	3–4	30–40
5. Seated Twisting	3–4	100

Note: Exercises 1–5 are performed as a giant set.

Mike Mentzer

Exercise	Sets	Reps
1. Roman Chair Sit-Ups (weighted)	2–3	25–10
2. Hanging Leg Raises	2	20–25
3. Side Sit-Ups	2	12–15

Richard Baldwin

Exercise	Sets	Reps
1. Roman Chair Sit-Ups	3	40–50
2. Hanging Leg Raises	3	15–20
3. Crunches	3	30–40
4. Rope Crunches	3	25–30

Bill Pearl

Exercise	Sets	Reps
1. Incline Sit-Ups	4–5	50
2. Hanging Leg Raises	4–5	20–30
3. Crunches	4–5	50
4. Leg Crossovers	4–5	50
5. Incline Leg Raises	4–5	50

Note: Exercises 1–5 are performed as a giant set.

Danny Padilla

Day 1

Exercise	Sets	Reps
1. Roman Chair Sit-Ups	4	25–50
2. Seated Twisting	4	50–100
3. Hanging Knee-Ups	4	25–30
4. Side Bends (no weight)	4	50–100
5. Crunches	4	25–30

Day 2

Exercise	Sets	Reps
1. Incline Sit-Ups	4	25–30
2. Seated Twisting	4	50–100
3. Hanging Leg Raises	4	15–20
4. Side Bends (no weight)	4	50–100
5. Rope Crunches	4	25–30

Note: Exercises 1–5 in each routine are performed as a giant set.

Ray Beaulieu

Day 1

Exercise	Sets	Reps
1. Crunches	3	30
2. Seated Twists	3	500

Note: Exercises are supersetted.

Day 2

Exercise	Sets	Reps
1. Roman Chair Sit-Ups	3	100
2. Seated Twists	3	500

Note: Exercises are supersetted. Abdominals are usually trained in the morning separate from the rest of the body.

Tim Belknap

Exercise	Sets	Reps
1. Crunches (weighted)	5	20–30
2. Bench Leg Raises	5	30–40
3. Side Bends	5	40–50

Note: Bracketed exercises are supersetted.

Ron Teufel

Exercise	Sets	Reps
1. High Incline Sit-Ups	5	20–30
2. Hanging Leg Raises	5	15–20
3. Crunches	4	30–40
4. Bench Leg Raises	4	30–40
5. Rope Crunches	3	20–30

Note: Bracketed exercises are supersetted.

Samir Bannout

Exercise	Sets	Reps
1. Hanging Leg Raises	3–4	15–20
2. Incline Sit-Ups	3–4	20–30
3. Incline Leg Raises	3–4	20–30
4. Roman Chair Sit-Ups	3–4	50
5. Seated Twisting	3–4	50

Note: Bracketed exercises are supersetted.

CONCLUSION

The information presented in this chapter will have given you plenty of food for thought as you use the Weider Instinctive Training Principle to develop your midsection. Adapt the exercises and routines of the champs to your own abilities and purposes, never miss a workout, and use a great deal of intensity in your ab programs, and you'll soon have your own set of washboard abdominals!

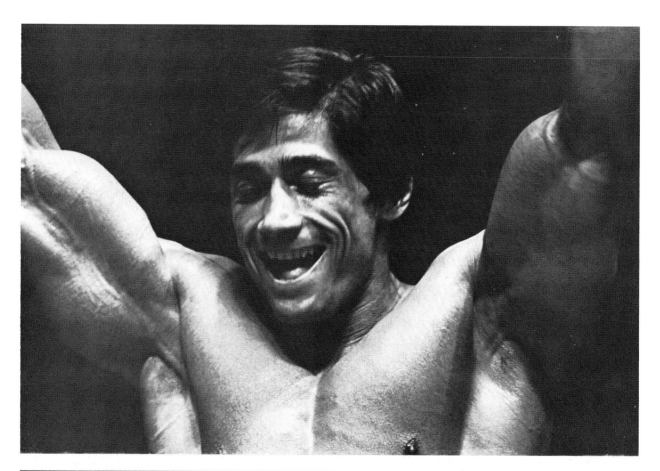

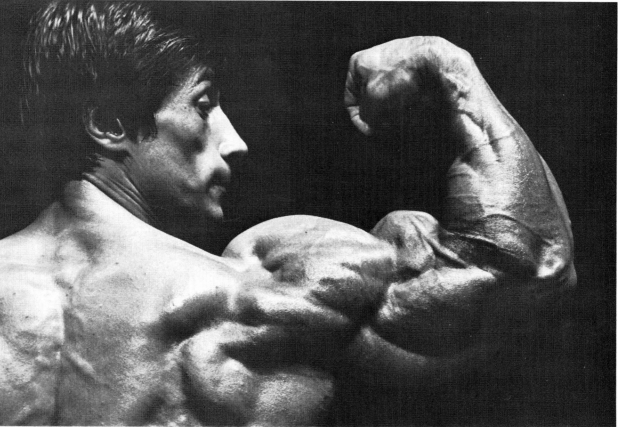

Danny Padilla, the Giant Killer.

7

Upper Arm Development

Bodybuilders across America, as well as around the world, are fascinated by the process of building huge, well-shaped, and supermuscular upper arms. Indeed, among the hundreds of letters I get each week at Weider Headquarters in southern California, a large percentage include requests for the arm routines of the sport's superstars.

As a result of the scores of letters I receive each week requesting upper arm training information, I consistently run the arm programs of the superstars in my two bodybuilding magazines, *Muscle & Fitness* and *Flex*. And, at the end of this chapter it will be my pleasure to give you the exact arm-building routines of more than 20 Weider-trained, IFBB superstars!

It almost seems as though a champion bodybuilder must have 20-inch upper arms in order to win a high-level national or international title these days. Much of this fascination that bodybuilders have with huge upper arm development stems from the superb upper arms of Larry Scott, who was widely publicized in my magazines during the mid- and late-1960s. The Great Scott won the first two Mr. Olympia titles,

and today, at the age of 45, his upper arms are as good as ever.

Following Larry Scott have come a flood of champion bodybuilders with super upper arm development. Virtually every IFBB champ has superb biceps and triceps development, but the best of these superstars include Arnold Schwarzenegger, Boyer Coe, Albert Beckles, Lou Ferrigno, Robby Robinson, Danny Padilla, Dennis Tinerino, Mike Mentzer, Jusup Wilkosz, Casey Viator, Tim Belknap, Bertil Fox, Lance Dreher, and Roy Callender.

With time, you may add your own name to this list of "heavily armed" IFBB superstars. But as you are building up your physique, don't allow your upper arm development to become so huge that your arms become out of proportion with the rest of your physique. Having evenly developed body proportions is the most important quality that a physique contestant can possess.

If your biceps and triceps are fully developed, your forearms must be equally well developed, or your lower arms will look like buggy whips. By the same token, your deltoids must also be quite massive, well-proportioned, and muscular, or your upper arms will dwarf your shoulders. And, of course, then every other section of your physique must also be massively developed, or your arms and shoulders will appear to be much too large for the rest of your body.

Some bodybuilders have extreme difficulty in developing their upper arms, but with persistence any serious bodybuilder can build impressive biceps and triceps. On the other side of the coin, a few bodybuilders hardly need to train their upper arms, since they grow so easily. Typical of this type of bodybuilder is Albert Beckles, winner of a number of IFBB professional bodybuilding titles.

Beckles' upper arms grow so easily that during the off-season, he seldom does any arm training whatsoever. Even close to a competition he does no more than 10–12 total sets of biceps or triceps work per week!

According to Albert Beckles, "All pressing exercises seem to sufficiently stimulate my triceps during the off-season. Similarly, the pulling exercises I do for my lats are sufficient to keep my biceps massive and muscular. Then, close to a contest, I will merely do a few sets of direct biceps and triceps movements two or three days per week to shape and striate my upper arm muscles.

"Keep in mind, however, that I have been blessed with genetics that allow my biceps and triceps to grow very easily and quickly. Additionally, I *have* trained my arms much harder in the past than I do now. Therefore, my type of arm-building philosophy may not work well for you. As in all facets of bodybuilding, you must utilize the Weider Instinctive Training Principle to evaluate the relative worth of each exercise, training routine, and workout tip."

Actually, my champs have found that pushing and pulling movements for the torso muscles strongly stimulate the triceps and biceps. If you were so short of time that you could only train three days

per week for 30 minutes, you could work virtually every muscle group in your body by doing only five sets of 6–10 reps in the Squat, Barbell Bent Rowing, and Bench Press movements. The Rows would keep your biceps in shape, while the Benches would keep your triceps bulging.

UPPER ARM ANATOMY AND KINESIOLOGY

There are three major muscle groups of the upper arm: the *biceps brachii* (usually called simply the *biceps*), the *brachialis*, and the *triceps brachii* (usually called the *triceps*).

The biceps are a two-headed muscle group that originates along the front part of the shoulder joint and inserts high on the lower arm bones. The biceps serve two basic functions. First, the muscle group contracts to bend the arm fully from a straight position. Secondly, the biceps help to supinate the hand.

You will read more about this supination function in the next section of this chapter, but essentially supination involves rotating the hand from a position with the palm down to one in which the palm faces upward when the arm is bent at a right angle while hanging down at the side of the body. Pronation is the opposite of supination (i.e., pronation involves rotating the hand from a position with the palm up to one in which the palm is facing the floor with the arm bent at a 90-degree angle).

The brachialis lies beneath the biceps muscles. It originates from near the middle of the upper arm bone and attaches to a lower arm bone. The brachialis can be seen vividly as a flat band of muscle between the biceps and triceps when a well-defined bodybuilder does a back double-biceps pose. As do the biceps, the brachialis functions to fully bend the arm from a straight position. While the biceps fully contract best when the hand is completely supinated, however, the brachialis fully contracts when the hand is completely pronated.

The triceps is a three-headed muscle

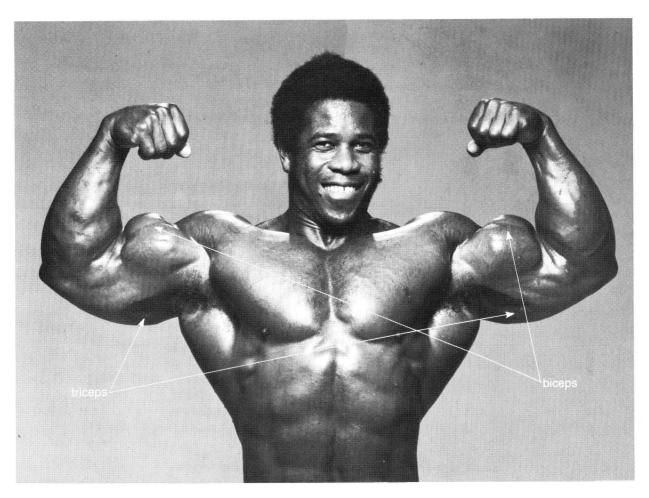

The Upper Arm Muscles.

group that originates under the rear deltoid and attaches via a common tendon that runs over the elbow to the lower arm bones. The triceps have one primary function—to completely straighten the arm from a fully bent position. Occasionally, though, the triceps will also contract in conjunction with the posterior deltoid to help move the upper arm bone directly to the rear.

SUPINATION AND THE CURL

To fully develop your biceps, you should always try to supinate your hands as you do various permutations of Dumbbell Curls. Obviously, you can't do this with a barbell or EZ-curl bar when doing Curls, because your hands are restricted to a set position and can't be rotated. Even though

bodybuilders, even a few superstars, frequently use an EZ-curl bar for Standing Barbell Curls and Barbell Preacher Curls, using this apparatus does less for the biceps than do Dumbbell Curls, since the hands are actually rotated *away* from a fully supinated position during a Curl movement.

To fully illustrate the supination movement, let's assume that you are simultaneously curling two dumbbells while standing erect, but we'll focus only on the orientation of your right hand. The movement and orientation of your left hand will merely be the mirror image of that of your right hand.

At the start of the movement, your right arm is hanging down at your side, your palm is facing the side of your leg. Without moving your upper arm, you bend your arm

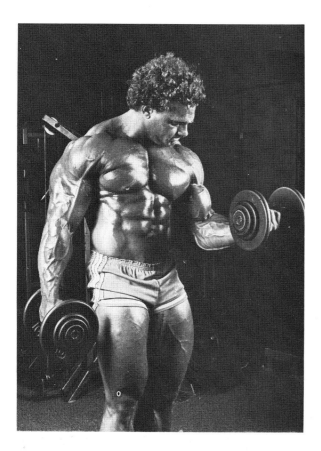

to move the dumbbell in a semicircle from the side of your thigh to your shoulder. But, as you curl the dumbbell upward, you must simultaneously rotate your thumb outward in a clockwise direction to bring your palm facing upward from about the middle position to the end of the movement.

Some bodybuilders with superior flexibility can actually supinate their hands so their palms almost face outward. And, as you lower the dumbbell in a Dumbbell Curl, you should pronate your hand until your palm is again facing your thigh before you begin another repetition.

You should supinate your hand (or hands) on every type of Dumbbell Curl, since this movement adds greater quality to your biceps development.

BICEPS PEAK

There are several types of Concentration Curls (with a dumbbell, barbell, or various types of pulleys) that help to accentuate the natural peak of a bodybuilder's biceps.

Regardless of how many hundreds of heavy sets of Concentration Curls that you do over the years, however, you will *not* build an Everest-peaked biceps unless you have the hereditary predisposition to possess such a high-peaked biceps.

Some bodybuilders, such as Boyer Coe, are blessed with the genetic ability to build a high-peaked biceps. And, over the years Boyer has done plenty of Concentration Curls to bring out the peaks on his biceps.

Other champion bodybuilders don't have the genetics to build a high biceps peak. Sergio Oliva didn't. Even though he has undoubtedly done thousands of sets of various types of Concentration Curls over the years, his biceps remained flat appearing. Granted, Sergio's biceps are *huge* beyond all comprehension, but they lack the peaks that a Boyer Coe reached easily.

I've even seen quite a number of champion bodybuilders (including one of the sport's all-time greats) who have one biceps with a high peak and another biceps that appears quite flat. And this situation is a perfect illustration of the role that genetics play in developing a high-peaked biceps. A bodybuilder will do the same exercises, sets, and reps for each arm, but he can still have one arm that does not acquire the same high-peaked biceps as his other arm.

COPING WITH SORE ELBOWS

Many bodybuilders end up developing sore elbows, which makes it difficult to train the triceps hard enough to build maximum mass and density. Therefore, you should be aware of how to prevent the development of sore elbows, how to train with sore elbows, and how to cure elbow soreness.

Prevention of elbow soreness is the best cure for this problem. To keep your elbows healthy, always warm them up thoroughly before training them. Some top bodybuilders prefer to train their biceps first as a way of indirectly warming up their elbows prior to bombing triceps. Others prefer to train their triceps after chest and/or deltoid work, which provides the elbows with a more direct type of warm-up.

Regardless of the type of indirect warm-up you provide to your elbows, you should also carefully warm up your elbows with light, high-rep sets of some type of triceps exercise. Lou Ferrigno, who has periodically had elbow problems, always does three or four light, high-rep sets of Pulley Pushdowns, going a little heavier on each succeeding warm-up set, as his elbows and triceps warm up.

If one or both of your elbows are sore, you can still do a fairly stiff triceps workout without too much pain or further aggravating the injury or injuries. To do so, first do a thorough warm up with Pulley Pushdowns as described in the preceding paragraph. Then you should do triceps exercises that don't *directly* stress the elbows. This means you should do Close-Grip Bench Presses or Parallel Bar Dips rather than Barbell or Dumbbell Triceps Extensions. And, it is a good idea to put ice on your elbows for 20–30 minutes after each triceps workout, a practice which helps to prevent pain the day after training them.

I'm often asked by rising bodybuilders if they should wrap their elbows when they have elbow pain. As far as elastic bandage wraps are concerned, my experience has been that it's not a good idea to use them. Neoprene rubber bands around the elbows, however, are quite good when you have elbow soreness. They don't provide more than a minimum of support during an exercise, but the rubber retains body heat quite effectively, which in turn keeps the elbows from being further injured during a triceps workout.

To cure an elbow injury, you may need to lay off of triceps training completely for a few weeks to allow the injury to heal. Or, you can follow the procedures outlined for training with an elbow injury until that injury finally heals. Normally, the elbows will heal up if you are careful to warm up thoroughly and avoid doing triceps exercises that in your experience tend to aggravate the injury.

In rare cases, you might require surgical repair of a torn elbow tendon, bone chips in your elbow, or other similar orthopedic injuries. Also, there are several prescription anti-inflammatory medicines that you can use if you have long-term tendinitis of the elbow. One of the best of these is a nonsteroidal, anti-inflammatory drug called *Motrin*. You can ask your physician about it.

THE CHAMPS' UPPER ARM EXERCISES

In this section I will present 17 of the greatest IFBB champs' upper arm exercises. Counting the variations I will give you for each of these upper arm movements, you will have more than 30 exercises to work with in making up your own individualized arm training programs.

Standing Barbell Curl

Main Area of Emphasis—Barbell Curls strongly stress the biceps muscles and

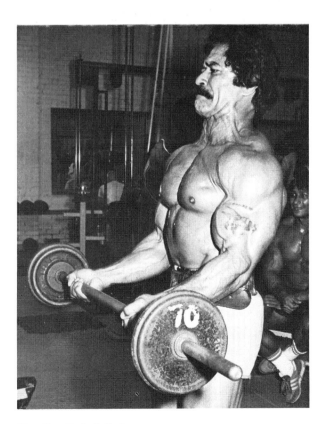

Standing Barbell Curl.

place secondary stress on the flexor muscles on the insides of the forearms.

Method of Performance—Take an undergrip on a barbell with your hands set 4–6 inches wider on each side than the width of your shoulders. Stand erect with the barbell, your arms running down the sides of your body and the barbell resting across your upper thighs. Press your upper arms against the sides of your torso, and keep them in this position throughout the movement. Being careful to keep your torso from swinging back and forth, slowly bend your elbows and curl the barbell in a semicircle from your thighs to a position under your chin. Slowly lower the barbell back along the same path it came up until it is back at the starting point. Repeat the movement for the required number of repetitions.

Variations—The main variation that you can use on Barbell Curls is to move the width of your grip inward for a narrow grip or outward for a wider grip. Arnold Schwarzenegger usually did his Barbell Curls with a wide grip, while Rick Wayne preferred to do them with a quite narrow grip. Both men had exceptional biceps development.

If you are having difficulty keeping your torso from swinging back and forth during the movement, you can do Standing Barbell Curls with your back pressed against a wall or the upright member of an exercise machine. This practice ensures that you will keep your torso motionless throughout the movement. You can also use a Weider Arm Blaster if you find that you have trouble with keeping your upper arms and elbows motionless.

Training Tips—Of all biceps movements, this is the easiest one on which to use the Weider Cheating Training Principle. I'd suggest that you use a weightlifting belt when you do Cheating Barbell Curls, however.

Standing Dumbbell Curl

Main Area of Emphasis—As with Barbell Curls, this movement strongly stresses the biceps muscles and secondarily stresses the flexor muscles on the insides of the forearms.

Method of Performance—Grasp two moderately weighted dumbbells and stand erect with them in your hands. Run your arms down the sides of your body, with your palms facing toward your legs. Pin your upper arms against the sides of your torso, and keep them in this position

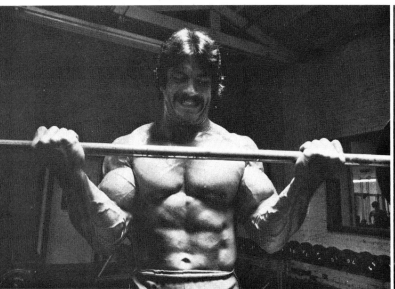
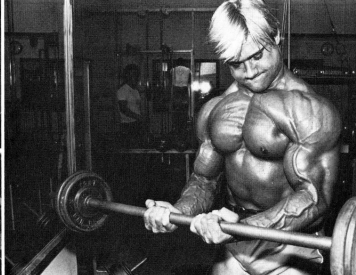

Standing Barbell Curl with wide grip, left; with narrow grip, right.

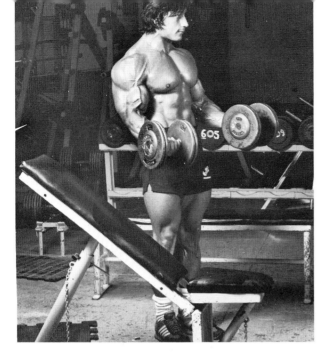

Standing Dumbbell Curl.

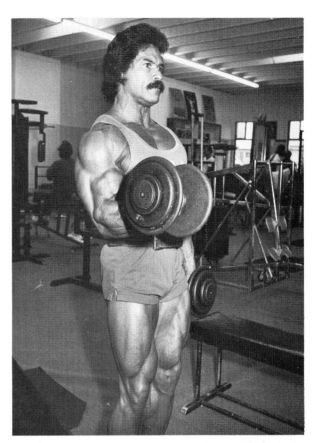

throughout the movement. From this basic starting position, slowly curl the dumbbells upward to your shoulders, being sure to supinate your hands as described earlier in this chapter. Slowly lower the dumbbells back to the starting position, pronating your hands in the process. Repeat the movement for the desired number of repetitions.

Variations—This movement is often done with alternate arms, one dumbbell beginning its upward journey as the other descends. This is called Alternate Dumbbell Curls. There is another variation called Hammer Curls used by many top bodybuilders in which the entire curling movement is done with the thumbs facing upward and the palms facing toward each other. Hammer Curls are an excellent movement for the brachialis muscles.

Training Tips—As with Barbell Curls, you can do this exercise while wearing a Weider Arm Blaster unit, or with your back pressed against a wall or the upright member of an exercise machine, to make the movement more strict. Another way to make Dumbbell Curls more strict is to sit at the end of a flat exercise bench while doing the Curls. Seated Dumbbell Curls can be performed either with both dumbbells going up simultaneously, or as Seated Alternate Dumbbell Curls.

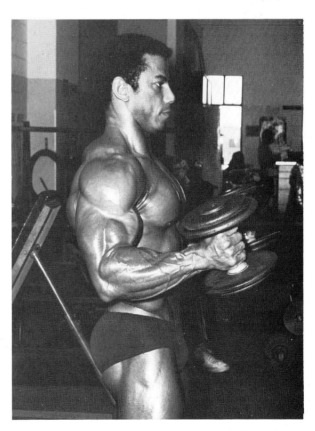

Alternate Dumbbell Curls, top; Hammer Curls, bottom.

Preacher Curl

Main Area of Emphasis—Preacher Curls strongly stress the biceps, particularly the lower insertions of the muscle. As a result, Preacher Curls develop a long, full, football-shaped biceps. Secondary stress is placed on the flexor muscles on the insides of the forearms.

Method of Performance—Set the preacher bench to a height where the top horizontal edge of the bench is about even with the lower edge of your rib cage as you are standing erect. Take an overgrip on a barbell, with your hands set only slightly wider than shoulder width. Lean over the preacher bench with your upper arms running down the padded and angled surface of the bench. The top edge of the bench should be against your arm pits, so you may need to bend your knees slightly. Your upper arms should run parallel to each other, which will mean that your hands on the barbell will be set slightly wider than the width of your elbow placement on the padded surface of the bench. Slowly straighten your arms fully. From this basic starting position, slowly curl the weight up to your chin by bending your elbows and allowing the barbell to travel in a semicircular arc upward. Lower the barbell back down to that starting point and repeat the movement for the desired number of repetitions.

Variations—This exercise is often done with two dumbbells rather than with a barbell. You can also use a low, floor pulley and a straight bar handle to do the movement. If you are using a barbell, try experimenting with a variety of grip widths when doing Preacher Curls.

Training Tips—Many bodybuilders call this movement the Scott Curl in honor of Larry Scott, the man who popularized its use. Larry won the first two Mr. Olympia titles, and his arms were amazingly full, particularly the biceps. One of Larry Scott's favorite training tricks when doing Preacher Curls was to do 6–8 slow burns at the bottom position of the movement once he could no longer do a full repetition.

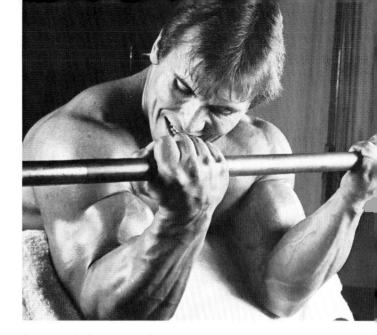

Preacher Curl with barbell.

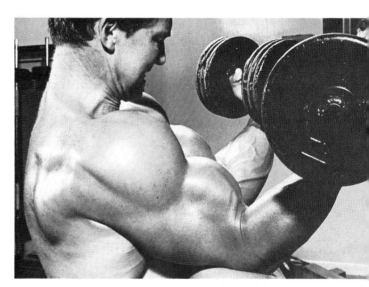

Preacher Curl with dumbbells.

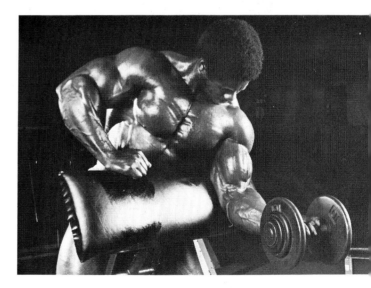

One-Arm Preacher Curl.

If you don't understand how to use the Weider Burns Training Principle, please refer to my discussion of burns in Chapter 3. If you do burns at the bottom of this movement, do them much more slowly than usual. The biceps are more vulnerable to injury in this position.

Incline Dumbbell Curl

Main Area of Emphasis—This movement strongly stresses the belly of the biceps, and it puts secondary stress on the flexor muscles on the insides of the forearms.

Method of Performance—Grasp two moderately weighted dumbbells and lie back on a 30-degree or 45-degree incline bench. If the bench has a seat on it, allow your body to slide down the bench until you are astride the seat. Hang your arms straight down from your shoulders with your palms facing toward each other. During the execution of the movement, your upper arms should remain as motionless as possible in this position. From the basic starting position, bend your elbows and slowly curl the weights directly forward in semicircular arcs up to your shoulders. As you are curling the weights upward, be sure to supinate your hands as previously discussed. Slowly lower the dumbbells back to the starting point, being sure to pronate your hands as you lower the weights. Repeat the movement for the desired number of repetitions.

Variations—One of the most common variations of Incline Dumbbell Curls involves curling the weights outward at either 45-degree or 90-degree angles from the shoulder joint. This type of curl tends to hit the outer head of the biceps more strongly than the rest of the muscle group. Another variation—and one in which you can achieve a peak contraction effect quite readily—is done lying facedown on the bench rather than faceup. This is a favorite biceps exercise of Boyer Coe, and he merely lies facedown on the bench, makes sure his upper arms are hanging directly down from his shoulder joints throughout the move-

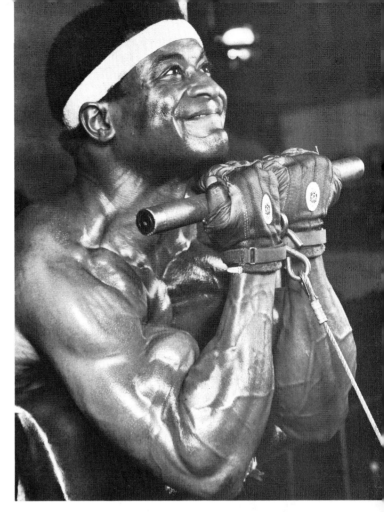

Pulley Preacher Curl.

Incline Dumbbell Curl.

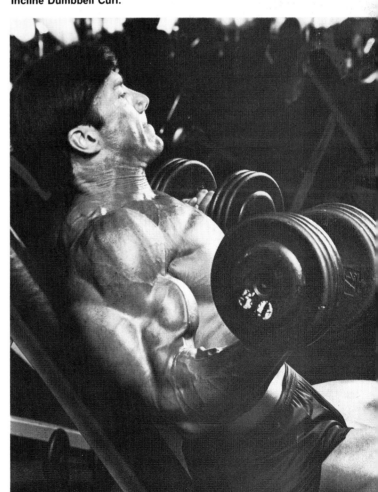

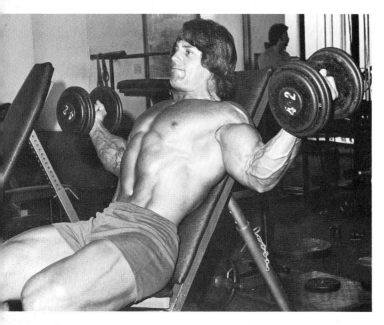

Incline Dumbbell Curl variation, curling outward.

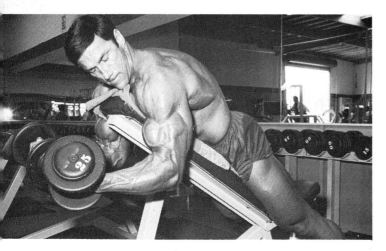

Facedown Incline Dumbbell Curl.

ment, and curls the dumbbells directly forward. Done this way, Incline Dumbbell Curls are great for adding to a bodybuilder's natural biceps peak.

Training Tips—Some bodybuilders use an incline bench one arm at a time as sort of a preacher bench for doing Dumbbell Curls. This is quite a convenient method of doing One-Arm Dumbbell Preacher Curls. Regardless of the variation of Incline Dumbbell Curls that you use, lying or running your arm down an incline bench braces your body and prevents you from cheating the dumbbell(s) up.

Nautilus Curl

Main Area of Emphasis—Most of the stress in this movement is placed on the biceps muscles, and very little goes on the flexor muscles on the insides of the forearms.

Method of Performance—Adjust the seat of the machine to a height so you can sit in it and run your upper arms up the angled pad without having to come out of the seat to do so. Supinate your hands, and place the parts of your wrists facing upward against the pads at the ends of the movement arms of the machine. Straighten your arms fully. From this basic starting position, merely bend your arms to curl the pads toward your head in semicircular arcs to a position in which your arms are bent as much as possible. Slowly allow your arms to return to the starting position, and repeat the movement for the required number of repetitions.

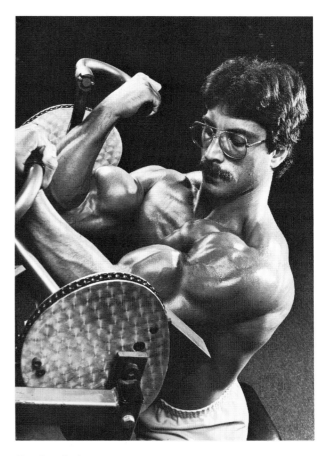

Nautilus Curl.

Variations—This movement can be done with one arm at a time, a favorite variation of massive Casey Viator. Or you can do it alternately. In the later variation, you must start moving one arm with both arms fully bent, and you must keep the top arm completely bent while the other is lowered to a straight-armed position and returned to full flexion. Alternate arms in this manner, and you will find that the movement has a particularly beneficial effect on your biceps, largely because you must maintain a static contraction of one biceps muscle while the other is extending and then contracting.

Training Tips—Many bodybuilders like to do Curls on a Nautilus machine, but I've seen very few who make this movement a dominant part of their training. Generally speaking, Nautilus machines are a good supplement to conventional barbell and dumbbell training, but it's not that good of an idea to train your body with more than about 20% of your movements on Nautilus apparatus. You'll soon become bored with doing the same old movements time after time on a Nautilus machine. Variety is very important in bodybuilding, because without it you will never have complete development in any body part.

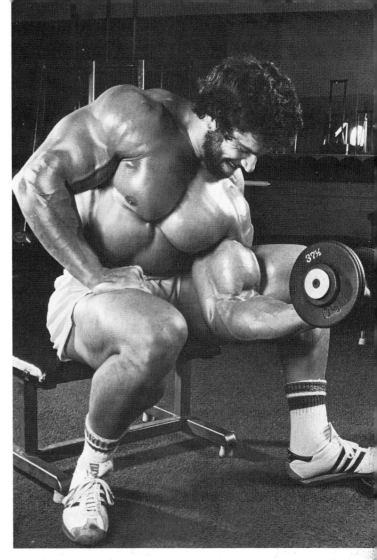

Dumbbell Concentration Curl.

Dumbbell Concentration Curl

Main Area of Emphasis—This is a shaping movement for the biceps, and particularly for the peak on each biceps muscle. It is of only minor importance for building mass into the biceps, and it stresses the forearm muscles only to a small degree.

Method of Performance—Sit at the end of a flat exercise bench or on a stool. Grasp a light dumbbell in your left hand, and place your feet a little wider than shoulder width in front of yourself. Bend over at the waist enough so you can brace the triceps of your left arm against the inside of your left knee. You can rest your free hand on your right leg, or you can use it as a brace behind your left arm. Straighten your left arm fully, and be sure your palm is down at the start of the movement. From this basic

starting position, slowly curl the dumbbell up to your shoulder, supinating your hand. Lower it slowly back to the starting position, and repeat the movement for the desired number of repetitions. Do the same number of sets and reps with your right arm.

Variations—There are a number of minor variations on the movement just described, which consist of different hand positions at the start of the movement (some bodybuilders start with their palm up, while others begin with the hand about halfway between full supination and full pronation). The main variation of Dumbbell Concentration Curls is the method of doing the movement advocated and used by Arnold Schwarzenegger. In this variation, Arnold stands erect, bends over at the waist so he can brace his free hand with his arm

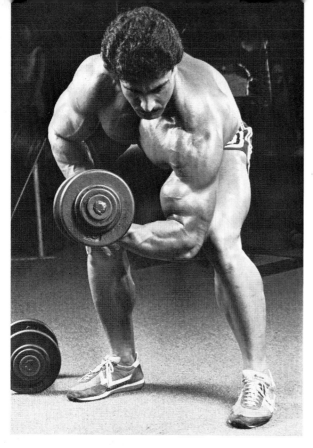

Crouching Dumbbell Concentration Curl.

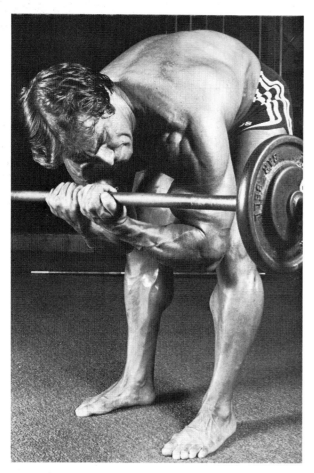

Barbell Concentration Curl with narrow grip.

straight on a dumbbell rack or high bench, and hangs his working arm straight down from his body. From this position, he keeps his upper arm steady and slowly curls the dumbbell up to his shoulder, making an arc across the midline of his body.

Training Tips—This is a good movement on which to practice peak contraction reps. To get a peak contraction effect in your biceps at the top of this movement, you should hold the fully flexed position for three or four seconds, tensing your working biceps as hard as possible. For more information on the use of peak contraction, please see the section on Peak Contraction in Chapter 3.

Barbell Concentration Curl

Main Area of Emphasis—This movement has the same effect on the biceps as does Dumbbell Concentration Curls.

Method of Performance—Take a narrow undergrip in the middle of a light barbell (there should be 4–6 inches of space between your little fingers). Place your feet a comfortable distance apart, and bend over at the waist until your torso is parallel to the floor. Hang your arms straight down from your shoulder joints, and maintain your upper arms in this position throughout the movement. If you have a problem with the barbell touching the floor at the bottom position of this movement, you should stand on either a thick block of wood or on the padded surface of a flat exercise bench as you do the exercise. From this basic starting position, slowly curl the barbell up to your chin. Lower it slowly back to the starting point, and repeat the movement for the desired number of repetitions.

Variations—You can play with the width of your grip on this movement, and some bodybuilders seem to prefer to use a shoulder-width grip rather than the narrow grip on the barbell, as just described. You can even use a reversed grip on the barbell, which more strongly stresses the forearm and brachialis muscles.

Training Tips—Barbell Concentration Curls are a favorite movement of Robby Robinson during his precontest phase. Robby likes to use a lot of peak contraction and continuous tension training to totally slice up his physique, and this movement is ideal for using these two Weider training principles.

Pulley Curl

Main Area of Emphasis—This is another excellent movement for shaping the biceps muscles.

Method of Performance—Attach a short bar handle to a low pulley on either a Universal Gym machine or a freestanding pulley. Place your feet a comfortable distance apart about a foot back from the pulley, your toes pointed at the pulley. Grasp the handle attached to the cable with a shoulder-width (or narrower) undergrip. Stand erect. Pin your upper arms against the sides of your torso and fully straighten your arms. From this basic starting position (and without moving your upper arms), slowly curl the handle attached to the cable from the tops of your thighs to your chin. Slowly lower the handle back to the starting position and repeat the movement for an appropriate number of repetitions.

Variations—A more strict variation of this movement can be done with the same handle while lying faceup on the floor, your feet a few inches away from the pulley. This variation is very similar to doing Standing Barbell Curls with your back against the wall. You can also do Cable Curls with one arm at a time by using a loop handle, or with both arms using two loop handles on pulleys located near the floor and close together. You can use a variety of body positions with one arm, ranging from a crouched position as in doing Dumbbell Concentration Curls to a position standing fully erect. The first of these variations is particularly good for enhancing the peak on your biceps. When you use two loop handles, you will be

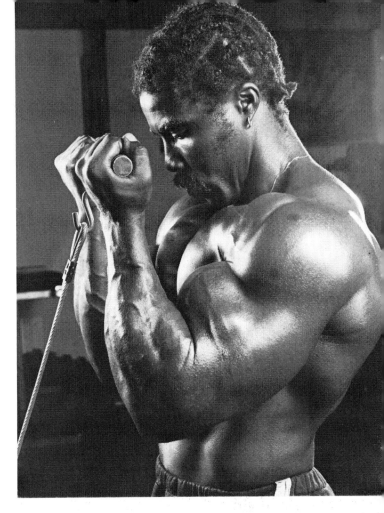

Pulley Curl.

One-Arm Pulley Curl.

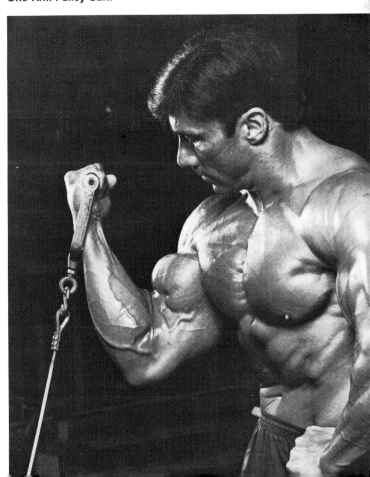

forced to stand pretty much erect, but still you can fidget with your body position to find the most effective curling arc.

Training Tips—Pulley movements for the arms (as well as for the rest of the body) are quite suited to using the Weider Continuous Tension Training Principle. This is because there are ususally no "dead" areas in which you feel very little resistance on the working muscles in most pulley exercises.

Pulley Pushdown

Main Area of Emphasis—Pushdowns stress the whole triceps muscle, with particular stress placed on the outer head of the muscle, which eventually imparts a "horseshoe" appearance to the outside rear portion of your arm. And, as mentioned earlier, Pushdowns are an excellent movement for warming up the elbows before more intense triceps training.

Method of Performance—You can use a variety of handles on a high pulley to do this movement. Up until the past five or six years, this movement was done by taking a narrow overgrip (index fingers either almost touching, or only two or three inches apart) in the middle of the normal lat machine handle. Recently, however, champion bodybuilders seem to prefer a shorter handle with grips that are angled slightly downward at the ends, since this appears to place the triceps muscles in their most powerful position for extending the arms. You can also do this movement with a rope handle looped around the pulley hook and dangling with two parallel strands from that hook. With this handle, you can assume a parallel grip, which provides variety to the movement.

For now, let's assume that you have taken a narrow overgrip on the short-angled handle. Set your feet at about shoulder width, your toes 6–8 inches back from the plane of the pulley and pointed toward the pulley. Bend your arms fully and press your upper arms to the sides of your torso (this position with the upper arms against the sides of your torso *must*

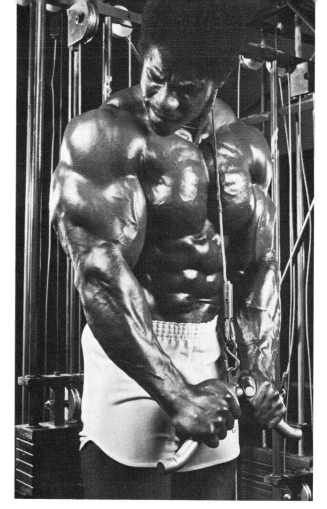

Pulley Pushdown.

be maintained throughout each set of the movement). From this basic starting position, slowly straighten your arms, tensing your triceps hard for a second or two at the finish position of the movement. Slowly allow your arms to return to the starting point of the exercise, and repeat the movement for the appropriate number of repetitions.

Variations—The main variations of this movement involve changes of grip position and width. Rather than using an overgrip, you can take an undergrip on the bar, a grip that seems to ease potential elbow pains in many cases. You can also use a variety of grip widths, ranging from a grip at about shoulder width to one in which your index fingers are touching each other in the middle of the handle you are using. And, as mentioned earlier in this description, you can use a parallel-handle grip by attaching a rope handle to the hook at the end of your cable.

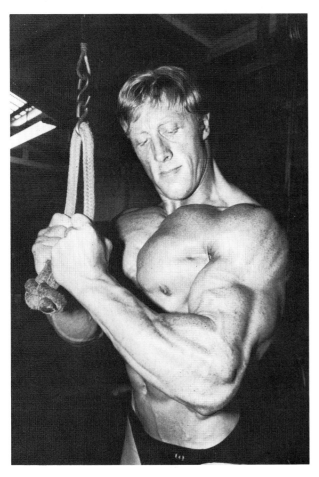

Pulley Pushdown with rope handle.

Reverse-Grip Pulley Pushdown.

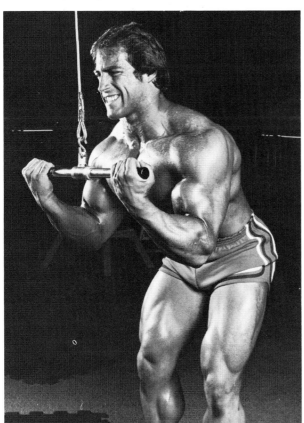

Training Tips—Under normal circumstances, you should always straighten your arms fully and tense your triceps hard at the bottom position of the movement. If you happen to have an elbow injury, however, you should not lock out your arms at the end of the movement, since this can aggravate an elbow injury. Instead, approach within about five degrees of full lockout before allowing your arms to return to the starting point of the movement. This comment holds true on all triceps exercises.

Behind Head Rope Triceps Extension

Main Area of Emphasis—This movement stresses the whole mass of the triceps muscles, but particularly the long, meaty, inner head of the triceps.

Method of Performance—Attach a rope handle to a pulley set a foot or two above the level of the top of your head. Grasp this rope with a parallel grip and face away from the pulley. Extend your arms directly overhead, then bend them fully while maintaining the same upper arm position (this position must remain the same during your entire set). Walk forward away from the pulley until you are at a point where you can lean your torso forward to a position slightly above an imaginary line drawn parallel to the floor. Once you are in this position, you should place one foot forward and bend your forward leg, the other foot to the rear and the leg straight. This leg and foot position will give you good balance as you do the movement.

From this basic starting position, slowly extend your arms. Hold the completely extended arm position for two or three seconds while tensing your triceps muscles as hard as possible. Return to the starting point by slowly flexing your arms. Repeat the movement for the required number of repetitions.

Variations—Some bodybuilders prefer to use the same handle for this movement as generally used for Pulley Pushdowns. I would suggest experimenting with each type of handle to see which is the most

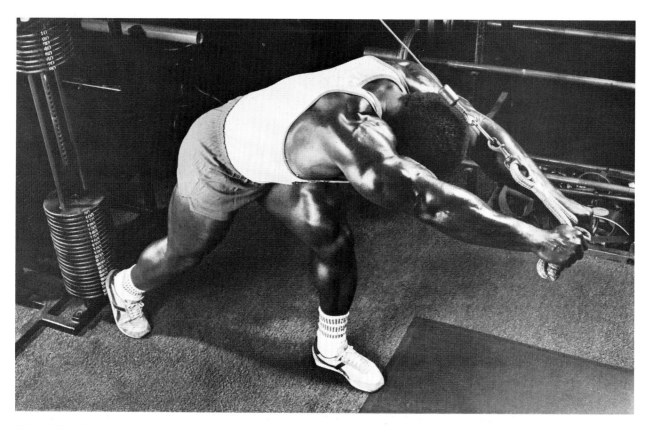

Behind Head Rope Triceps Extension.

comfortable and yields the best results. In another common variation, a bodybuilder will use a pulley set two or three feet from the floor. He will kneel on the floor facing away from the pulley and lean forward over a flat exercise bench, placing his elbows solidly on the padded surface of the bench. This position is much more secure than a standing position, and for this reason many bodybuilders prefer to use a kneeling stance for Rope Extensions. One man who popularized the kneeling stance was Larry Scott, the first Mr. Olympia winner, and his triceps were superbly developed.

Training Tips—Robby Robinson likes to do this movement one arm at a time with a loop handle. He cups the elbow of his working arm with his free hand to further steady his upper arm in position during the exercise. All one-arm (as well as one-leg) exercises allow for greater mental concentration on a movement. When using one arm at a time, you need not split your concentration between two sides of your body. You can focus it quite strongly just on the triceps of your working arm.

Close-Grip Bench Press

Main Area of Emphasis—This movement equally stresses the triceps, pectorals, and deltoids. Close-Grip Benches are an excellent triceps finishing-off movement, since you can use your delts and pecs to assist your nearly fatigued triceps to keep on pushing.

Method of Performance—Take a narrow overgrip in the middle of a moderately weighted barbell (there should be about six inches of space between your index fingers). Lie back on a flat exercise bench, place your feet flat on the floor to steady your body, and extend your arms so the weight is at straight arms' length directly above your shoulder joints. From this basic starting position, slowly bend your elbows and lower the barbell downward to touch your upper chest. As you lower and raise the barbell, your upper arms should travel outward along planes set at 45-degree angles from your torso. Push the barbell back to straight arms' length, and repeat the movement.

Variations—You can experiment with a variety of hand spacings, ranging from a

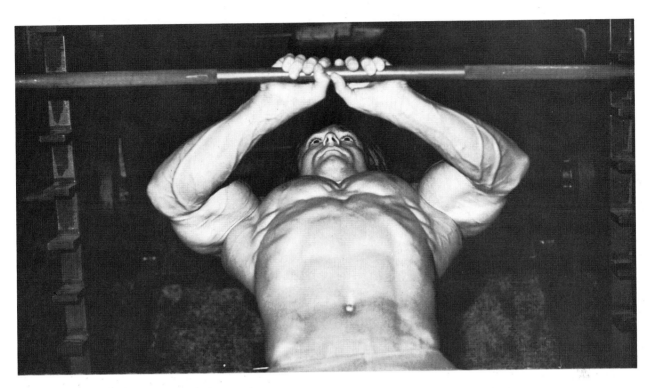

Close-Grip Bench Press.

grip set about 12 inches apart to one in which the index fingers are actually touching. Some bodybuilders have also found that they can feel this movement more readily if they do it on a bench set at a slight incline or decline. You can set your bench correctly by slipping a 2 x 4- or 4 x 4-inch block of wood under the foot or head end of the bench.

Training Tips—A small minority of bodybuilders (usually those who have had some prior shoulder injury) will find that Close-Grip Bench Presses cause shoulder joint pain. In such a case, you should avoid this movement. A good substitute for Close-Grip Bench Presses is Triceps Parallel Bar Dips.

Triceps Parallel Bar Dips

Main Area of Emphasis—This movement differs from the Parallel Bar Dips used for pectoral development. Done as a triceps exercise, Dips equally stress the triceps, deltoids, and pectorals.

Method of Performance—Stand between the bars and grasp them so when you jump

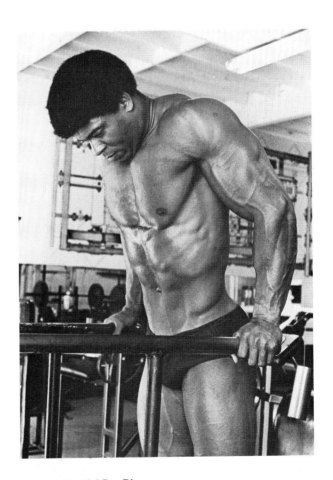

Triceps Parallel Bar Dips.

up to support yourself with straight arms on the bars your palms are facing inward toward each other. Jump up on the bars. Bend your knees to about a 90-degree angle and cross your ankles behind your body. Keeping your torso as upright as possible throughout the movement, slowly bend your arms and lower your body as far as you can. Ideally, your shoulder joints should be at almost the same level as your hands at the bottom point of the movement. Allow your elbows to travel directly to the rear a little as you lower yourself between the bars. Slowly push your body back to the starting position. Repeat the movement for the desired number of repetitions.

Variations—In most large gyms there are parallel bars that aren't actually parallel. They are angled inward at one end, which allows you to take a variety of grip widths on the bars. Experiment with every possible grip width to determine how each of them affects your triceps muscles when you do Dips.

Training Tips—On Dips for triceps development (as well as with Dips for pec-toral development), you will quickly grow strong enough so the movement becomes very easy to do. At that point you should add weight to your body by tying a light dumbbell to your waist with a rope, or by hanging a barbell plate or light dumbbell from a special belt used to add weight to Dips and Chins.

Dips Between Benches

Main Area of Emphasis—This movement is somewhat analagous to Triceps Parallel Bar Dips. As such, it stresses the triceps somewhat more strongly than Dips, but still places strong stress on the pectorals and deltoids.

Method of Performance—Place two exercise benches parallel to each other about 2½–3 feet apart. Place your hands 4 or 5 inches apart on the inner edge of one bench, your fingers pointed toward the opposite bench so your hips will be between your hands and the other bench. Walk your feet toward the other bench and place your heels on it. You may need to adjust the

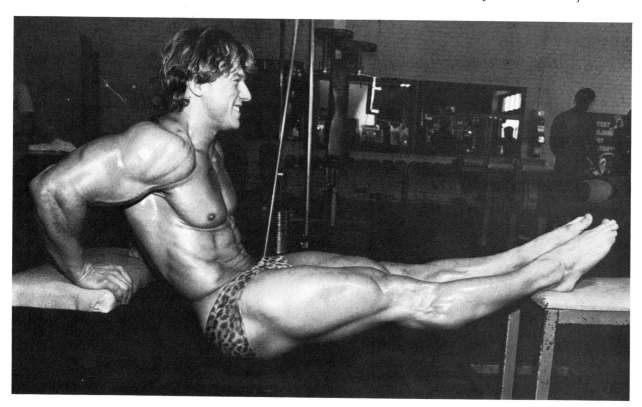

Dips Between Benches.

distance between the benches to assume the correct starting position. At the start of the movement, your legs should be straight and your torso should make an approximate 90-degree angle with your legs. Straighten your arms fully. From this basic starting position, slowly bend your arms as fully as possible. Straighten your arms to push your body back to the starting position. Repeat the movement for the desired number of repetitions.

Variations—You can adjust the width of your hand positioning. Some bodybuilders also prefer to have their feet on a somewhat higher bench than the one on which they place their hands.

Training Tips—You will grow strong enough in this movement to require extra resistance much more quickly than with Triceps Parallel Bar Dips, since much of your weight is off your arms and supported by the bench on which you rest your feet. There are two ways to add resistance to Dips Between Benches: have barbell plates or a dumbbell placed in your lap, or have your training partner stand behind you, place his hands on your shoulders and push downward with an appropriate degree of force.

Barbell Triceps Extension

Main Area of Emphasis—There is a wide variety of Barbell Triceps Extensions, and each permutation strongly stresses the whole triceps muscle, particularly the inner and middle heads of the muscle group.

Method of Performance—Take a narrow overgrip (there should be approximately six inches between your index fingers) in the middle of a barbell. Lie back on a flat exercise bench and place your feet flat on the floor to steady your body in position throughout the movement. Extend your arms directly above your shoulder joints. Being sure to keep your upper arms motionless throughout the movement, slowly bend your elbows and allow the barbell to move in a semicircular arc from the starting point down to touch lightly on your forehead or the bridge of your nose. Using triceps strength, slowly move the barbell back along the same arc to the starting point. Repeat the movement for the desired number of reps.

Variations—As previously mentioned, there are a large number of variations of Barbell Triceps Extensions. The easiest pair to master—once you have the hang of

Lying Barbell Triceps Extension.

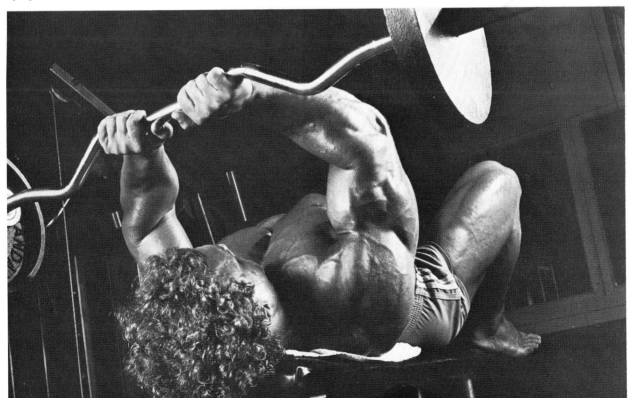

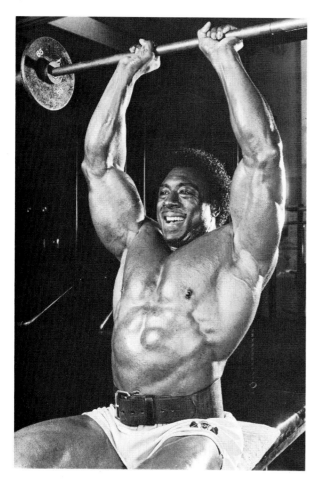

Seated Barbell Triceps Extension.

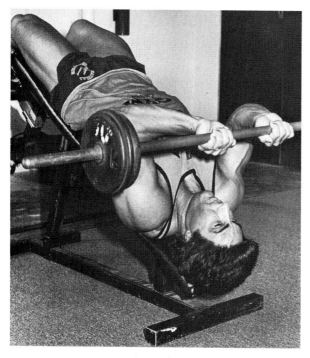

Decline Barbell Triceps Extension.

doing Lying Barbell Triceps Extensions—are done lying back on an incline or decline bench. The trick on these and all variations of Barbell Extensions is to have your upper arms perpendicular to the floor, regardless of the angle of your torso, and to maintain this arm position throughout the movement. Two other common variations of this exercise are done either standing erect, or while seated at the end of a flat exercise bench. You can also use an EZ-curl bar rather than a straight bar.

Training Tips—If you are having elbow problems, odds are good that Barbell Triceps Extensions will aggravate the problem. If so, you will need to avoid this movement for a period of time, if not for keeps.

Dumbbell Triceps Extension

Main Area of Emphasis—As with Barbell Triceps Extensions, there is a wide variety of Dumbbell Triceps Extensions. And, each variation of the movement strongly stresses the whole triceps muscle, particularly the inner and middle heads of the muscle complex.

Method of Performance—In the most fundamental type of Dumbbell Triceps Extension you will use one moderately weighted dumbbell held in both hands. Place your feet a comfortable distance apart and grasp the dumbbell. Bring the dumbbell up to your shoulder and then push it to straight arms' length directly above your head. At the start of the movement, your palms should be facing the ceiling and should be placed flat against the underside of the upper group of plates. For the sake of safety, your thumbs should encircle the dumbbell handle. You should also check to see that the collars are firmly placed if you are using an adjustable dumbbell.

From this basic starting position, and being sure that you don't move your upper arms from the basic position, slowly bend your elbows and allow the dumbbell to move downward and backward along a semicircular arc from the starting point to a position against your upper back. Slowly straighten your arms to move the dumbbell

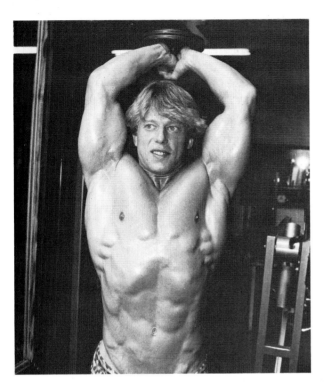

Dumbbell Triceps Extension.

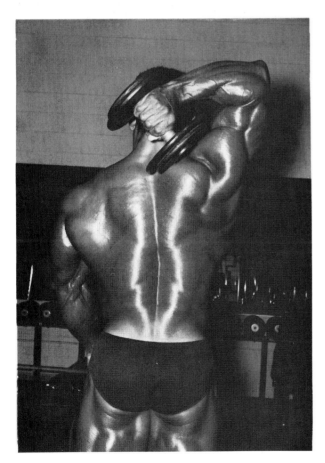

One-Arm Triceps Extension.

back along the same arc to the starting point, and repeat the movement.

Variations—Many bodybuilders prefer to do this exercise with one arm at a time while holding a light dumbbell in the working hand. Both this and the variation done with both hands can be performed seated at the end of a flat exercise bench, which isolates the legs from the movement, rather than standing.

Training Tips—If you feel uncomfortable with the act of pushing a dumbbell to arms' length for use with both hands, you can sit on the floor and use a flat exercise bench to get the dumbbell into position. Place the dumbbell on end on the bench. Sit with your back to the bench and close enough so you can lean backward slightly to grasp the dumbbell and then lean forward enough so you will clear the bench with the dumbbell in the bottom position of the exercise.

Nautilus Triceps Extension

Main Area of Emphasis—This exercise stresses the entire triceps muscle group, and particularly the large inner head of the muscle.

Method of Performance—Adjust the seat of the machine to a height so that when you sit in it your shoulder joints are slightly below the edge of the angled pad in front of your body. Turn your hands so your palms face inward toward each other. Run your arms up the angled pads, placing your elbows against the long upright side pads. The outsides of your wrists should be against the small pads attached to the movement arm of the machine as you place your upper arms on the pad. Sit on the machine seat and bend your arms fully. From this position, slowly extend your arms. Hold the extended position for two or three seconds, then slowly bend your arms to return to the starting position of the movement.

Variations—As with Nautilus Curls, you can do this movement with one arm at a time, or with alternate arms. The procedures for doing these variations are the same as for the Curls.

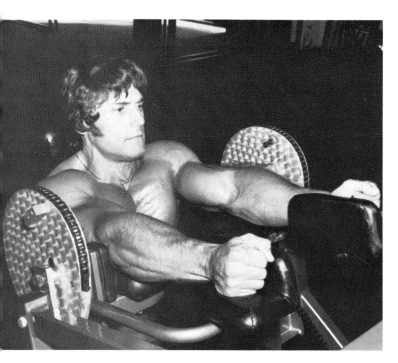

Nautilus Triceps Extension.

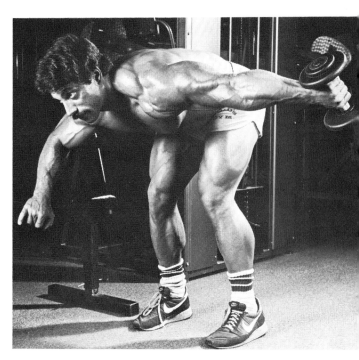

Dumbbell Kickback.

Training Tips—This is an excellent movement on which to use both the Weider Peak Contraction Training Principle and the Weider Slow, Continuous Tension Training Principle.

Dumbbell Kickbacks

Main Area of Emphasis—This movement stresses the entire triceps muscle complex.

Method of Performance—Grasp a light dumbbell in your right hand. Bend over at the waist until your torso is parallel to the floor, and place your free hand on a flat exercise bench to brace your body in this position. Press your upper arm against your torso and parallel to the floor. Bend your left arm fully. From this basic starting position, slowly extend your arm fully. Hold this extended position, flexing your triceps as hard as possible, for two or three seconds. Lower the dumbbell slowly back to the starting position, and repeat the movement.

Variations—Some bodybuilders like to do this movement standing on their own and with two dumbbells held in their hands. In

this variation, you can extend your arms either alternately or simultaneously.

Training Tips—This is the best free-weight movement on which to practice the Weider Peak Contraction Training Principle on your triceps.

THE CHAMPS' UPPER ARM ROUTINES

In this section I will present the upper arm training programs of more than 20 Weider-trained IFBB champions. Keep in mind that each of the routines presented in this section is extremely strenuous, and you should adapt each one to your own purposes and training ability level.

Beginning bodybuilders should do only one or two sets of each listed exercise and a total of no more than 4–5 total sets for biceps and 5–6 total sets for triceps. Intermediate bodybuilders should do a total of 6–8/8–10 sets of arm work, while advanced men can do 8–10/10–12 total sets in the off-season and a few more sets for each muscle group when in a precontest cycle.

Lou Ferrigno

Exercise	Sets	Reps
1. Dumbbell Curls	5	8–10
2. Close-Grip Barbell Preacher Curl	5	8–10
3. Incline Dumbbell Curls	5	8–10
4. Pulley Pushdowns	5	8–10
5. Lying Barbell Triceps Extensions	5	8–10
6. Seated Barbell Triceps Extensions	5	8–10

Arnold Schwarzenegger (biceps)

Exercise	Sets	Reps
1. Barbell Curls	4–6	10
2. Dumbbell Curls	4–6	10
3. Dumbbell Concentration Curls	4–6	10

Boyer Coe (triceps)

Exercise	Sets	Reps
1. Pulley Pushdown	3–4	8
2. Lying Barbell Triceps Extension	3–4	8
3. One-Arm Dumbbell Triceps Extension	3–4	8
4. Dumbbell Kickback	3–4	8

Boyer Coe (biceps)

Exercise	Sets	Reps
1. Barbell Preacher Curl	4–5	8–10
2. Face-Down Incline Dumbbell Curls	4	8–10
3. Dumbbell Concentration Curls	4	10–12
4. One-Arm Cable Curls	2–3	10–15

Bertil Fox (biceps)

Exercise	Sets	Reps
1. Cheating Curl (EZ-curl bar)	6	6–8
2. Incline Dumbbell Curls	6	6–8
3. Dumbbell Concentration Curls	6	6–8
4. Barbell Preacher Curls	6	6–8
5. One-Arm Cable Curls	6	6–8

Steve Davis (triceps)

Exercise	Sets	Reps
1. Pulley Pushdowns	4	12
2. Lying Triceps Extension (EZ-curl bar)	3	10
3. Behind Head Rope Extensions	3	8–12
4. Parallel Bar Dips (weighted)	3	8–12
5. Dips Between Benches	3	15–20

Larry Scott (biceps)

Exercise	Sets	Reps
1. Incline Dumbbell Curl	2–3	6–8
2. Dumbbell Preacher Curl	3–4	6–8
3. Barbell Preacher Curl	3–4	6–8
4. Reverse Curl (EZ-curl bar)	3–4	6–8
5. Zottman Curl	3	8–10

Note: Bracketed exercises are performed as a triset.

Robby Robinson

Exercise	Sets	Reps
1. Standing Barbell Curl	4	6–8
2. Barbell Preacher Curl	4	6–8
3. Dumbbell Concentration Curl	4	6–8
4. Behind Head Rope Extensions	4	8–10
5. One-Arm Dumbbell Triceps Extentions	4	8–10
6. One-Arm Cable Pushdowns	4	8–10

Bob Jodkiewicz

Exercise	Sets	Reps
1. Lying Triceps Extension	4	8–10
2. Barbell Preacher Curl	4	8–10
3. Pulley Pushdown	2	8–10
4. Nautilus Curl	2	8–10
5. One-Arm Dumbbell Triceps Extension	2	8–10
6. Dumbbell Concentration Curls	2	8–10
7. One-Arm Cable Triceps Extensions	2	8–10
8. One-Arm Cable Curls	2	8–10

Note: Bracketed exercises are supersetted.

Mike Mentzer (triceps)

Exercise	Sets	Reps
1. Pulley Pushdown	1–2	6–8
2. Parallel Bar Dips	1–2	6–8
3. Lying Barbell Triceps Extensions	1–2	6–8
4. Nautilus Triceps Extensions	1–2	6–8

Note: On all exercises, one or two forced reps are done at the end of each set.

Roy Callender

Exercise	Sets	Reps
1. Barbell Curl	5–6	8–10
2. Incline Dumbbell Curl	5–6	8–10
3. Dumbbell Concentration Curl	4–5	10–12
4. Pullover and Press	6–8	8–10
5. Incline Cable Triceps Extension	5–6	8–10
6. Lying Dumbbell Triceps Extension	5–6	8–10
7. Behind Head Rope Extensions	4–5	10–12

Tom Platz

Exercise	Sets	Reps
1. Standing Alternate Dumbbell Curl	4–5	8–10
2. Close-Grip Bench Presses	4–5	8–10
3. Seated Barbell Triceps Extensions	4–5	8–10
4. Standing Barbell Curls	5–6	8–10
5. Pulley Pushdowns	4–5	8–10

Note: Bracketed exercises are supersetted.

Lance Dreher

Exercise	Sets	Reps
1. Incline Dumbbell Curl	5	6–10
2. Dumbbell Concentration Curl	5	6–10
3. Nautilus Curls	5	6–10
4. Lying Barbell Triceps Extension	5	6–10
5. Seated Barbell Triceps Extension	5	6–10
6. Pulley Pushdown	5	6–10

Danny Padilla (biceps)

Exercise	Sets	Reps
1. Dumbbell Curls	5	6–8
2. Dumbbell Concentration Curls	4	10
3. Incline Dumbbell Curls	4	8–10
4. Standing Barbell Curls	4	8–10

Dennis Tinerino (biceps)

Exercise	Sets	Reps
1. Alternate Dumbbell Curls	4	5–6
2. Barbell Preacher Curls	4	5–6
3. Standing Barbell Curls	4	5–6

Ron Teufel

Exercise	Sets	Reps
1. Close-Grip Bench Press	5	10–12
2. Incline Dumbbell Curls	5	10–12
3. Pulley Pushdowns	5	10–12
4. Cable Curls	5	10–12
5. Behind Head Rope Extensions	4	8–10
6. Standing Barbell Curls	4	8–10
7. Lying Triceps Extensions	4	8–10
8. Barbell Preacher Curls	4	8–10

Note: Bracketed exercises are supersetted.

Ed Corney (biceps)

Exercise	Sets	Reps
1. Standing Barbell Curls	3–4	8–10
2. Dumbbell Preacher Curls (one arm)	3–4	8–10
3. Cable Concentration Curls	3–4	10–12

Casey Viator (biceps)

Exercise	Sets	Reps
1. Dumbbell Concentration Curls	4–5	10–12
2. One-Arm Standing Cable Curls	4	10–12
3. Standing Barbell Curls	4	10–12
4. Standing Alternate Dumbbell Curls	4	10–12

Casey Viator (triceps)

Exercise	Sets	Reps
1. Lying Barbell Triceps Extensions	4–5	10–12
2. One-Arm Dumbbell Triceps Extension	4	10–12
3. Dumbbell Kickbacks	4	10–12
4. Seated Barbell Triceps Extension	4	10–12

Bronston Austin, Jr.

Exercise	Sets	Reps
1. Barbell Reverse Curls	6	10
2. One-Arm Dumbbell Triceps Extensions	4	10
3. Lying Barbell Triceps Extensions	4	10
4. Pulley Pushdowns	4	10
5. One-Arm Pulley Pushdowns	2–3	10
6. Standing Barbell Curls	6	10
7. Seated Dumbbell Curls	6	10
8. Barbell Preacher Curls	6	10

Note: Bracketed exercises are supersetted.

Tim Belknap

Exercise	Sets	Reps
1. Close-Grip Bench Presses	3	10–12
2. Decline Barbell Triceps Extensions	3	10–12
3. Pulley Pushdowns	3	10–12
4. Standing Barbell Curls	3	10
5. Seated Dumbbell Curls	3	10
6. One-Arm Cable Curls	3	10

Ray Mentzer

Exercise	Sets	Reps
1. Nautilus Curls	1–2	6–8
2. Barbell Preacher Curls	1–2	6–8
3. Dumbbell Concentration Curls	1–2	6–8
4. Pulley Pushdowns	1–2	6–8
5. Parallel Bar Dips	1–2	6–8
6. Nautilus Triceps Extensions	1–2	6–8

Jusup Wilkosz

Exercise	Sets	Reps
1. Incline Dumbbell Curls	5	10–12
2. Barbell Preacher Curls	5	10–12
3. Dumbbell Concentration Curls	5	10–12
4. Pulley Pushdowns	5	10–12
5. Parallel Bar Dips (weighted)	5	10–12
6. One-Arm Dumbbell Triceps Extension	5	10–12
7. One-Arm Cable Triceps Extension	5	10–12

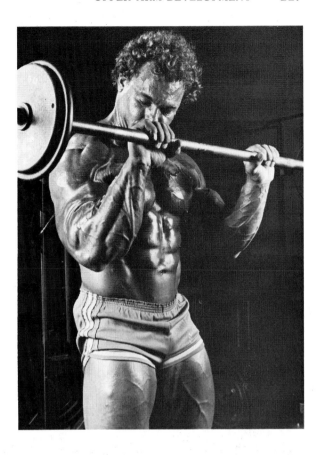

CONCLUSION

This chapter will have given you plenty of food for thought as you use the Weider Instinctive Training Principle to formulate your own unique upper-arm training routines. Be patient, however, since it takes many years to develop a quality physique. Be patient, but go for a superbly developed pair of upper arms.

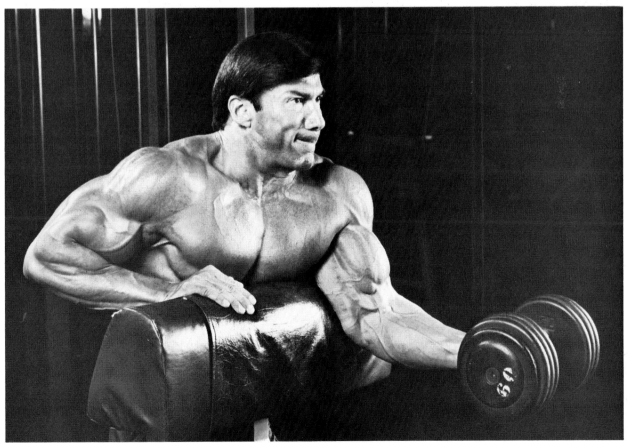

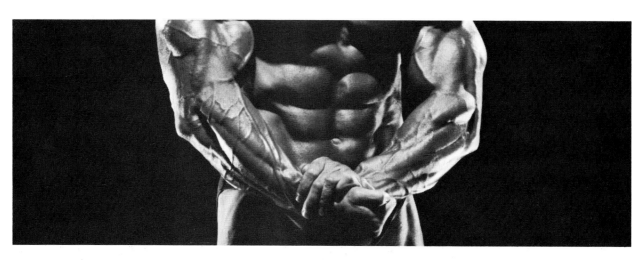

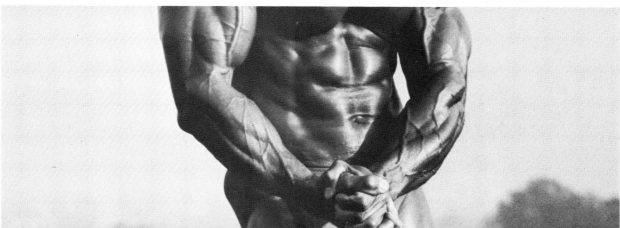

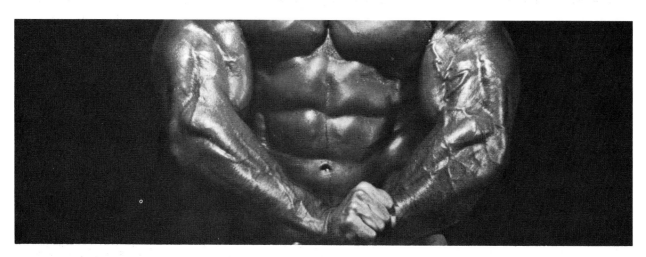

The forearms of Scott Wilson, Chris Dickerson, and Mike Mentzer.

8

Formidable Forearms

The forearm muscles are frequently ignored in workouts by most bodybuilders, even though the muscle group should be blasted with high-intensity exercises on a regular basis if the forearms are to remain proportionately equal with the rest of a bodybuilder's physique. A few champs do little or no forearm exercise and still look like they have had bowling pins surgically inserted under the skin of their lower arms. Most bodybuilders, however, must train their forearms quite regularly and intensely to maintain perfect physical proportions.

Unfortunately, the forearms are normally a rather stubborn muscle group to develop. Since you are constantly grasping things with your hands throughout the day, your forearm muscles must contract and relax hundreds of times each day. And, even though these contractions are of quite low intensity, they make the forearm muscles very tough and resistant to increases in mass and quality.

Because the forearm muscles are composed of such tough and resistant tissue, as are the calves which contract every time you take a step, you will probably discover that they respond best to higher reps (in the range of 15–20). And, again like the calves, you can probably profit from daily (or near-daily) forearm training. In essence, you will need to shock the forearms into growth by attacking them frequently with heavy training poundages and relatively high reps.

To supplement your bodybuilding movements with weights, there are several other activities that will add to the muscle mass and quality in your forearms. One time-tested activity is squeezing a rubber ball throughout the day. Buy one of the inexpensive balls made of solid rubber that can be found in dime stores and toy shops. Alternatively, you can squeeze one of the hand grips found in sporting goods stores. Regardless of the apparatus, squeeze it for several minutes with each hand three or four times a day.

Other gripping-related activities include rope climbing, hanging from a chinning bar, and crumpling up sheets of newspaper with only one hand. Or, with thick barbell plates, you can grasp them with a "pinch grip" and hold them clear of the floor for up to a minute. Once you become good at holding a single plate, try to hold two or more plates. The thicker and heavier the plate(s) you pinch grip, the greater the degree of intensity applied to the flexor muscles of your forearms.

In addition to actually performing direct exercises for the muscles of your forearms, many of the movements you do for other muscle groups will stimulate your forearm muscles. As an example, your forearms work quite hard when gripping the heavy barbells and dumbbells used in back training. Mike Mentzer (Mr. America, Mr. Universe, and runner-up in the Mr. Olympia) claims he sufficiently stimulates his massive forearm muscles simply by "gripping the barbell and dumbbell handles hard."

Unless you are as lucky as Mike Mentzer, who apparently has superior genetic ability for building massive forearms, you will be forced to follow an eclectic forearm development program. This means that you will do regular hard forearm training with weights, plus some type of supplementary forearm-building activity on a near-daily basis. And, if you follow such an eclectic program, you will eventually have bowling pin forearms of your own.

SHOCK BOMBING FOREARMS

You can make great progress in developing your forearms over a short period of time by shock bombing them with several brief workouts every day. This shock bombing technique virtually always jolts the stubborn forearm muscles into a dramatic growth spurt, but it doesn't work for more than five or six days at a time. Still, once you have put in three or four weeks of "normal" forearm training, you can again shock bomb them for another week. And, you can shock bomb your forearms once per month for a long period of time, or until they are up to par with the rest of your physique.

In order to conveniently shock bomb your forearms, you will need to have a barbell set in your home, since it will be

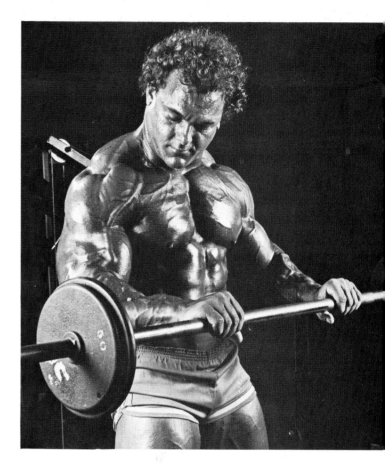

exceedingly inconvenient to drive to a gym several times each day. You should do the routine I will recommend in a moment at least five times per day, allowing an hour or more of rest time between each workout. And, you can profitably do up to 8–10 such "mini-workouts" for your forearms each day.

The following is a sample forearm program that you should do each time you train your forearms in a shock bombing cycle:

1. Reverse Curl: 1 x 8–12
2. Barbell Wrist Curl: 1 x 15–20
3. Barbell Reverse Wrist Curl: 1 x 15–20

Emphasis in this routine should be less on the amount of weight you handle in each exercise than on the pump you receive from the brief triset.

Just for your reference, shock bombing also works quite well for the calves and other muscle groups. As with the forearms, you can shock bomb your calves for up to five or six consecutive days. For all of the other muscle groups of your body, however, you won't be able to profit from more than two or three days of shock bombing.

FOREARM ANATOMY AND KINESIOLOGY

The muscles of the forearms are very complex in their structure and function. This is because the hand and its fingers are motivated by the forearm muscles, and the hand complex is a precision instrument capable of a myriad of delicate to powerful functions.

The muscles of the forearm can, however, be divided into three groupings. The grouping largest in mass is the flexors, which include the *flexor carpi radialis, flexor carpi ulnaris, flexor digitorum superficialis, flexor digitorum profundis,* and *flexor pollicis longus* muscles. The flexor muscles of the forearms contract to close the fingers into a fist.

A second forearm muscle group is the extensors, which contract to extend the fingers from a closed position. The extensor muscles include the *extensor carpi ulnaris, extensor digitorum, extensor digiti minimi, extensor indicis,* and *extensor pollicis brevis.*

The third group consists only of the *brachioradialis,* the large muscle on the upper outside of the forearm. This muscle contracts to help bend the arm fully when the hand is pronated, as when doing Reverse Curls with a barbell.

There are also groups that help to rotate the forearm in relation to the upper arm, but they are very difficult to isolate with weight movements. For your reference, however, a couple of these are the *abductor pollicus longus* and *pronator quadratus.*

CHAMPIONSHIP FOREARM EXERCISES

In this section I fully describe the four primary forearm exercises performed by all of the Weider-trained IFBB champs. There are, however, enough variations on these four exercises to give you more than 15

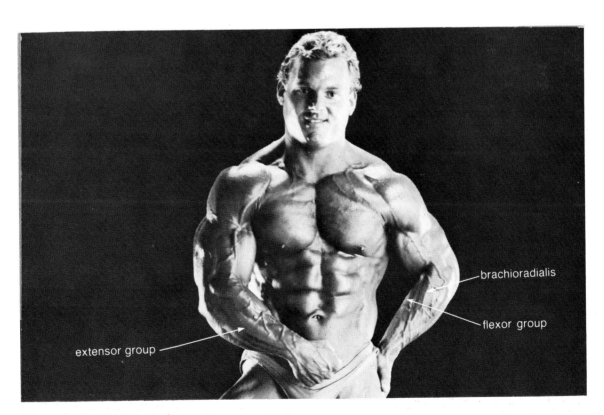

extensor group · brachioradialis · flexor group

The Forearm Muscles.

movements with which to experiment in your own forearm routines. As with each exercise presented in this book, you should experiment with every possible bodybuilding movement, using the Weider Instinctive Training Principle to determine which ones are of the greatest value to you.

Reverse Curl

Main Area of Emphasis—This exercise stresses the biceps, brachialis, and brachioradialis muscles.

Method of Performance—Take a shoulder-width overgrip on a moderately weighted barbell, set your feet a comfortable distance apart, and stand erect with your arms straight down at your sides and the barbell resting across your upper thighs. Press your upper arms against the sides of your torso, and keep them in this position throughout the movement. Being sure to keep your torso upright, slowly curl the barbell in a semicircle from your thighs to the underside of your chin. Slowly lower the barbell back along the same arc to the starting point, and repeat the movement for the required number of repetitions.

Variations—You can do this movement standing erect and using a floor pulley with a bar handle attached to it. Many bodybuilders like to utilize the continuous tension afforded by cable movements. You can use an EZ-curl bar for your Reverse Curls, and you can do any Reverse Curl variation on a preacher bench.

Training Tips—Experiment with narrower and wider grips on the handle of the barbell. Many top bodybuilders seem to prefer a relatively narrow grip in which the index fingers are five or six inches apart.

Zottman Curl

Main Area of Emphasis—As with Reverse Curls, this movement stresses the biceps, brachialis, and brachioradialis muscles.

Variations—To isolate the legs from this movement, you can do it either seated at

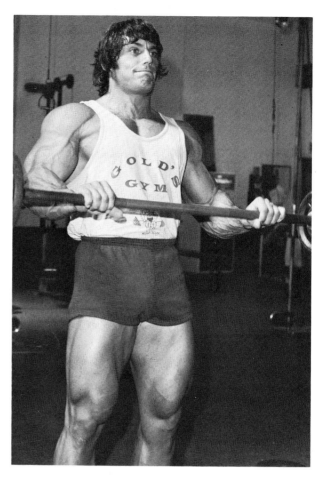

Reverse Curl.

Reverse Curl on preacher bench.

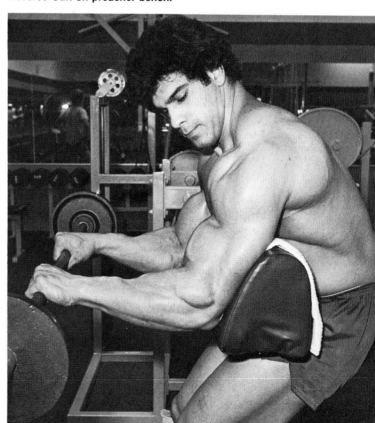

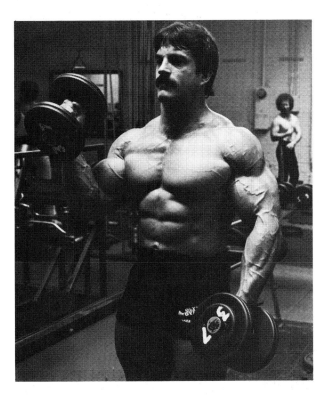

Zottman Curl.

hands and wrists hang off the edges of your knees. Sag your wrists downward as far as possible, then curl the barbell upward in a small semicircular arc by flexing your wrists as completely as possible. Lower the weight back to the starting point, and repeat the movement for the desired number of repetitions.

Variations—Be sure to do some sets of this movement with your palms down. You can do this exercise with a floor pulley and a bar handle attached to the cable running through the pulley. You can also do it with two dumbbells, or with a single dumbbell, held in your hands. All variations can be done with your forearms supported (i.e., with them running along the padded surface of a flat exercise bench, your wrists and hands running off the end of the bench).

Training Tips—To achieve a peak contraction effect on supported Wrist Curls, you should elevate the end of the bench toward your elbows, so your forearms are running downward at an angle toward your hands. Or, instead of elevating the bench, you can simply do your Wrist Curls while your arms are resting on a decline bench.

the end of a flat exercise bench or lying back on a high incline bench.

Training Tips—You will find it difficult to coordinate this movement at first, so I will suggest a good way to help remember your hand orientation. Think "dumbbell up, palm up—dumbbell down, palm down." This is to say that your palm will be facing upward as you curl one dumbbell upward, and it will be facing downward as you lower the weight.

Wrist Curl

Main Area of Emphasis—When done with the palms facing upward, this movement strongly stresses the flexor muscles on the insides of your forearms. And, when done with the palms downward, Wrist Curls stress the extensor muscles on the outsides of the forearms.

Method of Performance—Take a shoulder-width undergrip on a barbell and sit at the end of a flat exercise bench. Place your feet shoulder-width apart, and run your forearms down your thighs so your

Wrist Curl.

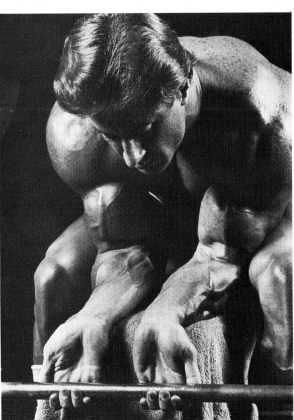

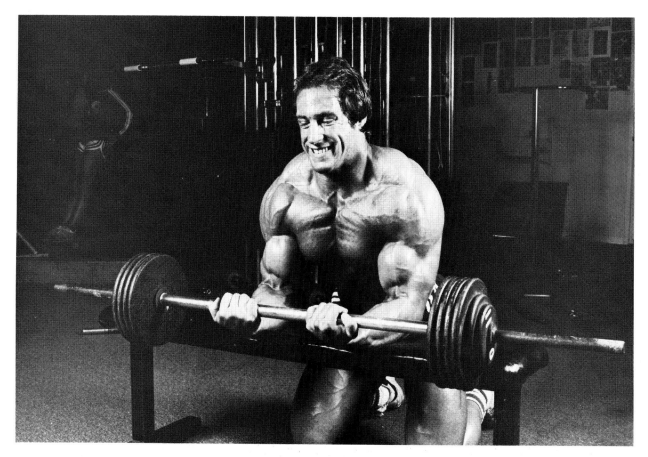

Wrist Curl variation.

Reverse Wrist Curl.

One-Arm Wrist Curl.

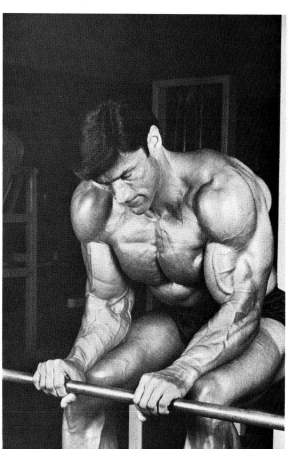

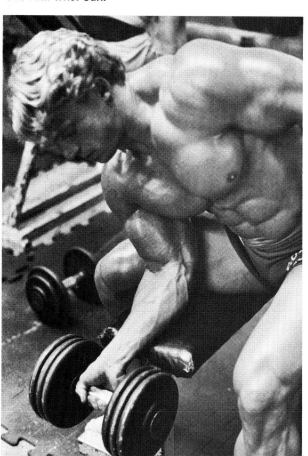

Standing Wrist Curl

Main Area of Emphasis—This exercise strongly stresses the powerful flexor muscles on the insides of the forearms.

Method of Performance—Place a barbell on a barbell rack so the barbell is a little lower than waist level. Back up to the barbell and grasp it at shoulder width, your palms facing toward the rear. Lift the barbell off the rack and straighten your arms, so your arms hang down at the sides of your body and the barbell handle is resting across the upper rear section of your thighs. From this starting position, flex your wrists to curl the barbell backward and upward in a small semicircle as high as possible. Slowly return the barbell to the starting position. Repeat the movement.

Variations—You can do a very similar movement by holding two dumbbells at your sides, your palms facing each other, and curling the dumbbells upward and inward by flexing your wrists.

Training Tips—Since there will still be a heavy weight on your flexor muscles when the dumbbells have been wrist-curled up as high as possible, this is a good movement on which to experience a peak contraction effect in your forearm muscles.

Standing Wrist Curl.

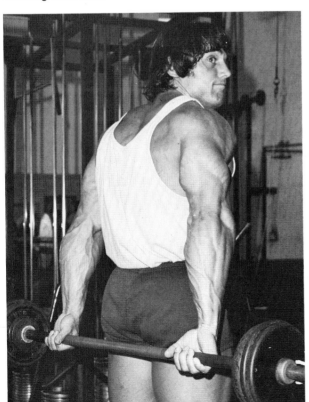

THE CHAMPIONS' FOREARM ROUTINES

In this section I will present the forearm training routines of 15 IFBB superstar bodybuilders. Bear in mind as you read these routines, however, that they are of very high intensity and suitable for use as written by only very advanced bodybuilders. If you are a relative beginner to bodybuilding, you should do only one or two sets of each listed movement, and perform no more than 6–8 total sets. At the intermediate level, you should do 8–10 total sets of forearm work, while at the advanced level you can profitably perform up to 12–15 total sets in each forearm workout.

Casey Viator

Day 1

Exercise	Sets	Reps
1. Zottman Curls	5	6–10
2. Barbell Wrist Curls	5	15–20
3. Barbell Reverse Wrist Curls	5	15–20

Day 2

1. Barbell Reverse Curls	5	6–10
2. Barbell Wrist Curls	5	15–20
3. Barbell Reverse Wrist Curls	5	15–20

Note: On a heavy day Casey uses up to 225 pounds on his Wrist Curls with palms up.

Jusup Wilkosz

Exercise	Sets	Reps
1. Barbell Reverse Curls	4	10–12
2. Barbell Wrist Curls	4	10–12

Samir Bannout

Exercise	Sets	Reps
1. Zottman Curl	4–5	8–10
2. One-Arm Dumbbell Wrist Curl	4–5	10–15
3. Barbell Reverse Wrist Curl (supported)	4–5	10–15

Roy Callender

Exercise	Sets	Reps
1. Barbell Reverse Curl	6–8	8–10
2. Standing Barbell Wrist Curl	6–8	10–12
3. Barbell Reverse Wrist Curl (supported)	6–8	10–12

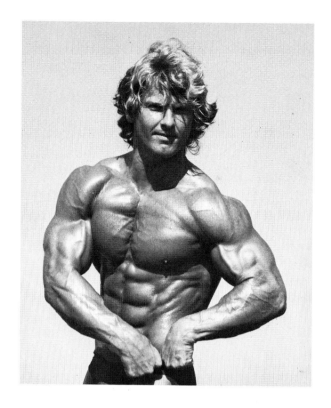

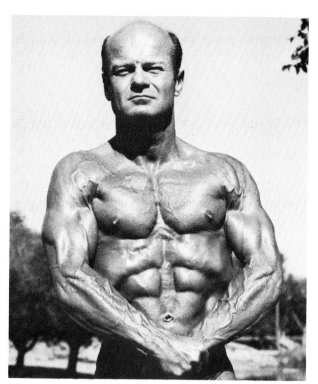

Forearms of Ulf Bengtsson (top left), Roy Chaves (bottom left), and Clarence Bass (above).

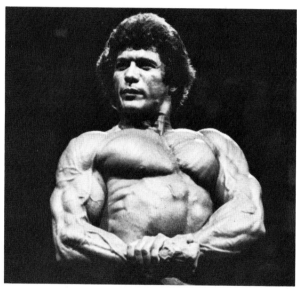

Mike Mentzer

Exercise	Sets	Reps
1. Reverse Curl	2–3	8–10
2. Barbell Wrist Curl	2–3	10–15

Tom Platz

Exercise	Sets	Reps
1. Barbell Wrist Curl (supported)	5–8	10–12

Ray Beaulieu

Exercise	Sets	Reps
1. Reverse Curls	3	40
2. Barbell Wrist Curls	3	15
3. Reverse Wrist Curls	3	10
4. Standing Dumbbell Wrist Curls	3	15

Note: Forearms are trained totally separately from the rest of the body, usually at night before retiring.

Lou Ferrigno

Exercise	Sets	Reps
1. Barbell Wrist Curl	5	15–20
2. Barbell Reverse Wrist Curl	5	15–20

Bob Birdsong

Exercise	Sets	Reps
Monday–Wednesday–Friday		
1. Reverse Curl	5	8–10
2. Dumbbell Wrist Curl (supported)	5	15
3. Standing Barbell Wrist Curl	5	15
Tuesday–Thursday		
1. Barbell Wrist Curl	5	15
2. Barbell Reverse Wrist Curl	5	15

Bill Pearl

Day One

Exercise	Sets	Reps
1. Barbell Wrist Curl	5	15

Day Two

Exercise	Sets	Reps
1. Barbell Reverse Wrist Curl	5	15

Bronston Austin, Jr.

Exercise	Sets	Reps
1. Barbell Reverse Curl	6	10
{ 2. Barbell Wrist Curl (supported)	6	15
{ 3. Barbell Reverse Wrist Curl (supported)	6	15

Note: Bracketed exercises are supersetted.

Boyer Coe

Exercise	Sets	Reps
1. Barbell Reverse Curl	4–5	8–10
2. Barbell Wrist Curl	4–5	15–20
3. Barbell Reverse Wrist Curl	4–5	15–20

Tim Belknap

Exercise	Sets	Reps
{ 1. Barbell Reverse Curl	5	10
{ 2. One-Arm Dumbbell Wrist Curl	5	10–12

Note: Exercises are supersetted.

Lance Dreher

Exercise	Sets	Reps
1. Barbell Reverse Curl	5	6–10
{ 2. Barbell Wrist Curl	5	6–10
{ 3. Barbell Reverse Wrist Curl	5	6–10

Note: Bracketed exercises are supersetted.

Danny Padilla

Day 1

Exercise	Sets	Reps
1. Barbell Reverse Curl	4–5	8–10
2. Barbell Wrist Curl (supported)	4–5	10–15

Day 2

Exercise	Sets	Reps
1. Zottman Curl	4–5	8–10
2. One-Arm Dumbbell Wrist Curl (supported)	4–5	10–15

CONCLUSION

The contents of this chapter should have given you considerable food for thought as you develop routines to build your own pair of massive and powerful forearms. Adapt the routines of the champs to your own abilities and requirements, train consistently hard in good form, and soon you'll have championship forearm development.

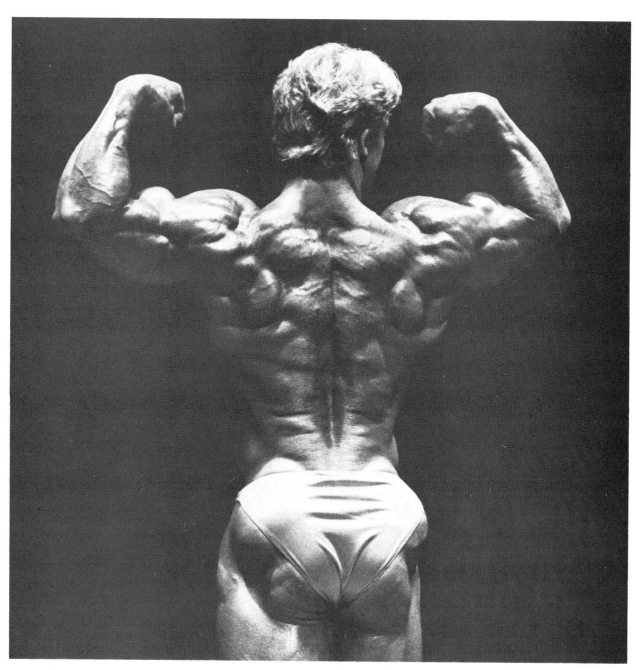

Andreas Cahling.

9

Building a Humongous Back

Fully, massively, powerfully and deeply developed, from the base of the skull to the top of the pelvis and from armpit to armpit, the back is one of a bodybuilder's greatest assets. Viewing the back of a Roy Callender, Casey Viator, Arnold Schwarzenegger, Danny Padilla, Albert Beckles, Roger Walker, Tom Platz, Robby Robinson, Mike Mentzer, Chris Dickerson, Greg De-Ferro, Franco Columbu, Bertil Fox or Frank Zane posed in top shape at a Mr. Olympia competition can be absolutely awe-inspiring!

There is such a myriad of sharp ridges and deep valleys in a fully developed back that it can cause roars of delight from the audience at a major competition. Massive Albert Beckles (a consistent winner of IFBB pro contests, despite being in his mid-forties) has an incredibly ripped upper back, and he takes full advantage of it by making the first pose in his routine a back shot with his arms held straight out from his shoulders in a crucifix position. When Beckles snaps his arms up from his sides into this position, there's such a large number of muscular details across his

upper back that it drives an audience wild.

Frank Zane has a similarly ripped-to-shreds back, which has been a big plus for him over the many years that he's competed, and which has helped him to win three consecutive Mr. Olympia titles. Arnold Schwarzenegger has combined considerable muscular detail with huge mass to win a record *seven* Mr. Olympia titles. And all of the remaining Mr. Olympia winners—Larry Scott, Sergio Oliva and Dr. Franco Columbu—have also had superb back development.

Then, there's the gorillalike back of Casey Viator! The Case has trained so heavily over the years that his spinal erector muscles are as thick as two huge writhing pythons under his skin. His lats are so thick that you could make enough steaks from them to feed a family of cannibals for a month, and his traps look like someone sliced cannon balls in half and inserted them under the skin! Viator has then ripped this writhing and super-powerful mass of muscle to perfection, so when he does a back double-biceps shot, it's simply an unbelievable sight.

Many of the back muscles are also visible from the front. The traps, for example, hump up like mini-mountains on each side of the neck when a Robby Robinson, Arnold Schwarzenegger or Scott Wilson does a "most muscular" pose. And in relaxation, when viewed from the front, the trapezius muscles slope in powerful masses downward from the ears to the points of the shoulders.

As impressive as the traps may appear from the front, the lats are the back muscles that really add to the impressiveness of many front poses. Standing semi-relaxed, the lats give the body its V-shape that denotes superior symmetry. And in a front double-biceps or front lat spread shot, the lats of a Roy Callender give a tremendous wedge shape to the torso.

It takes heavy and consistently hard work to develop a championship back. And since it's such a large muscle group, you must expend huge quantities of energy to train your back. This means that there will be considerable fatigue-related pain associated with building your back, but your efforts will be well rewarded, for thick and muscular back development will add considerably to your winning physique!

BACK ANATOMY AND KINESIOLOGY

In discussing back anatomy, bodybuilders usually deal with three main areas—the upper back (*trapezius*), the mid-back (*latissimus dorsi*) and the lower back (*erector spinae*). And, generally speaking, top bodybuilders train their backs in these three groupings. Some train all three groups in one session, while others train only one or two of the groups each workout. Still, to have a fully developed back, it is impossible to ignore any of these three areas.

Starting from the top and working down, the trapezius is a kite-shaped muscle in the upper back. The top point of this kite is at the base of the skull, the lower point about halfway down the spine, and the two side points attach to the backs of the shoulder points. The function of the trapezius mus-

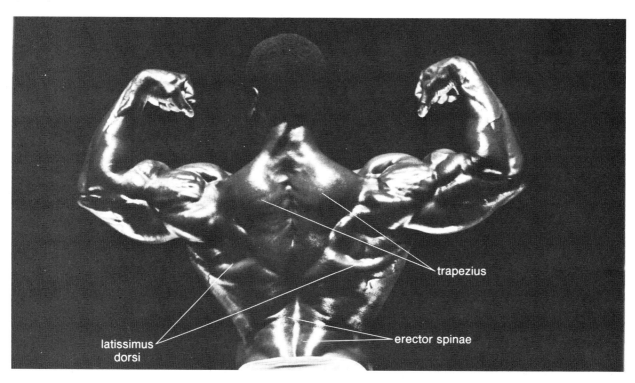

The Back Muscles.

cle is primarily to pull the points of the shoulders upward and backward.

The main muscle in the middle of the back is the latissimus dorsi, which originates along the sides of the rib cage and attaches via a large tendon to the humeri (upper arm bones). The main function of the latissimus dorsi muscle is to pull the upper arm bones downward and backward. A secondary function is to rotate the scapulae (shoulder blades), in which smaller mid-back muscles such as the infraspinatus, teres major and teres minor assist.

The erector spinae (sometimes called the spinal erectors) run like two rivers of muscle on each side of the spinal column in the lower back. They run upward from the top edge of the pelvis to about the middle of the back, where the trapezius has its lower insertion. The main function of the erector spinae is to straighten the torso from a position where it is bent over in relation to the thigh bones. The erector spinae also act to arch the spine.

HELPFUL TRAINING TIPS

Training the trapezius and lower back muscles is rather straightforward, so I will confine my discussion of "Helpful Training Tips" to working the lats. And there are several little tricks that you can use to improve the intensity and effectiveness of your latissimus dorsi exercises.

The first tip is to always do your lat exercises with your spine arched as much as possible. Due to the unique structure and function of the latissimus dorsi muscles, they can be fully contracted only when your back is arched and your upper arm bones are pulled completely down and to the rear. At first this will be a somewhat difficult skill to master, but once you have learned to arch your back on each lat movement, it will become second nature to you and you probably won't even need to think about it.

The most crucial lat exercises in which to have your spine arched are Front Chins and Front Lat Pulldowns (see the exercise descriptions later in this chapter). But you should also keep your back arched as you do Chins and Pulldowns Behind the Neck, Seated Pulley Rowing, other forms of Pulley Rowing, Barbell Bent Rowing, and Dumbbell Bent Rowing.

Grip width is a second crucial factor in developing the lats, as well as the pectorals (Chapter 11) and deltoids (Chapter 12). Many bodybuilders do their lat work, such as Front Lat Pulldowns, with a wide grip. Unfortunately, such a wide grip on the lat bar doesn't allow for a large degree of articulation of the upper arm bones in relation to the shoulder joints. And the wider the range of motion over which your upper arm bones travel on Lat Pulldowns, the greater the degree of stimulation you apply to your lats.

A relatively narrow grip (something at shoulder width, or slightly wider) gives you a much greater degree of articulation of your upper arms bones. You can prove this to yourself with a mirror and a broomstick. Stand in front of the mirror with a wide grip (hands 12–14 inches wider than your shoulders on each side) on the broomstick, which will be held overhead, as in the starting position of a Lat Pulldown. Then slowly move the stick down to the base of your neck, taking careful note of how many degrees of articulation your upper arm bones achieve in relation to your shoulder joints. This articulation will be roughly 90 degrees.

Next, take a shoulder-width grip on the broomstick and perform the same experiment. With that grip, your upper arm bones will articulate approximately 160 degrees, or about 70 degrees more than when you use a wide grip. Therefore, when you use the narrower grip on Front Lat Pulldowns (or any other lat exercise) you will be both stretching your lats to a greater degree and contracting them more thoroughly. And *that* gives you larger lats with a much better quality of muscle development.

The grip you take on a chinning bar, lat machine handle, or barbell bar has considerable bearing on how efficiently you train your lats as well. This is primarily because certain types of grips place your biceps in

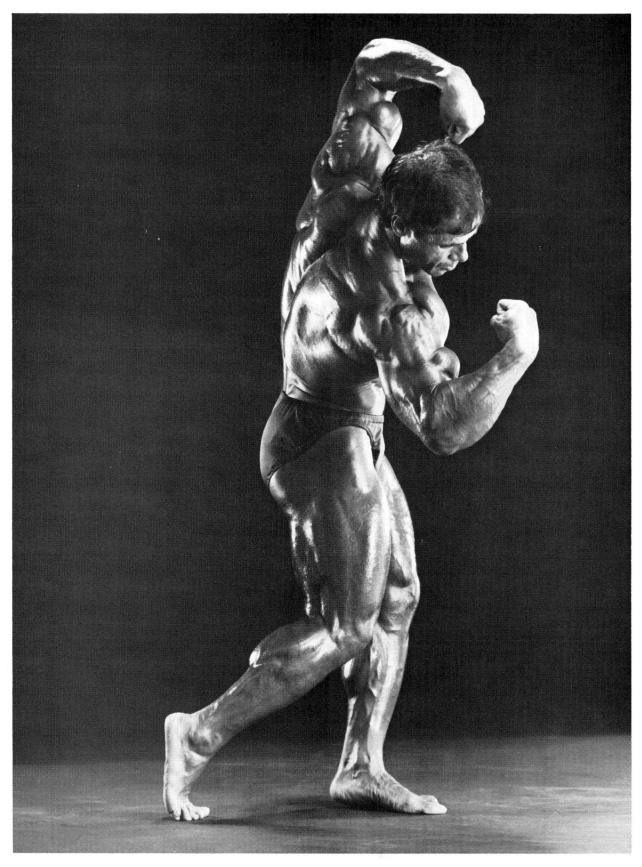

Awesome back and shoulders of Franco Columbu.

more mechanically stronger positions than other types. And since your smaller and weaker biceps will fatigue and fail on a rep before your larger and stronger lats will fail, it's an advantage to use a grip orientation that places your hands in a position to make your biceps as strong as possible.

The grip that places your biceps in the weakest position for Chins, Pulldowns and Rows is an overgrip (one in which your palms are facing away from you as you do Chins). Still, this grip is used in many lat exercises, because it allows your back to assume a more favorable mechanical position for pulling a weight with the lats. Thus, the weakness of an overgrip is compensated for by the better mechanical position of your back in certain movements.

The biceps can be put in a much stronger mechanical position by using an undergrip on the bar or handle of whatever apparatus you are using for lat work. This type of grip is particularly useful when doing Chins and Front Lat Pulldowns, but Lat Pulldowns Behind the Neck are usually done with an overgrip, since it's difficult to do this movement with an undergrip.

The final type of grip that is frequently used when doing lat work is one in which the palms of the hands face each other, which is called a "parallel grip." The use of a parallel grip for lat work places your biceps in the strongest possible mechanical position for pulling on a weight.

Chins can be done with a V-bar attachment that rests over a chinning bar, allowing you to assume a narrow parallel grip. A similar type of handle, with narrow parallel handles, can be used for Seated Pulley Rowing and Lat Pulldowns. And, there is a handle frequently used for Pulldowns that has parallel grips set at about shoulder width.

My advice on grip use when doing lat work is to use the maximum possible variety of grips, just as you would use the maximum possible variety of exercises for your back. But, try to do more of your lat exercises with a grip that puts your biceps muscles in a strong mechanical position.

THE CHAMPS' BACK EXERCISES

In this section, I will describe and illustrate 14 major back exercises that are used by all of the Weider-trained IFBB superstars. Counting grip variations, types of equipment used, methods of performance, etc., you will have approximately 25 back movements with which you can experiment while using the Weider Instinctive Training Principle to make up your own back workouts.

Shrugs

Main Area of Emphasis—All variations of the Shrug movement strongly stress the trapezius muscles.

Method of Performance—Grasp a heavy barbell with a shoulder-width overgrip and lift it up to your upper thighs with your arms straight. Your arms should remain straight, just as if they were cables attached to the points of your shoulders and with hooks on the opposite ends with which to hold the weight. Your feet should be set a comfortable distance apart, and your body should remain upright throughout the movement. From this basic position, sag your shoulders as far downward and forward as possible. Then, shrug them as far upward and backward as you can, actually trying to touch your ears with the points of your shoulders. Lower the barbell back to the stretched position, and repeat the movement for the desired number of repetitions.

Variations—You can do this movement with two dumbbells held in your hands, or at the Bench Press station of a Universal Gyms machine. With dumbbells, Rotation Shrugs are usually done, in which the shoulders are shrugged upward and then lowered in what would appear from the side to be a circle, which can be both clockwise and counterclockwise. When doing Shrugs on the Universal machine, you can do them facing toward the weight stack or facing away from the stack.

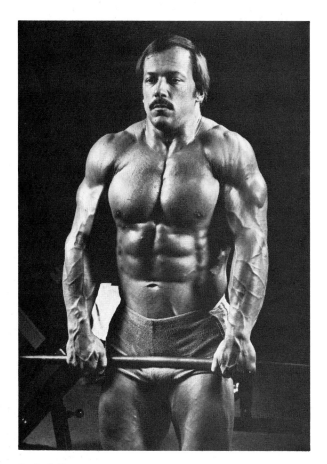

Barbell Shrug.

Dumbbell Shrug.

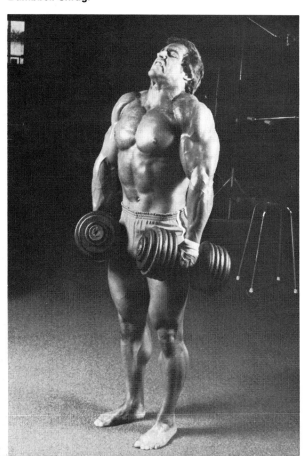

Training Tips—You can work up to using very heavy weights in this movement by placing your barbell across the pins of a power rack at a level a little below where the barbell will usually descend when doing the movement, which saves you the effort of having to lift a heavy weight to your waist. You will also profit from learning how to use straps to assist your grip when doing Shrugs with very heavy weights.

Upright Rowing

Comment—This excellent trapezius movement is fully described in Chapter 12 in the discussion on deltoid training.

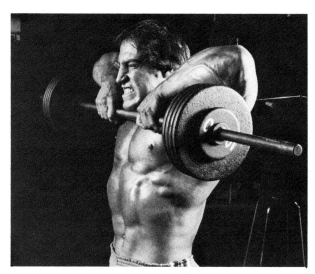

Upright Rowing.

Deadlift

Main Area of Emphasis—Deadlifts strongly stress the muscles of the lower back, thighs and forearms. Secondary stress is placed on the upper back muscles and the muscles of the hips and buttocks.

Method of Performance—Stand up to a heavy barbell as it rests on the floor and place your feet at about shoulder width, your toes pointed directly ahead. Bend over and grasp the barbell with a shoulder-width overgrip. Flatten your back and bend your legs, so your hips are above your knees and your shoulders are above your hips. Look slightly upward and maintain this eye focus throughout the movement. Straighten your arms and keep them straight throughout the movement. From this basic starting position, simultaneously straighten your legs and back to fully straighten your body. At the conclusion of the movement, the barbell will be resting across your thighs, and your shoulders will be held slightly back. Return the weight to the floor by reversing the sequence of leg and back bend that was used to raise the barbell. Repeat the movement for the desired number of repetitions.

Variations—Some bodybuilders will stand on a block of wood four inches thick to gain a longer range of motion when doing Deadlifts. You should also investigate the use of straps when using heavy weights, or you can use a reversed grip (one palm facing forward and one palm facing backward) as you do Deadlifts. A reversed grip keeps the bar from rolling out of your hands, because as it rolls out of one hand, it rolls into the other.

Training Tips—Deadlifts can become a real "ego" exercise in which bodybuilders compete against each other to see who can use the most weight for a single repetition. This practice is very dangerous and sooner or later it will result in an injury. Deadlifts are a good back-building tool, but only if sufficient reps are used to obviate the chance of injury. I recommend always doing five or more reps.

Stiff-Leg Deadlift

Main Area of Emphasis—This movement stresses primarily the spinal erectors, thigh biceps and the gripping muscles of the forearms. Secondary emphasis is placed on the upper back muscles and the muscles of the hips and buttocks.

Method of Performance—Place a moderately weighted barbell across the padded surface of a flat exercise bench. Stand on the bench with your toes up to the barbell and bend over to grasp the barbell with a

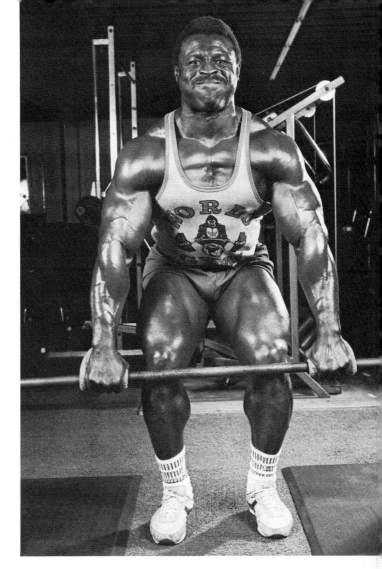

Deadlift.

Reversed-Grip Deadlift.

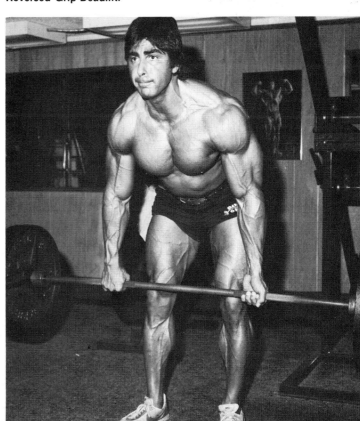

shoulder-width overgrip. Bend your legs and deadlift the weight up to a position where your body is completely straight and the barbell is resting across your upper thighs. Lock your knees and keep them locked throughout the movement. From this basic starting position, slowly bend forward at the waist until the handle of your barbell lightly contacts the bench. Then slowly straighten your body until you are back to the starting position. Repeat the movement for the required number of repetitions.

Variations—This movement can be done standing flat on the floor, but the plates of your barbell would contact the floor and terminate the movement far short of its possible range of motion. To avoid this, some bodybuilders stand on a block of wood four inches thick and use smaller-diameter plates on their barbell.

Training Tips—Always do this movement slowly and with moderate weights, since doing Deadlifts with your legs straight puts your back in a weak mechanical position. Your lower back could easily be injured if you used weights that were very heavy or did the movement in a quick and bouncing manner.

Hyperextension

Main Area of Emphasis—This exercise strongly stresses the erector spinae muscles and puts secondary stress on the thigh biceps and the muscles of the buttocks.

Method of Performance—Most gyms have a special bench on which hyperextensions are done. On one end of it there is a board about 1½ x 3 feet in width and length, and this board is padded on the top surface. At the other end of the machine are two much smaller pads that are facing the floor. Stand between the two different types of pads, facing the larger pad. Lean forward and place your hips and upper thighs on the front padded surface while placing your heels under the rear set of pads. Slide far enough forward so that the top of your pelvis is at the front end of the padded surface. Keep your legs slightly

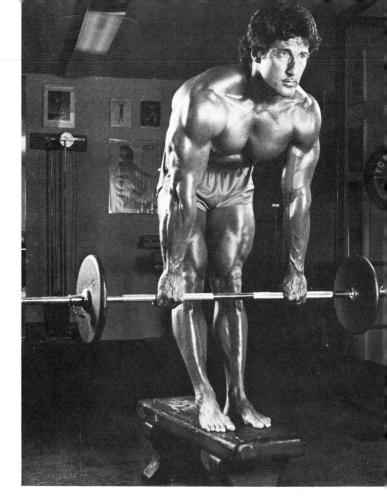

Stiff-Leg Deadlift.

Hyperextension.

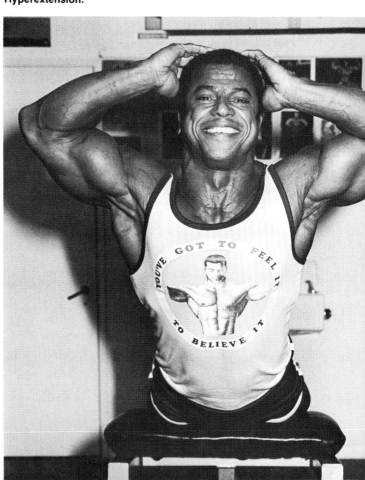

bent throughout the movement. Sag your torso forward until it is perpendicular to the floor. Place your hands behind your head as if doing a Sit-Up (actually, a Hyperextension is a sort of Sit-Up in reverse). From this starting position, contract your lower back muscles to move your torso up to a position slightly above an imaginary line drawn parallel to the floor. Don't arch backward much farther than this, however, since doing so can be injurious to your back. Return to the starting position, and repeat the movement for the required number of repetitions.

Variations—If you don't have this Hyperextension bench available, you can improvise the movement with the use of a training partner and a high (and *sturdy*) table or a high padded bench. Simply lie across the table or bench with your torso completely off it and your legs on the bench or table. Have your training partner hold down on your ankles as you do the Hyperextension movement just described.

Training Tips—This is a good exercise to use for building up your spinal erectors when you have a sore lower back. Also, you will soon become strong enough in the movement to use additional weight in it. This can be accomplished by either holding a barbell plate behind your head or holding a light barbell across your shoulders and keeping it in position by grasping the bar out toward the plates.

Good Mornings

Main Area of Emphasis—This exercise strongly stresses the erector spinae muscles and puts secondary emphasis on the thigh biceps and buttocks.

Method of Performance—Place a light barbell across your shoulders and behind your neck, balancing it in this position throughout the movement by grasping the bar on each side out near the plates. Place your feet at about shoulder width, your toes pointed directly ahead. Unlock your legs slightly and keep them in this position throughout the movement. From this basic starting position, slowly bend forward at

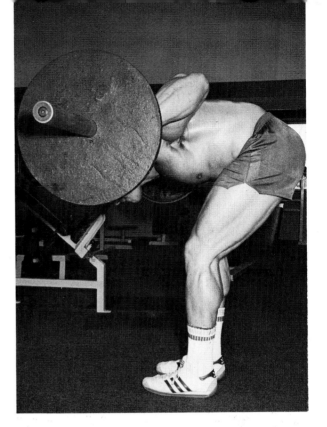

Good Mornings.

the waist until your torso is slightly below an imaginary line drawn parallel to the floor. Using the strength of the muscles of your lower back, slowly return to the starting position.

Variations—Some bodybuilders prefer to use a longer range of motion in this exercise, actually bending over until their torsos rest on their thighs.

Training Tips—If you find that resting the barbell across your neck is a bit painful, you can relieve this pain by wrapping a towel around the barbell handle.

Chins

Main Area of Emphasis—This is one of the favorite latissimus dorsi movements of all bodybuilders. It also strongly stresses the biceps muscles and the gripping muscles of the forearms. Pulling yourself up so that the bar touches the front of your neck (Front Chins) hits primarily the lower lats, while pulling yourself up to touch the bar behind your neck (Chins Behind the Neck) stresses primarily the upper lats.

Method of Performance—Set a low stool to the side of the chinning bar so that you can stand on it to take your grip, then swing off the stool to hang directly beneath the bar to do your exercises. Grasp the bar with an overgrip, your hands set four or five inches wider on each side than the width of your shoulders. Hang below the bar. Most bodybuilders then bend their legs at right angles and cross their ankles. Being sure to keep your back arched throughout the movement, slowly pull your body up to the bar by bending your arms. As you pull yourself up, be sure that your elbows travel downward *and* backward to duplicate the kinesiology of your lats. Pull yourself up to touch the bar either on your upper chest or on your trapezius muscles at the back of your neck. Slowly lower yourself back to the starting position, being sure to stretch your lats as fully as possible by completely straightening your arms and trying to slightly rotate your scapulae outward. Repeat the movement for the desired number of repetitions.

Variations—The main variations on this movement are ones of grip width. You can use a very wide grip, or one in which your hands are only 4 or 5 inches apart. You can also use an undergrip of varying widths, or hang a triangle attachment over the bar so that you can use a narrow parallel grip as you do your Chins. Finally, some bodybuilders like to lean back in a somewhat exaggerated manner as they do Front Chins.

Training Tips—Eventually, you will need added resistance attached to your body when you do Chins. The best way to do this is to make a loop of canvas webbing. The webbing will be about five feet long and tied together at both ends to make the loop. Then you hang the loop around your body and hang a light dumbbell on the loop of webbing and between your legs. There are also a number of commercial chinning/dipping belts available which have a chain to which you can attach a dumbbell to add resistance to the movement.

Lat Pulldown

Main Area of Emphasis—This movement is very similar in function to Chins, and it

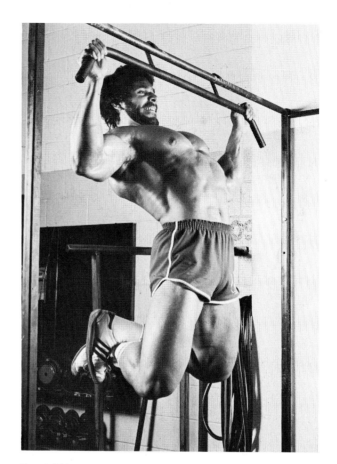
Front Chins.

Chins Behind the Neck.

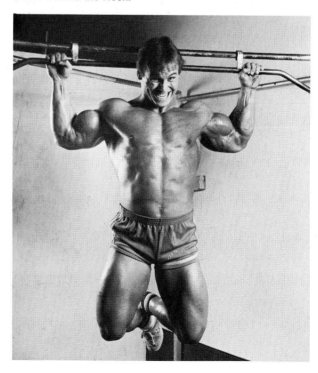

affects exactly the same muscle groups. The main difference is that you can conveniently use a lighter weight on Pulldowns if you aren't strong enough to do Chins properly.

Method of Performance—On a Universal Gyms machine, you will be forced to do Pulldowns while either sitting or kneeling on the floor. In most large commercial gyms, however, the lat machines are equipped with a seat and a cross bar about a foot above the seat against which you can rest your thighs to keep your body from moving upward when you are using very heavy weights for Pulldowns. Many of these machines have pins that you can adjust to move this cross bar upward or downward according to your body dimensions.

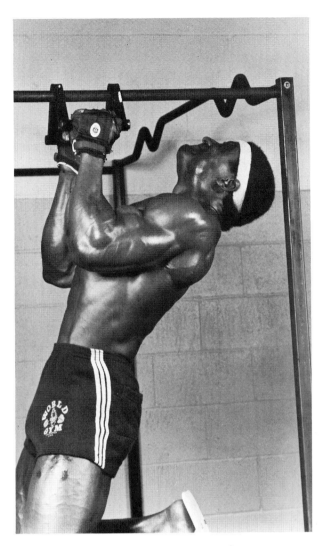

Narrow V-Grip Chins, above; Wide-Grip Chins, below.

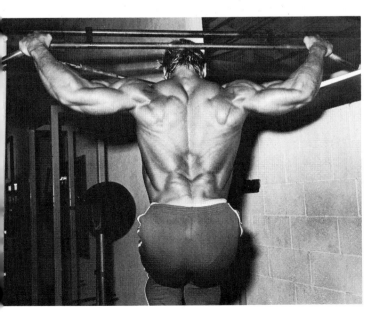

Lat Pulldown in front of neck.

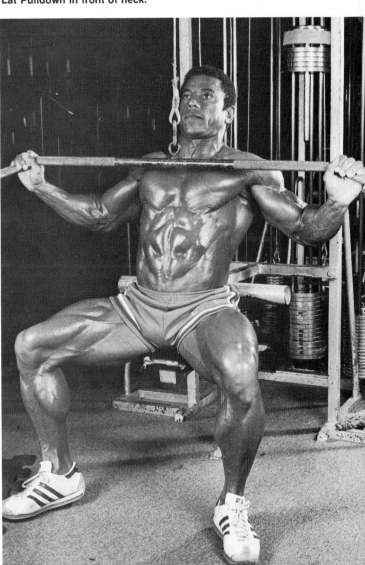

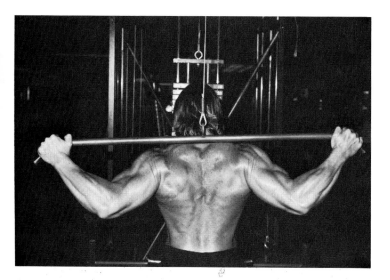

Lat Pulldown behind the neck.

Take an overgrip on the lat pulley bar with your hands set four or five inches wider on each side than the width of your shoulders. Slide your thighs under the cross bar and sit on the seat. Stretch your lats by fully straightening your arms and trying to slightly rotate your scapulae outward. Being sure that your back is arched throughout the movement, bend your arms and pull the lat bar down to touch your upper chest. Return to the starting position and repeat the movement for the desired number of repetitions.

Variations—You can also pull the bar down behind your neck, use an undergrip, vary the width of your hand spacing on the lat bar, or use the lat bar described earlier in this chapter which has parallel handles set at about shoulder width.

Training Tips—If you have to use a lat machine that does not have a cross bar to restrain your thighs, your training partner can keep your body from moving upward by standing behind you and pushing down on your traps on each side of your neck. It's also very easy to give someone forced reps on Lat Pulldowns when he is using a machine with a restraining cross bar. All you need to do is stand behind him with your hands on the lat bar, pulling down just enough to allow him to finish two or three forced reps past his point of normal muscular failure.

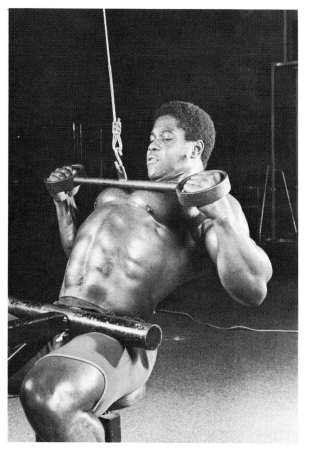

Parallel-Grip Lat Pulldown.

Lat Pulldown with a narrow grip.

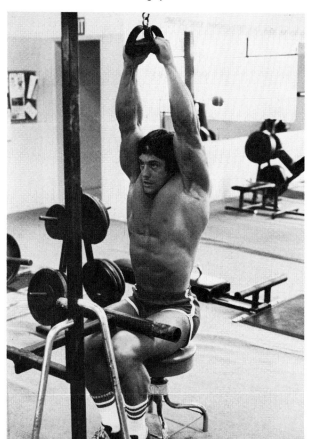

Seated Pulley Rowing

Main Area of Emphasis—This is one of the very best back exercises, since it both thickens and widens the lats, plus stresses the traps and spinal erectors. Secondary emphasis is placed on the biceps and the gripping muscles of the forearms.

Method of Performance—Use the handle that allows you to take a narrow parallel grip. Grasp this handle and place your feet against the cross bar close to the weight stack. If the cable on the seated rowing machine is of correct length, you won't be able to sit on the padded surface of the machine with your feet on the restraining bar and your torso bent fully forward without the weight stack—or whatever part of the stack you are using—sliding several inches up its rails. At any rate, sit in this position with your legs slightly bent to take potential strain off your lower back, your arms completely straight, and your body bent forward as fully as possible to fully stretch the lats. From this basic starting position, simultaneously lean backward until your torso is perpendicular to the floor, arch your back and bend your arms to pull the handle of the machine in to touch your lower rib cage. As you pull the handle toward your torso, be sure that your elbows travel backward quite close in to the sides of your torso. Return to the fully stretched starting position, and repeat this movement for the desired number of repetitions.

Variations—The main variations in this movement involve using various alternative types of handles. Many bodybuilders use the lat machine bar with the shoulder-width parallel handles, while others use a shorter straight-bar handle.

Training Tips—The most common mistake made when doing Seated Pulley Rows is to lean too far backward as you are pulling on the handle of the machine to complete the movement. When you do this, the exercise emphasis is shifted from the lats more to the trapezius muscles.

Barbell Bent Rowing

Main Area of Emphasis—This is one of the most basic lat movements. It also strongly stresses the lower back muscles, the trapezius muscles, the biceps, the rear delts and the gripping muscles of the forearms.

Method of Performance—Stand up to a moderately heavy barbell and grasp it with a shoulder-width overgrip. Your feet should be set at about shoulder width, and your legs should be slightly bent to take potential stress off your lower back as you do the movement. Fully straighten your arms and raise your torso up until it is parallel to the floor. This should raise the barbell just clear of the floor. Arch your back. From this basic starting position, pull the barbell directly up to touch the lower part of your rib cage by bending your arms. As you bend your arms, be sure that your upper arms travel upward at about 45-degree angles away from your torso. Slowly lower the barbell back to the starting position, and repeat the movement for the desired number of repetitions.

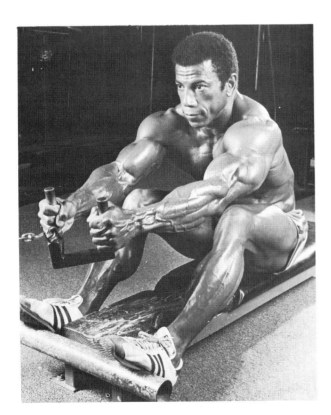

Seated Pulley Rowing.

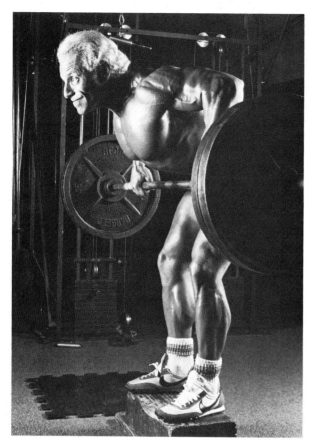

Barbell Bent Rowing.

Variations—You can vary the width of your grip from one clear out to the edges of the plates to one so narrow that your index fingers are only three or four inches apart. Many bodybuilders stand on a block of wood four inches thick when doing Barbell Bent Rows, because this allows them to get a better stretch at the bottom of the movement without the barbell's plates touching the floor. You can also accomplish the same effect by standing on the padded surface of a flat exercise bench.

Training Tips—I would definitely recommend that you wear a weightlifting belt when you do this movement. And if your lower back is slightly sore, you can rest your forehead on the padded surface of a flat exercise bench to take pressure off your lower back.

One-Arm Dumbbell Bent Rowing

Main Area of Emphasis—This movement strongly stresses the lats, rear delts, biceps and the gripping muscles of the forearms.

Method of Performance—I will describe how to do this movement with your left hand, and you can simply reverse the description to do it with your right hand. Stand with your right side toward a flat exercise bench. Place your right hand on the bench to steady your upper body in position during the movement. Place your right foot near the bench about a foot in front of your right hand, and place your left foot on the floor a bit more away from the bench and about 2–2½ feet back from your hand. In both cases, your feet should be pointed directly forward. Your right leg should be bent about 45 degrees and your left leg should be held relatively straight throughout the movement. Hold a moderately weighted dumbbell in your left hand and fully straighten your arm. The dumbbell should be held so that its handle is parallel to your torso. Stretch your left lat by allowing the dumbbell to travel slightly forward in the bottom position of the movement. From this basic starting position, slowly pull the dumbbell directly upward until it touches the side of your rib cage. As you are pulling the dumbbell upward, be sure that your upper arm bone travels out a little away from your torso. Lower the dumbbell back to the starting

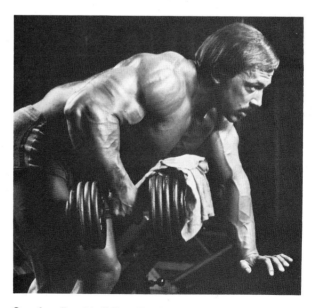

One-Arm Dumbbell Bent Rowing.

position and repeat the movement for the desired number of repetitions. Be sure to do an equal number of sets and repetitions with each arm.

Variations—Some bodybuilders have been doing this movement by placing the right knee and lower leg on the exercise bench, but still extending the left leg to the rear as they pull the dumbbell with their left hand.

Training Tips—Using straps, you can pull very heavy dumbbells up in this movement. I've seen many bodybuilders use dumbbells weighing at least 150 pounds in this movement when wearing straps to reinforce their grips.

T-Bar Rowing

Main Area of Emphasis—This movement strongly stresses the lats and spinal erectors, with secondary emphasis on the biceps and the gripping muscles of the forearms. Most of the bodybuilders whom I know that do this movement regularly have very deeply developed spinal erectors.

Method of Performance—There will be two little platforms on which to stand on either side of the hinged bar. Stand on these platforms and bend over to take an overgrip on the T-bar's handles. Bend your legs slightly to take potential stress off your lower back. Fully straighten your arms, arch your back and pull your shoulders upward just enough so that the plates of the T-bar machine are clear of the floor at the start of the movement. From there, simply pull the handles upward until the plates contact your chest, the same as you would be pulling on the handle of a pulley for Seated Pulley Rows. Return the handles of the T-bar to the starting position and repeat the movement for the required number of repetitions.

Variations—There is a T-bar machine in many gyms now that has a pulley running from the end of the bar with the handles back to a weight stack. Using this type of machine allows you to use a much longer range of motion in the exercise, since there will be no plates to contact your chest and

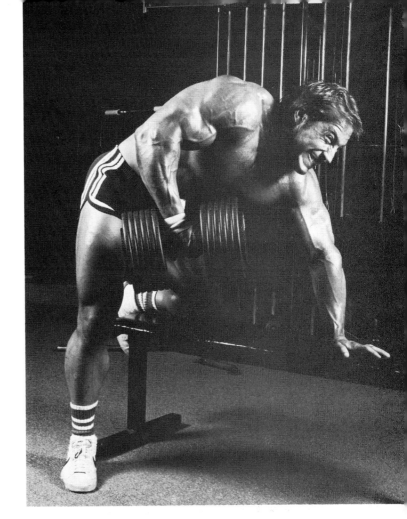

One-Arm Bent Row with one leg on a bench.

T-Bar Rowing.

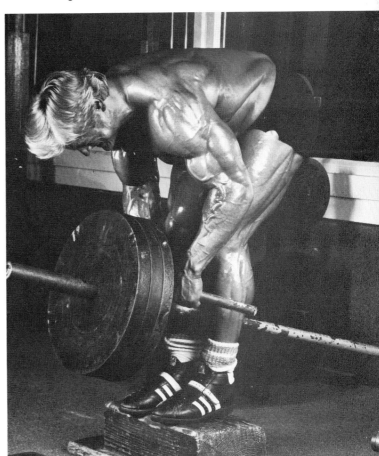

prematurely stop the movement.

Training Tips—Be careful not to allow your torso to rock back and forth as you do T-Bar Rows.

One-Arm Pulley Rowing

Main Area of Emphasis—This is a good lower-lat movement, which secondarily stresses the rear delts, biceps and the gripping muscles of your forearms.

Method of Performance—Grasp the loop handle of a floor pulley in your left hand and back up enough so that there will be tension on the cable at the beginning of the movement. Face directly at the floor pulley, extend your right leg slightly forward and bend it at about a 45-degree angle, extend your left leg 2½–3 feet to the rear and keep it held straight. Then straighten your arm fully. At the start of the movement, your palm should be down, since this helps to stretch your lat. Bend your torso over so that it is just above an imaginary line drawn parallel to the floor. From this basic starting position, pull the pulley handle directly in to touch the side of your rib cage as near to the bottom of the rib cage as possible. As you are pulling the handle in,

rotate your hand so that your palm is facing upward at the contracted position of the movement. Allow your arm to return to the starting position, rotating your hand so that your palm is again facing downward in that position. Repeat the movement for the desired number of sets and repetitions. Be sure to do an equal number of sets and reps with each arm.

Variations—Some bodybuilders do this exercise with their right side to the pulley and the cable running under their torso. At the start of the movement, their left arm is straight and crossing under their torso. Then the movement consists of fully bending their arm until their left hand is directly beneath their left shoulder. This is almost exactly the movement you would use to pull on the starter rope or cable of a lawn mower.

Training Tips—This is a very good "finishing off" movement for the lats, so it should be scheduled either last in your lat routine or toward the end of the program.

One-Arm Pulley Rowing while crouching, below; while sitting, bottom.

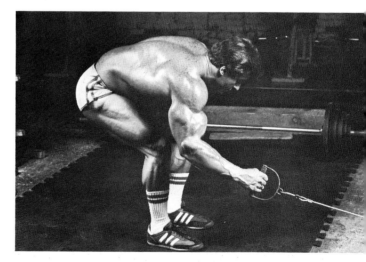

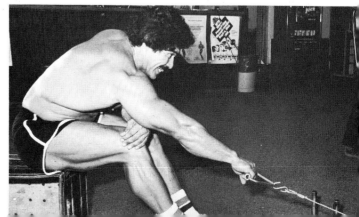

One-Arm Pulley Rowing.

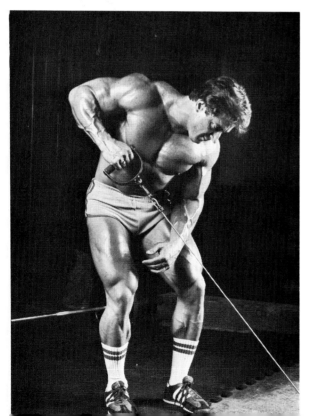

Nautilus Pullover

Main Area of Emphasis—Although some bodybuilders consider this to be a pectoral muscle builder, it is a very good isolation movement for the lats. Secondarily, it stresses the serratus muscles.

Method of Performance—Adjust the seat of the machine upward or downward so that when you sit on it your shoulders are directly level with the pivot points of the movement arms of the machine. Fasten the lap belt around your hips. Push down with your feet on the foot bar to bring the pads at the end of the movement arms of the machine into a position where you can place your elbows against them. Grasp the cross member between the movement arms to steady your elbows in position against these pads for the duration of your set. Release foot pressure on the foot bar and cross your legs beneath the seat. Allow your elbows to travel in semicircular arcs backward as far as is comfortably possible. Then, using your lat strength, pull your elbows forward in semicircular arcs until they are well past the plane of your waist. In doing this, you will have moved your elbows over an arc of more than 180 degrees. Slowly return your elbows to the fully stretched starting position and repeat the movement for the desired number of repetitions. When you are finished with your set, step on the foot bar to pull the padded lever arms far enough forward so that you can comfortably remove your elbows from the pads. Slowly let pressure off the foot bar to allow the weight stack to return to its normal position, unbuckle your lap belt, and step out of the machine.

Variations—There are a few Nautilus pullover machines in which you can pull over one arm at a time. You can also do the movement holding on to the cross member between the lever arms, rather than with your elbows against the pads of the machine.

Training Tips—You can very productively do burns in the fully contracted position of the movement. Or, you can have a partner help you with forced reps by pull-

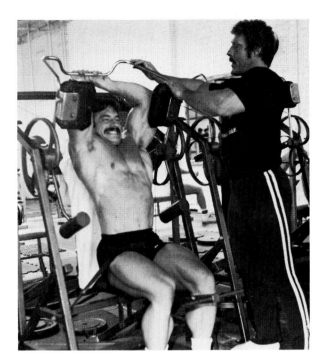

Nautilus Pullover.

ing down on one of the lever arms just enough to help you force out two or three more reps than you would normally be able to do on your own.

CHAMPIONSHIP BACK ROUTINES

In this section, I will present the back training programs of 22 IFBB superstar bodybuilders. In most cases, these are primarily lat routines, but in instances where a program is intended just for the trapezius or lower back muscles, that will be noted.

Keep in mind as you read these routines that they are of very high intensity and suitable for use as written only by very advanced Olympian bodybuilders. You must adapt these programs to your own ability levels.

If you are a novice bodybuilder, you should do only one or two sets of each exercise and perform a total of only 6–8 sets. At the intermediate level of bodybuilding training, you can do 10–12 total sets of back work, while more advanced bodybuilders can profitably do up to 15 total sets of back training.

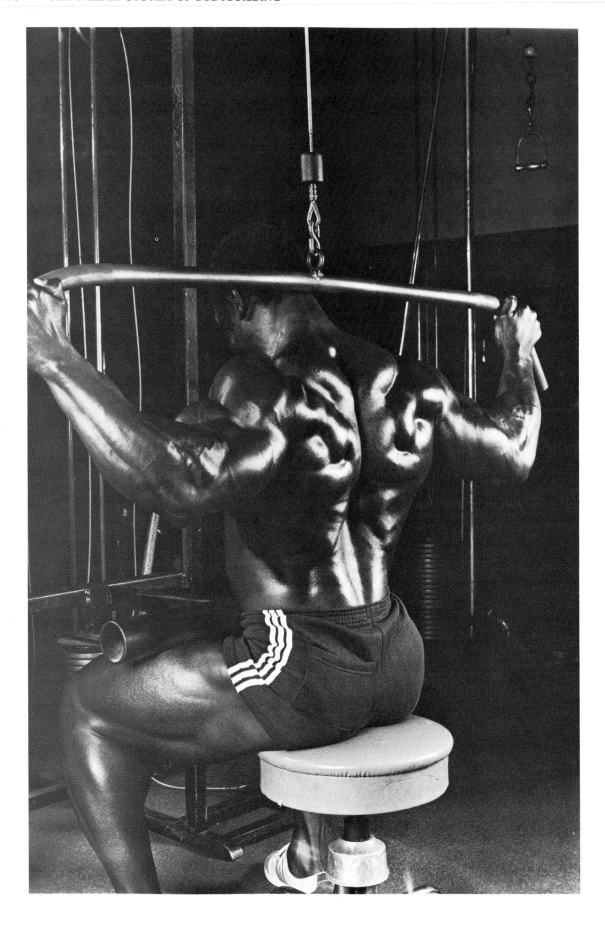

Roy Callender

Exercise	Sets	Reps
1. Barbell Bent-Arm Pullovers	10–15	10–12
2. Chins Behind Neck (weighted)	8–10	8–10
3. Front Chins (weighted)	8–10	8–10
4. Close Grip Triangle Chins (weighted)	6–8	8–10
5. Front Lat Pulldowns	8–10	8–10
6. Lat Pulldowns Behind Neck	8–10	8–10
7. T-Bar Rowing	8–10	8–10
8. Seated Pulley Rowing	8–10	8–10

Arnold Schwarzenegger

Exercise	Sets	Reps
1. Wide-Grip Front Chins	4–5	8–10
2. Pulldowns Behind Neck	4–5	8–10
3. Barbell Bent Rowing	4–5	8–10
4. T-Bar Rowing	4–5	8–10
5. Seated Pulley Rowing	4–5	8–10

Robby Robinson

Exercise	Sets	Reps
1. Barbell Bent Rowing	5	10–15
2. Narrow-Grip Chins	5	10–15
3. Seated Pulley Rowing	5	12–15
4. Pulldown Behind Neck	5	10–15

Roger Walker

Exercise	Sets	Reps
1. Barbell Bent Rowing	6–8	6–8
2. T-Bar Rowing	6	6–8
3. Front Chins	4	8–10
4. Pulldown Behind Neck	6	10–15
5. One-Arm Dumbbell Bent Rows	6	10–15

Mike Mentzer
(trapezius only)

Exercise	Sets	Reps
1. Power Cleans	3	8–5
{ 2. Dumbbell Shrugs	2–3	6–8
{ 3. Upright Rowing	2–3	6–8

Note: Bracketed exercises are supersetted.

Bronston Austin, Jr.

Exercise	Sets	Reps
1. Seated Pulley Rowing	5–8	5–8
2. T-Bar Rowing	5–8	5–8
3. Barbell Bent Rowing	5–8	5–8
4. One-Arm Dumbbell Bent Rowing	5–8	5–8
5. Nautilus Pullovers	5–8	5–8
6. Front Lat Pulldowns	5–8	8–10

Casey Viator

Exercise	Sets	Reps
1. Deadlifts	4–6	8–5
2. Nautilus Pullovers	4–6	10–15
3. Lat Pulldowns Behind Neck	4–6	10–15
4. One-Arm Dumbbell Bent Rowing	4–6	10–12
5. Chins Behind Neck (weighted)	6–8	10–15
6. Front Chins (weighted)	6–8	10–15
7. Barbell Shrugs	6–8	15–20

Tony Pearson

Exercise	Sets	Reps
1. Front Chins/Chins Behind Neck	8	10–12
2. T-Bar Rowing	5	8–10
3. Barbell Bent Rowing	5	8–10
4. Hyperextensions	3–5	10–15

Bill Pearl
(trapezius only)

Exercise	Sets	Reps
1. Upright Rowing	4	8–12
2. Rotating Dumbbell Shrugs	4	10–15
3. Shrugs on Universal Bench Press	4	10–15

Chris Dickerson

Exercise	Sets	Reps
1. Front Chins (weighted)	4–5	10–15
2. One-Arm Dumbbell Bent Rowing	4–6	8–10
3. Pulldowns Behind Neck	4	8–10
4. One-Arm Pulley Rowing	4	8–10
5. Seated Pulley Rowing	4	8–10

Steve Michalik

Exercise	Sets	Reps
1. Seated Pulley Rowing	8–10	8–10
2. Seated Close-Grip Lat Pulldowns	8–10	8–10
3. Nautilus Pullovers	8–10	8–10
4. Close Parallel-Grip Lat Pulldowns	8–10	8–10
5. Seated Front Lat Pulldowns	8–10	8–10
6. Bent Laterals (head supported)	8–10	8–10

Andreas Cahling

Exercise	Sets	Reps
1. Front Chins	2–3	10–15
2. Reverse-Grip Lat Pulldowns (medium grip)	2	8–12
3. Medium-Grip Front Lat Pulldowns	2	8–12
4. Wide-Grip Front Pulldowns	2	8–12
5. Wide-Grip Pulldowns Behind Neck	2	8–12
6. One-Arm Dumbbell Bent Rowing	2	8–12
7. Hyperextensions	2–3	8–12

Tim Belknap

Exercise	Sets	Reps
1. Wide-Grip Front Chins (as warm-up)	2–3	10–15
2. Wide-Grip Front Lat Pulldowns	3	12–15
3. Wide-Grip Seated Pulley Rowing	3	12–15
4. Narrow-Grip Seated Pulley Rowing	3	12–15
5. Nautilus Pullovers	3	10–12
6. Stiff-Leg Deadlifts	3	10–12
7. Hyperextensions	3	20–30

Bertil Fox

Exercise	Sets	Reps
1. Lat Pulldown Behind Neck	5	8–10
2. Front Lat Pulldowns	5	8–10
3. One-Arm Dumbbell Bent Rowing	6	8–10
{ 4. Chins (weighted; various types)	6	8–10
5. Cross-Bench Dumbbell Pullover	6	8–10
6. Seated Pulley Rowing	6	8–10

Note: Bracketed exercises are supersetted.

Tony Emmott

Exercise	Sets	Reps
1. Dumbbell Shrugs	3	8–10
2. Hyperextensions	4	10–15
3. Front Chins (weighted)	4	6–8
4. Seated Pulley Rowing	4	6–8
5. Pulldowns Behind Neck	4	6–8

Frank Zane

Exercise	Sets	Reps
1. Top Deadlift (in power rack)	4	10
2. Lat Pulldown Behind Neck	4	10
3. Front Lat Pulldown	4	10
4. Seated Pulley Rowing	4	10
5. One-arm Dumbbell Bent Rowing	4	10

Greg DeFerro

Exercise	Sets	Reps
{ 1. Wide-Grip Front Lat Pulldowns	3	8–12
2. Bench Bent Rowing	3	8–12
{ 3. Medium-Grip Front Lat Pulldowns	3	8–12
4. T-Bar Rowing	3	10
5. Seated Pulley Rowing	3	10
6. High Pulley Rowing	3	10
7. Hyperextensions	4	10–12

Note: Bracketed exercises are supersetted.

Dr. Franco Columbu

Exercise	Sets	Reps
1. Wide-Grip Front Chins (weighted)	6	10–15
2. T-Bar Rowing	4	10
3. Seated Pulley Rowing	4	10
{ 4. One-Arm Dumbbell Bent Rowing	3	10
5. Close-Grip Chins	3	10

Note: Bracketed exercises are supersetted.

Boyer Coe

Exercise	Sets	Reps
1. Hyperextensions	4–5	10–15
2. Dumbbell Shrugs	4–5	10–15
3. Front Chins (weighted)	2–3	10–15
4. Lat Pulldown Behind Neck	2–3	10–15
5. Seated Pulley Rowing	2–3	10–15
6. One-Arm Dumbbell Bent Rowing	2–3	10–15

Samir Bannout

Exercise	Sets	Reps
1. Wide-Grip Front Chins	4–5	10–12
2. Lat Pulldowns Behind Neck	4–5	10–12
3. Seated Pulley Rowing	4–5	8–10
4. One-Arm Dumbbell Bent Rowing	4–5	8–10
5. Nautilus Pullovers	4–5	10–15

Scott Wilson

Exercise	Sets	Reps
1. Deadlifts	5	5
2. Barbell Bent Rowing	5	6–8
3. T-Bar Rowing	5	6–8
4. Front Lat Pulldown	5	8
5. One-Arm Dumbbell Bent Rowing	5	8
6. Barbell Shrugs (in power rack)	5	8
7. Upright Rowing	5	8

Danny Padilla

Exercise	Sets	Reps
1. Chins Behind Neck	4	10–15
2. Front Chins	4	10–15
3. Barbell Bent Rowing	4	8–10
4. Seated Pulley Rowing	4	8–10
5. One-Arm Dumbbell Bent Rowing	4	8–10
6. Nautilus Pullovers	4	8–10

CONCLUSION

The information presented in this chapter will have given you plenty of food for thought as you use the Weider Instinctive Training Principle to build your own humongous back. Adapt the routines of the champs to your own abilities and purposes, never miss a workout, use heavy weights in good form in all of your exercises, and you'll soon have your own humongous back to display at your next bodybuilding competition!

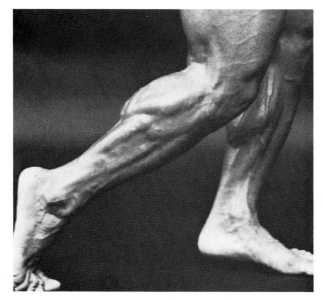

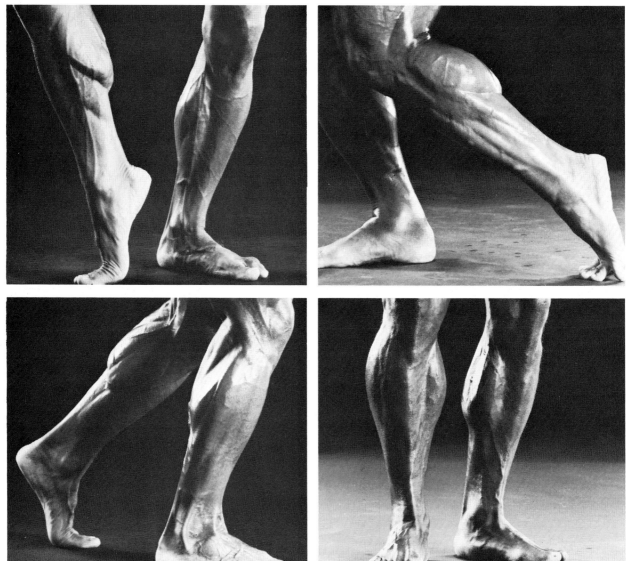

The calves of Franco Columbu (left), Tim Belknap (below left), Tom Platz (below), Boyer Coe (bottom left), and Bertil Fox (bottom). Note the many aspects that calves display when flexed in different poses.

10

Calves Like Diamonds

Large, high-quality, diamond-shaped calves are as rare as unflawed 100-carat diamonds, and just as valuable to a serious competitive bodybuilder. Of all the body's muscle groups, the calves seem to be most adamant about resisting heavy exercise and remaining relatively underdeveloped. Indeed, more champion bodybuilders suffer from slight to major deficiencies of calf development than of any other muscle group.

Among contemporary IFBB champs, Chris Dickerson is the King of Calves, although many of the superstars have phenomenal calf development, or they wouldn't be considered superstars. Among these men are Mike Mentzer, Tom Platz, Arnold Schwarzenegger, Casey Viator, Dr. Franco Columbu, Boyer Coe, Tim Belknap, Dennis Tinerino, Johnny Fuller, Jusup Wilkosz, Frank Zane, Danny Padilla, Samir Bannout, and several others.

SHOCK BOMBING

One reason why the calves are so difficult to develop is that you have been walking and running every day since you were very young, which has caused your calf muscle tissue, which is brought into play each time you take a step, to become very tough and resistant to exercise. As a result, you must shock bomb—or train them extremely heavily and frequently—in order to push your calves to grow.

You must also use the Weider Muscle Priority Training Principle on your calves if they are weakly developed. I remember when Arnold Schwarzenegger came to America in the late 1960s to be trained by me, and his calves were pitifully developed compared to the rest of his body. But by utilizing the Weider Muscle Priority and Overload Training Principles, Arnold was able to bring his calves up phenomenally within only a couple of years.

Arnold not only trained his calves first in his routine with the Muscle Priority Principle, but he also cut off at the knees the lower legs of all of his sweat pants. This way he kept his calves in high *mental priority*, because he was constantly reminded that they were weak every time he happened to glance into a gym mirror. This trick really works for weakly developed calves, as well as for any other weak body part, so give it a try! Remember, your mind must be your strongest muscle.

When Arnold first came to America, he was using a mere 400 pounds for Toe Raises on the standing calf machine. But, he had always idolized massively developed Reg Park, who had great calves during his heyday in the 1950s and early 1960s. When Arnold visited Reg in South Africa for an exhibition, he trained with his hero and was astounded to notice that Park used up to 1,000 pounds for his Toe Raises on the standing calf machine.

So, the day Arnold returned to California, he began adding plates to his standing calf machine. Gradually, he overloaded his calves more and more, and with each new overload they gradually grew in mass as they grew in strength. Soon, Arnold too was using more than half a ton on his standing calf machine (he even had to have other bodybuilders stand on the lever arms of the machine to make the weight heavier!). And, Arnold's calves had grown to be unbelievably massive and muscularly dense!

Another aspect of shock bombing the calves involves training them more than every other day, as you train most muscle groups. Many champion bodybuilders blast their calves six days a week, a few of them even twice a day. You should train your calves at least four days a week. One good way to do this is to bomb them very heavily one day, hit them moderately heavily the second day, rest them on the third day, then resume your three-day cycle on the fourth day.

Blasting the calves from all angles with a maximum variety of exercises is also important. Use the Weider Muscle Confusion Training Principle by never using the same exercises, combinations of movements, sets, reps, poundages or training tempo twice in a year. This will keep your calves constantly off balance and unable to grow accustomed to a single type of workout. When a muscle is kept off balance like this, it is much more likely to grow.

Shock bombing your calves also occasionally involves using very high reps (e.g.,

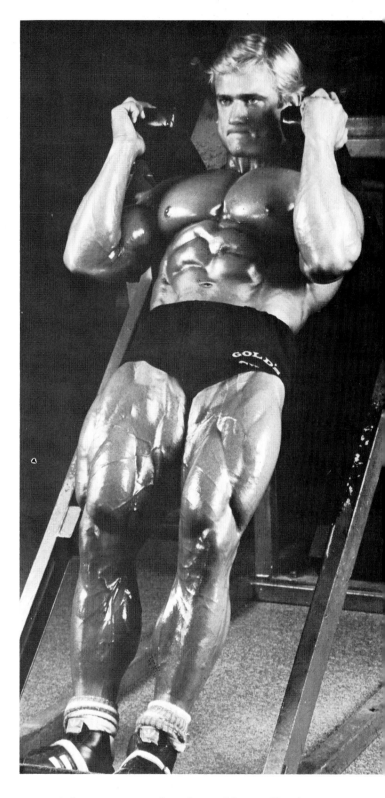

30–50) in some sets for them. Normally the calves are high-rep muscles that require 15–20 repetitions per set anyway. But from time to time you should do up to 50 reps with either a light weight in some exercise or another, or simply do one or two sets of

weightless One-Legged Toe Raises at various times during the day. Incidentally, doing these One-Legged Toe Raises at least five or six times a day for the final three weeks before a competition is a good way to really cut your calves to ribbons.

The calf muscles will also frequently respond to very low reps, in the range of 8–10. This is particularly true of exercises for the soleus muscles, so you can occasionally shock bomb your soleus muscles with 8–10 sets of 8–10 reps of Toe Raises with a very heavy weight on a seated calf machine.

The final element of calf shock bombing that I'd like to recommend involves frequent use of nonbodybuilding exercises. Occasionally sprinting in deep sand at the beach, for example, will give you a super calf pump. So will sprinting up the steps of a football stadium or basketball arena.

You can also constantly stretch your calf muscles throughout the day, a favorite calf-building technique of Boyer Coe (World Professional Grand Prix Champion). Boyer suggests either making yourself a calf block by nailing a 4 x 4-inch block of wood to a thin sheet of plywood to keep the block from rolling under your feet, or use the riser of a stairwell for your stretching.

Put the toes and ball of one foot at a time on the block of wood or stair riser and spend several minutes alternately stretching each heel as far below the level of your toes as possible, holding each stretch for 30–60 seconds at a time. Do this two or three times a day in addition to your normal calf-training routine, and you'll see results!

Finally, those bodybuilders who have taken ballet lessons—men such as Chris Dickerson, Casey Viator, and Joe Nazario—have gotten great calf stimulation from their dance classes. Ballet involves plenty of explosive leaping, rising on the toes, and a form of static stretching that is very beneficial in shock bombing the calves.

CALF ANATOMY AND KINESIOLOGY

All of the calf muscles at the back of the lower leg act to extend your toes, as when rising up on your toes. The main muscle of the calf is the *gastrocnemius*, which is a large and powerful diamond-shaped muscle originating in the upper regions of the lower leg bones and running into the Achilles tendon, which attaches to the heel bone. When the gastrocnemius contracts, it pulls upward on the heel bone, which in turn forces your toes downward.

When the gastrocnemius muscle is fully developed, it projects outward in a sharply sweeping curve on the inner side of your calf complex. It's what many bodybuilders call the "inner head" of the calf. Mike Mentzer and Chris Dickerson have maximized this type of gastrocnemius development.

The muscle that adds sweep to the outer greatly to the width of the calf, is the *soleus*. It is a broad, flat muscle lying under leus. It is a broad, flat muscle lying under the gastrocnemius. The origins and insertions of the soleus muscle are roughly the same as those of the gastrocnemius, but the soleus can be fully contracted only when the leg is bent at a 90-degree angle, while the gastrocnemius fully contracts when the leg is held straight or slightly bent.

Due to the kinesiology of the soleus, a seated calf machine was developed within the past 10 years in order to conveniently place stress on that muscle group when the leg is bent at 90 degrees. Prior to the development of that machine, the only way a bodybuilder could fully develop his soleus muscles was to heavily pad a barbell and rest it across his knees while seated at the end of a flat exercise bench and with his toes on a block of wood. Then he could do a movement that is exactly like that done on a seated calf machine, except that it is much more complicated to get the loaded barbell into position across the knees than it is to use this machine.

Due to the development of a seated calf machine, virtually all bodybuilders now do heavy and direct soleus training. And as a result, today's champs have calf width that the old-timers would envy. They also have much greater muscular detail on the outside of their calves, so they can do a wider

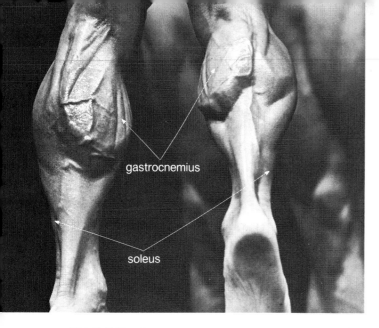

gastrocnemius

soleus

The Calf Muscles.

variety of side-calf poses than body-builders of earlier eras.

FOOT POSITIONS

In all calf exercises, you should vary the angle of your feet in order to hit the calf muscles from slightly different angles. In standard practice, there are three foot angles that are used: toes pointed straight ahead, toes angled outward at 45 degrees on each side, and toes angled inward at 45 degrees on each side.

Angling your toes inward tends to stress the inner section of your calf more, while angling your toes outward tends to put more stress on the outer part of your calf. Pointing your toes straight ahead seems to have a general effect on calf development. While some bodybuilders use only one or two of these toe positions, most use all three, in the firm belief that they need to use three toe angles to develop maximum calf mass, shape and quality.

In addition to toe angles, there is another toe position variable that most body-builders ignore. That variable is the distance between your feet as you place them on a toe block. You can have your feet very close together, or wider apart than shoulder width as you do your calf movements, although most bodybuilders use a stance that puts their feet a little more narrow than shoulder width.

I am positive that you will notice a very beneficial effect on your calf development if you vary the distance between your toe placements—in addition to angling your feet in the three standard directions—as you do your calf exercises. In general, variety is definitely the spice of life in calf training.

TO SHOE OR NOT TO SHOE?

Many bodybuilders, including a couple of the champs, like to do their calf exercises barefoot. However, after talking to every possible champion and experimenting with bare feet and wearing shoes, I have concluded that you will get much better results wearing shoes as you do your calf training.

The soles of athletic shoes are well-padded, so you can use much heavier weights while wearing them than you can barefoot. Can you imagine Arnold Schwarzenegger doing Toe Raises on a standing calf machine loaded with a half ton of weight while barefoot?

The soles of good-quality athletic shoes also have treads that will grip a calf block very securely, allowing you to use a greater range of motion—particularly in the downward stretched position—when wearing shoes than when barefoot.

THE CHAMPS' CALF EXERCISES

In this section you will find six calf exercises that are used by all of the champions. Generally speaking, there are far fewer calf exercises than exercises for any other part of the body. Still, with variations in equipment, toe position, etc., you will have more than 20 calf movements with which you can work in making up your own calf-building programs.

Standing Calf Machine

Main Area of Emphasis—This is the most basic of all calf exercises, and it stresses all of the muscles at the backs of your lower legs. It hits the gastrocnemius particularly hard.

Method of Performance—Stand up to the yoke of the machine and place your shoulders under the padded surfaces of the yoke. Grasp the handles (if provided on the machine that you are using) or the sides of the movement arms of the machine, and maintain this hand position throughout the movement. Bend your legs and place your toes and the balls of your feet on the toe block. For this first set, place your heels about 8–10 inches apart and point your toes directly forward. Straighten your body completely, and sag your heels as far below the level of your toes as possible to stretch your calf muscles. Then rise up as high as you can on your toes. Lower your heels back down to the starting position and repeat the movement for the desired number of repetitions.

Variations—Before the development of a standing calf machine, this movement was done by simply resting a barbell across the shoulders as if preparing to do a set of Squats, placing your toes on a block, and trying to do Toe Raises from this position. Obviously, you will have severe balance problems if you try to do this movement, which is why the standing calf machine was invented. Still, in many outdated bodybuilding courses you will see this Barbell Calf Raise recommended.

Training Tips—Some bodybuilders seem to feel the movement a little more in their calves if they do Standing Calf Machine Toe Raises with their legs slightly bent. If you use this method, however, be sure that you don't kick with your legs a little to get the weight up. A training partner can conveniently give you forced reps on this exercise by pushing up on the ends of the yokes across your shoulders. As on all calf exercises, experiment with foot angles and varying widths of toe placement.

Seated Calf Machine

Main Area of Emphasis—As discussed a little earlier in this chapter, this exercise works the soleus muscles quite strongly and directly. It also stresses the gastrocnemius muscles fairly strongly.

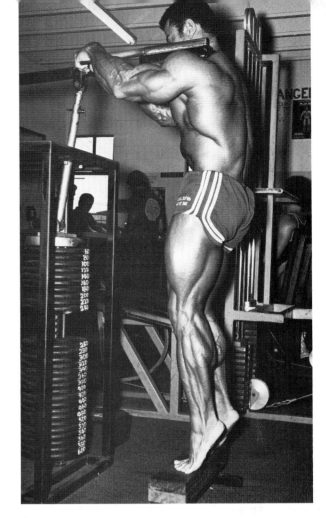

Standing Calf Machine.

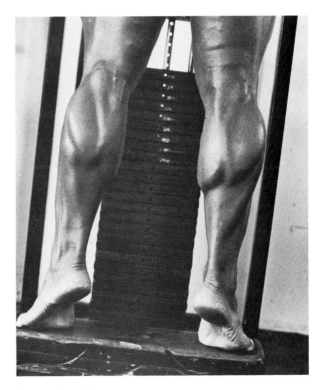

Toes out position.

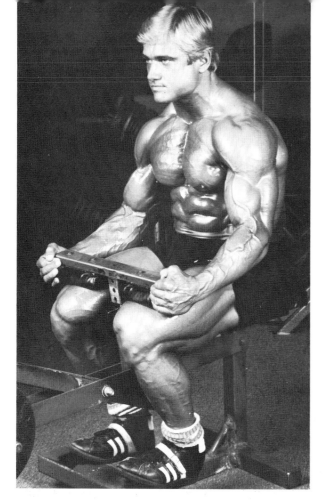

Seated Calf Machine.

of metal tubing that runs from the bar attached to the weights up to the knee pads. With a little experimentation, you can easily learn which holes in which to insert the pin so the machine is adjusted correctly to your relative lower leg length. Your training partner can easily give you forced reps in this movement by pulling up slightly on the weights at the end of the lever arm of the machine. Or, if you desire to do some forced negative reps, he can push down on the weights rather than lifting up on them.

Donkey Calf Raise

Main Area of Emphasis—This is a very direct gastrocnemius movement.

Method of Performance—Arrange a toe block close enough to the padded surface of a leg extension machine so that you can place your toes on the block, lean over so your torso is parallel to the floor, and rest your head and arms on the padded surface

Method of Performance—Sit on the machine's seat and place the toes and balls of your feet on the toe bar attached to the machine. Force your knees under the movable pads of the machine, rise slightly up on your toes, and push the machine's stop bar forward to release the weight for use in the exercise. Stretch your heels as far below the level of your toes as possible, and then rise up as high as you can under resistance on your toes. Lower your heels back down to the starting position, and repeat the movement for the required number of repetitions. Replace the stop bar to its original position at the end of each set.

Variations—As mentioned earlier in this chapter, you can pad the middle of a barbell handle and rest the barbell across your knees to simulate this movement.

Training Tips—Many seated calf machines have a pin and several holes through which you can insert this pin in the column

Donkey Calf Raise.

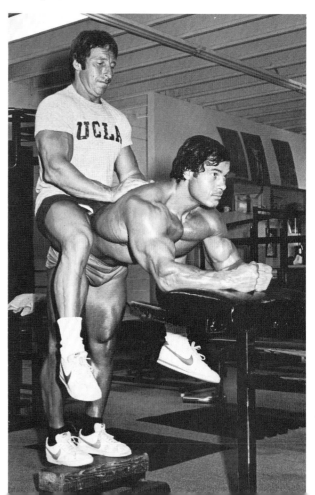

of the machine. Have a heavy training partner jump up astride your hips and grasp the sides of your waist to steady himself in position across your hips throughout the movement. Keeping your legs straight, sag your heels as far below the level of your toes as possible. Then rise up as high as you can on your toes. Lower your heels back down to the starting position and repeat the movement for the desired number of repetitions.

Variations—This exercise can be done on a Nautilus Multi machine by placing the hip belt around your hips and lower back, attaching it to the movable arm of the machine, placing your toes and the balls of your feet on one of the steps of the machine, and simply rising up and down on your toes while bent slightly over and holding on to the cross bar at the front of the machine for balance. In this type of movement, you can also do the exercise with one leg at a time, a favorite variation of Frank Zane's three times Mr. Olympia).

Training Tips—Some very strong bodybuilders can use two training partners across their hips and lower backs as resistance during this movement. Be sure, however, that these training partners sit as far back as possible, since having them sit on your shoulders will place no additional resistance on your calf muscles. Another way to add resistance to your calves would be to have your training partner astride your hips hold a dumbbell or a couple of heavy barbell plates.

Calf Press

Main Area of Emphasis—This movement hits the entire calf muscle complex, and particularly the gastrocnemius muscles.

Method of Performance—Lie on your back under a vertical leg press machine with your hips directly beneath the sliding platform. Place your toes and the balls of your feet on the edge of the platform that is away from your head. Maintaining this foot position, push your legs straight. Allow the weight of the platform to push your toes as far as possible past your heels to-

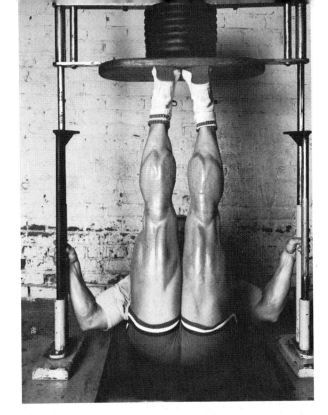

Calf Press on a vertical machine.

ward your hips to stretch your calves. Then extend your toes as far as you can. Return your heels to the starting point of the movement, and repeat the exercise for the desired number of repetitions.

Variations—You can do this same movement while seated in a Universal Gyms leg press apparatus, as well as on a 45-degree angled leg press machine.

Calf Raise on a 45-degree-angled machine.

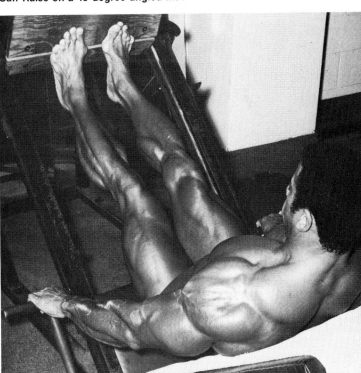

Training Tips—As long as you keep the stops of the machines in place, there will be no problem with becoming pinned by the weight if it slips off your feet. And, as previously discussed, you should wear a good-quality athletic shoe with a good tread when doing calf movements.

One-Leg Toe Raise

Main Area of Emphasis—This exercise builds up the entire calf muscle complex, but particularly the gastrocnemius muscle.

Method of Performance—Place a calf block up close to any sturdy upright. Grasp a moderately heavy dumbbell in your right hand and place the toes and ball of your left foot on the toe block. Hold the dumbbell directly down at your side throughout the movement, and grasp the upright with your left hand to steady your body in position throughout the movement. Bend your right leg to at least a 90-degree angle to keep it out of the way during the movment. Allow your left heel to travel as far as possible below the level of your left foot's toes. Then rise up as high as you can on the toes of your left foot. Allow your left heel to return back to the starting position, and repeat the movement for the desired number of repetitions. Be certain that you do an equal number of sets and repetitions for each calf.

Variations—As mentioned earlier in this chapter, you can do this movement on a stair riser, either while holding a dumbbell in your hand or without additional resistance added to the movement.

Training Tips—The mistake that most bodybuilders make is to pull up too much on the upright that they are holding to balance their bodies in position. You can pull up on it a little toward the end of a set to give yourself two or three forced reps, but avoid pulling up on the upright any sooner than this.

Hack Machine Toe Raise

Main Area of Emphasis—This is a movement that Tom Platz uses a lot, and it is

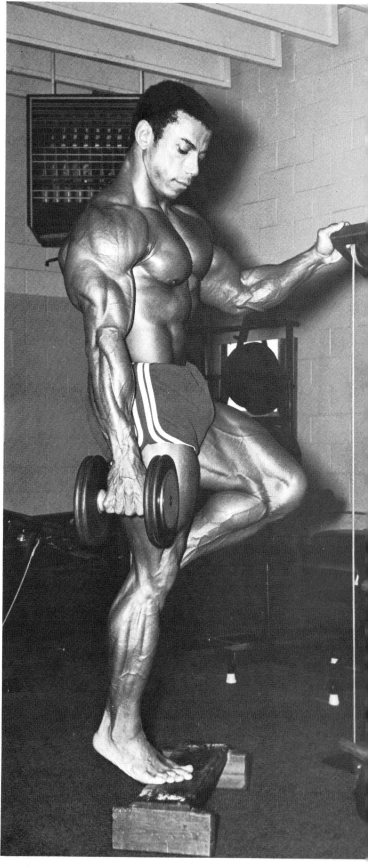

One-Leg Toe Raise.

excellent for building up the gastrocnemius muscle from a slightly different angle than any of the previous exercises that I have discussed.

Method of Performance—This exercise is best done on the type of hack slide machine that has handles at the bottom of a sliding platform. Lie facedown on this platform and grasp the handles. Straighten your legs, and place the toes and balls of your feet on the edge of the small angled platform at the bottom of the machine on which you normally place your feet as you do Hack Squats. Allow your heels to travel as far below the level of your toes as possible to stretch your calves, then extend your toes as far as you can. Lower your heels back down to the starting point and repeat this movement for the desired number of repetitions.

Variations—This exercise can also be done on the type of hack slide machine that has yokes that pass over your shoulders, although it's a little more difficult, since this machine doesn't have a padded surface against which you can rest your body.

Training Tips—The easiest way for your training partner to give you forced reps on this movement is for him to kneel at your feet and pull up on the heels of your shoes just enough to get your feet to the fully extended position for two or three forced reps.

CHAMPIONSHIP CALF ROUTINES

In this section I will give you the calf-training routines of 15 Weider-trained IFBB superstar bodybuilders. Keep in mind as you read these routines, however, that they are of very high intensity and suitable for use as written by only very advanced bodybuilders. If you are a relative beginner

Hack Machine Squat, prone position.

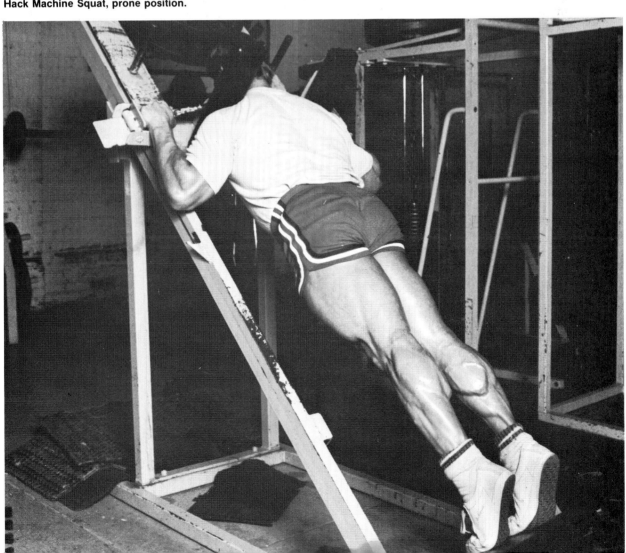

to bodybuilding, you should do only one or two sets of each listed exercise, and perform no more than 5–6 total sets. At the intermediate level of bodybuilding training, you can do 8–10 total sets of calf work each training session, and more advanced bodybuilders can profitably perform 12–15 total sets of calf training.

Chris Dickerson

Exercise	Sets	Reps
1. Calf Press (45-degree machine)	3–5	25–30
2. Seated Calf Machine	3–5	25–30
3. Standing Calf Machine	3–5	25–30

Arnold Schwarzenegger

Exercise	Sets	Reps
1. Standing Calf Machine	5	8–10
2. Donkey Calf Raise	5	15–20
3. Calf Press	5	10–15

Lou Ferrigno

Day 1

Exercise	Sets	Reps
1. Seated Calf Machine	10–12	6–10

Day 2

1. Standing Calf Machine	10–12	15–20

Casey Viator

Exercise	Sets	Reps
1. Standing Calf Machine	6–8	10–15
2. Seated Calf Machine	6–8	10–15
3. Calf Press	4–6	15–20

Mike Mentzer

Exercise	Sets	Reps
1. Toe Press	2	8–12
2. Seated Calf Machine	2	8–12
3. Standing Calf Machine	1	8–12

Robby Robinson

Exercise	Sets	Reps
1. Standing Calf Machine	8	15
2. Calf Press	8	15
3. Seated Calf Machine	8	10
4. Donkey Toe Raise	8	20

Tom Platz

Exercise	Sets	Reps
1. Standing Calf Machine	3–4	10–15
2. Seated Calf Machine	3–4	10–15
3. Calf Press	3–4	10–15
4. Hack Machine Toe Raise	3–4	10–15

Dr. Franco Columbu

Day 1

Exercise	Sets	Reps
1. Standing Calf Machine	4–5	15–20
2. Donkey Calf Raise	4–5	15–20

Day 2

1. Seated Calf Machine	4–5	15–20
2. Calf Press	4–5	15–20

Boyer Coe

Day 1

Exercise	Sets	Reps
1. Calf Press (vertical machine)	6	10–12
2. Standing Calf Machine	6	10–12

Day 2

1. Calf Press (45-degree angled machine)	8–10	10–15
2. Donkey Calf Raise	8–10	10–15
3. One-Leg Calf Raise	4–5	10–15

Ed Corney

Day 1

Exercise	Sets	Reps
1. Seated Calf Machine	5	15
2. Donkey Calf Raise	5	15
3. One-Leg Calf Raise	5	15

Day 2

1. Standing Calf Machine	5	20
2. Calf Press	5	20

Dennis Tinerino

Exercise	Sets	Reps
1. Standing Calf Machine	4–6	15–20
2. Seated Calf Machine	4–6	15–20
3. Donkey Calf Raise	4–6	15–20

Tim Belknap

Exercise	Sets	Reps
{ 1. Standing Calf Machine	5	10–15
{ 2. Donkey Calf Raises	5	10–15

Note: Exercises are supersetted.

Frank Zane

Exercise	Sets	Reps
1. One-Leg Toe Raise on Nautilus Multi Machine	4–5	20
{ 2. Seated Calf Machine	4–5	15
{ 3. Calf Presses (45-degree machine)	4–5	15

Note: Bracketed exercises are supersetted.

Samir Bannout

Day 1

Exercise	Sets	Reps
1. Standing Calf Machine	5–6	10–15
2. Donkey Calf Raise	5–6	15–20

Day 2

Exercise	Sets	Reps
1. Seated Calf Machine	4–5	10–15
2. Calf Presses (horizontal machine)	4–5	15–20

Danny Padilla

Day 1

Exercise	Sets	Reps
1. Seated Calf Machine	4	10–15
2. Donkey Calf Raise	4	15–20
3. One-Leg Calf Raise	4	15–20

Day 2

Exercise	Sets	Reps
1. Standing Calf Machine	4	10–15
2. Donkey Calf Raise (on Nautilus Multi machine)	4	15–20
3. Calf Press	4	15–20

MY FAVORITE CALF ROUTINE

Through considerable experimentation, I have arrived at a calf workout that will probably put muscle on the calves of a skeleton. It consists of five workouts a week, and you must scale it according to your experience level as a bodybuilder. If you are a relative beginner to the sport's hard training, do only about five sets of each recommended movement. Interme-

diates can do 6–8 sets of each exercise, while advanced bodybuilders can profitably perform up to 10 sets of each recommended movement.

Here is a calf routine that I am confident will give you great results:

Monday and Thursday

Seated Calf Machine — 5–10 sets — 8–10 reps

Tuesday and Friday

Standing Calf Machine — 5–10 sets — 15–20 reps

Wednesday

Take a total rest from calf training.

Saturday

One-Leg Calf Raise (no added resistance on the exercise)—do 5–10 sets of maximum reps each leg, rapidly alternating legs until desired number of sets has been completed.

Sunday

Take a total rest from calf training.

I have put a great number of bodybuilders of various experience levels on this routine at the Weider Research Clinic, and they have invariably received tremendous results from using this routine. Over a three-month period of time, one bodybuilder put slightly over one inch of new muscle mass on his calves, and every bodybuilder on the program added at least one half inch to his calf girth. So, give this routine a try!

CONCLUSION

The contents of this chapter will give you plenty to think about as you develop personalized routines using the Weider Instinctive Training Principle to develop the diamond-shaped and huge calves of an IFBB champ. Adapt the routines of the champs as I have presented them in this chapter, be sure to train consistently, use plenty of weight with good form in all of your calf exercises, and soon you'll have a super pair of calves!

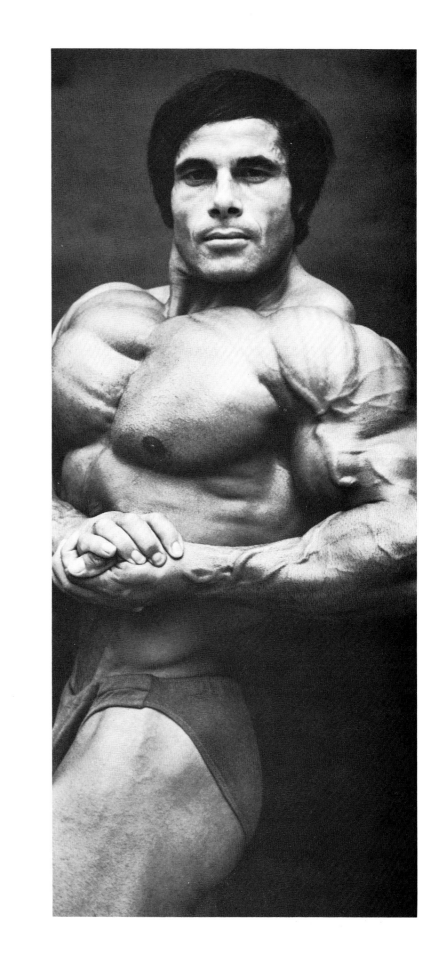

11

Championship Chest Development

Virtually all bodybuilders would enjoy having a huge chest with thick and deeply striated pectorals. But unfortunately many of them incorrectly go about developing their chests, and they fall far short of their goals. They want chest development comparable to that of Arnold Schwarzenegger, Franco Columbu, or Roy Callender, but they aren't willing to pay the price for such incredible development. As a result, their chests appear flat and unimpressive.

There are two aspects of the chest to which you must give emphasis if you wish to develop a huge and deeply muscled chest. You must build a good foundation for chest development by expanding your rib cage. Then you must attack your chest muscles from every possible angle and with great training intensity in order to thicken, balance, shape and striate the pectoral muscles that lie over the upper rib cage. Only then will you have developed a championship chest.

Be careful, however, as you work at building your chest that you don't go overboard and allow it to get disproportionately large, ruining the balance of your physique as a whole. Many bodybuilders fall in love with training their chests and make this elementary mistake. Carefully avoid this mistake—but still fully develop your chest—and you will more quickly build a winning physique.

RIB CAGE EXPANSION

While it would seem to be impossible to lengthen the ribs (they're *bones*, aren't they?), in order to expand the volume of your rib cage, you *can* effectively lengthen your ribs by stretching the cartilages that connect the ribs to your sternum (breast bone). And this can be accomplished by combining an exercise that stimulates deep breathing with a movement that stretches the rib box.

It is easiest to expand the rib cage if you are still in a body maturation cycle, i.e., you are between the ages of about 14 or 15 and 20 or 21. Then, the cartilages that attach your ribs to the sternum are quite pliable and can be more easily stretched. It's not uncommon for bodybuilders in their late teens to increase their chest expansion by six to eight inches during a six-month period of rib cage expansion specialization.

As you grow older, however, the rib cartilages slowly harden and lose their pliability. As a result, it becomes much more difficult and is a considerably slower process to increase the rib box expansion. Still, with persistence and hard work, a man in his twenties, thirties or even forties *can* add several inches to his chest expansion.

It is very advantageous for any serious bodybuilder to have a large rib cage. With a huge rib box like that of Casey Viator, your expanded side-chest poses from each side will be very impressive. A large rib cage also gives you a better foundation on which to build all of your torso muscles, so it's not surprising that a fellow like Viator not only has a huge chest, but also a large torso in general.

There is also a health advantage to having an expanded rib cage, because it gives your internal organs, particularly your lungs, more room in which to operate. Your lungs can also expand in size. It's almost like the case of a goldfish in a small bowl of water. In such a cramped environment, it won't grow much in size. But goldfish turned loose in large, decorative lawn or garden pools, rapidly grow to a huge size!

I often think of chest-building in general as being the same as building a house. First you must have a solid foundation poured, and then you build the house on that foundation. No building contractor in his right mind would put up a house without first laying a solid foundation. If he did, the house would soon crumble into a useless heap of boards.

In bodybuilding, your rib cage is your building foundation and your pectorals are the house that rests on this solid foundation. A bodybuilder who concentrates solely on building his pectorals won't find them crumbling away to nothing in the first storm of winter, but he certainly will never have the type of chest development that wins titles. His chest will always have a flat and incompletely developed appearance.

I hope that I am convincing you that you should spend time specializing on rib cage expansion, because it will undoubtedly be time well-spent if you have competitive aspirations in bodybuilding. If you happen to be a teenager just beginning bodybuilding training, you should place more of your chest-training emphasis on rib cage expansion than on exercises that build thicker pectorals.

If you have been training for several years and have already developed thickly muscled pectorals, you can still greatly benefit from a few months of rib-box expansion specialization, even if your pecs shrink a little while working on your rib cage. Once you resume training your pectorals intensely, they will be back to their former high level of development within a few weeks.

Experienced bodybuilders should objectively evaluate the volume of their rib cages. And if you are unable to do this for yourself, seek the advice of qualified coaches or other experienced bodybuilders. Should you discover that your rib cage could do with a bit more expansion, use the Weider Muscle Priority Training Principle in your chest program by cutting back on your pec work to conserve energy for rib cage expansion training.

Teenage bodybuilders will benefit substantially from 4–6 months of rib cage expansion specialization. Older and more experienced bodybuilders should probably stay on such a specialized program for at least 6–8 months. In either case, I would suggest continuing with chest expansion specialization for as long as you continue to see improvement in your expanded chest measurement from month to month. But once you fail to see such an increase in measurement, you can cease expansion specialization and concentrate your chest-building efforts on perfecting your pectoral development.

Your rib cage expansion program should be followed three nonconsecutive days a week. Since part of the program consists of light-weight, high-rep Squats, you might find it best to perform your rib cage expan-

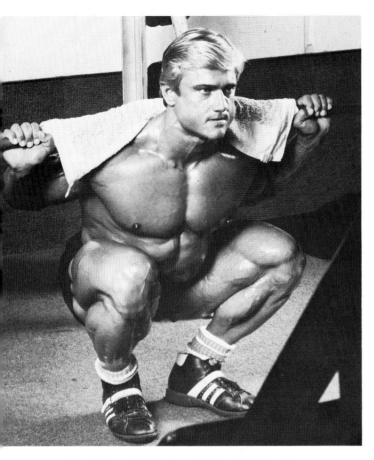

Tom Platz at the bottom of a Breathing Squat.

sion routine on your leg workout days. Work at expanding your rib box first in your workout, and then concentrate on your thigh routine after you have finished rib cage work.

The rib cage expansion specialization program that I recommend consists of supersetting 25 reps of Breathing Squats with 25 reps of Breathing Pullovers using a barbell. Novice bodybuilders can perform two such supersets, taking a minimum pause between exercises and resting for three or four minutes between supersets. Intermediate bodybuilders will benefit from three supersets of these chest-expansion movements, and advanced men can do four or five such supersets.

In this superset, the Breathing Squats will greatly stimulate your respiration rate. At the end of a set of Breathing Squats, you will usually be huffing and puffing like one of those huge steam locomotives that you

see in old Western films. Then you immediately do Breathing Pullovers to stretch your rib cage. And it's the combination of deep breathing and stretching that will do the job in expanding the volume of your rib box.

Breathing Squats are basically like the regular Squats you do in your thigh workout. But since emphasis is more on breathing than on how much weight you can use in your Squats, restrict your Breathing Squat poundage to a weight equal to or less than your own body weight. You will also follow a particular breathing pattern between reps of your Breathing Squats, but other than breathing differently and using a light weight, this movement is exactly like a normal Squat.

To begin a set of Breathing Squats, rest the bar across your shoulders, lift it off the rack, step back, and set your feet in a comfortable position for squatting. Standing erect, exhale as fully as possible and then inhale as deeply as you can. Follow this deep in-and-out breathing pattern for three breaths, holding the third one as you squat down. Exhale as you return to the starting position, then repeat the breathing pattern.

Between each of the first 10 reps of your Breathing Squats take in three huge, gasping breaths. For the next 10 reps breathe out and in four times between each repetition. And between each of the final five reps take five maxed-out breaths. Even with the strictly regimented heavy breathing during this exercise, you will probably find yourself somewhat out of breath at the conclusion of a 25-rep set of Breathing Squats.

Take advantage of this breathless condition by immediately lying back on a flat exercise bench to do 25 repetitions of Breathing Pullovers. Emphasis in this type of Pullover should be on stretching rather than on using muscle strength to do the movement, so use a light weight for the exercise. A barbell weighing 30–40 pounds should be perfect.

Grasp the barbell with a shoulder-width grip and lock your arms straight for the duration of your set. Begin with the barbell supported at straight arms' length directly above your shoulder joints, as in the finish position of a Barbell Bench Press.

Simultaneously breathe in as fully as possible and slowly lower the barbell in a semicircular arc to as low a position behind your head as is comfortably possible. Hold this deep breath as you slowly return the barbell to the starting position, then exhale. Repeat this Breathing Pullover for a full set of 25 repetitions.

For variety, you can use a narrow grip (about six inches between your index fingers) on the barbell. Sometimes it's a good idea to vary your grip width on each set of Breathing Pullovers in order to stretch your rib cage from a variety of angles. You can also perform this movement holding two dumbbells, or with a single dumbbell held in both hands.

After three or four minutes of rest, you can repeat this superset of Breathing Squats and Breathing Pullovers. And, with sufficient time, you will discover that these two movements will substantially expand your rib cage, adding greatly to your chest and torso impressiveness.

PECTORAL MUSCLE ANATOMY AND KINESIOLOGY

The *pectoral* muscles are two large fan-shaped muscles covering the upper rib cage. Each pectoral muscle originates from attachments along the sternum and rib cage, and it runs into a large tendon that attaches to the upper part of the *humeris* (upper arm bone).

To approximate the kinesiology of your pectoral muscles, stand erect, bend your arms at a 90-degree angle, and raise your elbows up to shoulder level, your palms toward the floor. Move your elbows directly to the rear parallel to the floor in semicircular arcs until they are as close to each other behind your back as possible. This approximates the fully extended function of your pectorals.

Next, move your elbows forward in semicircular arcs parallel to the floor as far as

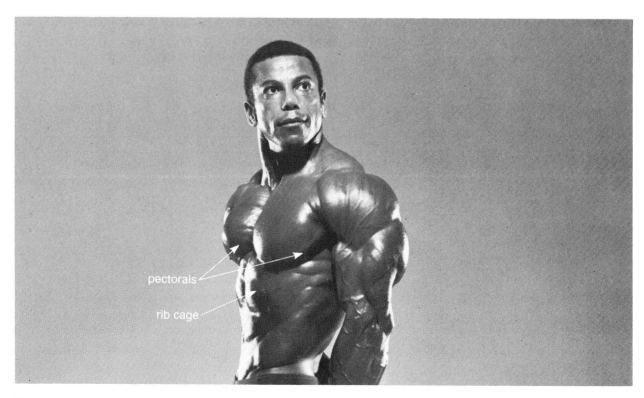

The Chest.

you can (your upper arms should actually cross each other in front of your body). This final position approximates the fully contracted function of your pectorals.

As you perform these movements forward and backward, you will notice that the full range of motion your pectorals can impart to each upper arm bone is an arc exceeding 180 degrees. The key in maximizing pectoral extension and contraction in the full range of motion is how much of an arc through which your upper arm bones travel.

By varying the angle at which you move your upper arms above or below a plane horizontal to the floor, you can stress different sections of your pectorals more intensely than others. With your arms above the horizontal plane, you will place greater stress on the upper sections of your pectorals. And with your arms below the horizontal plane, you shift stress more to the lower sections of your pectorals.

THE BENCH PRESS CONTROVERSY

During the 1950s, 1960s, and early 1970s, virtually all bodybuilders used the Bench Press as their basic pectoral exercise, occasionally performing up to 20 sets of the movement each chest workout. While there are still staunch advocates of the Bench Press for pectoral building, a great many bodybuilders today believe that the Bench Press is either totally worthless as a chest movement or, at best, "just another chest exercise."

Dr. Franco Columbu is one of the sport's leading proponents of using Bench Presses for pectoral building. Franco comments, "You have five or six good chest exercises, and the Bench Press with a barbell is far and away the best. Number two is the Incline Press, and number three is the Parallel Bar Dip. These three exercises would make a very good chest routine.

"Flyes, which all bodybuilders do, are almost useless for chest development, even when done with pulleys, because tension is on the pectorals for only part of the movement. Bench Presses involve the whole pectoral mass, as well as the deltoids and triceps. If I did no other chest exercise, I would always do the Bench Press."

Arnold Schwarzenegger has consistently done Bench Presses in his chest workouts, and he notes, "Doing a Bench Press correctly is not an easy skill to learn. You have to find the grip that suits you. If you hold your hands too close together, your triceps will be doing most of the work. And your pectorals will be doing more of the work if your hands are set too wide apart. You'll have to experiment to discover how to hold the bar to suit your own anatomy.

"The value of Bench Pressing for a bodybuilder is a highly individual matter. If you have the correct anatomical characteristics, it can be an excellent pectoral mass-building movement. For most bodybuilders, however, it is no better than any other exercise."

Massive Casey Viator believes that Bench Presses are not only a good pectoral exercise, but also an excellent movement for adding mass to most of the upper body. "I consistently do repetitions with over 500 pounds in my Bench Press workouts," Casey stated. "Of course, this movement has considerably thickened my pectoral muscles, but it has also added mass to my front deltoids, triceps, and even to my lats and other upper back muscles.

"Doing a heavy Bench Press repetition involves a coordinated effort from many muscle groups to move the barbell upward from the chest. And as a result, the movement adds mass to all of these muscle groups. It's one of the best upper body mass-builders that I know of."

Carlos Rodriguez, Mr. Universe, takes a more moderate stance on the value of the Bench Press for building the pectorals: "Bench Presses are usually the first exercise I do in my chest routine, because it's a good basic exercise and it gives a thorough warm-up to my pectoral muscles before I do my other chest exercises. Although I do the Bench Press all of the time, I don't feel that it's a much better chest-building movement than any other."

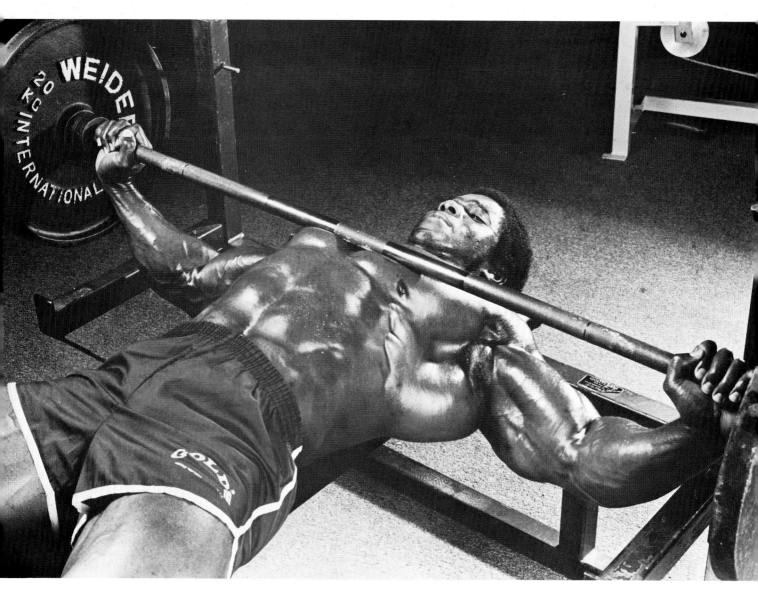

Bench Press with widest possible grip.

Boyer Coe concurs with Rodriguez: "The Bench Press is a good basic chest movement, but not that much better than any other pectoral exercise. I did a great deal of Bench Pressing in my first three or four years of bodybuilding training, but since then I haven't done it much.

"The Bench Press is an excellent basic chest exercise for beginning and intermediate bodybuilders. As such, it builds chest and shoulder muscle mass, and it adds considerably to a bodybuilder's pressing power. This in turn allows him to use much heavier poundages in his other chest and

shoulder exercises. And this is one of the most valuable by-products of using the Bench Press extensively in the first couple of years of bodybuilding training.

"I don't, however, feel that Barbell Bench Presses are that valuable to an advanced-level bodybuilder. There are numerous other exercises that stress the pectorals more directly, over a longer range of motion, and in greater isolation from the rest of the body. I personally do most of my chest exercises, including pressing movements, on machines, which help to keep continuous tension on my pecs throughout the complete range of motion of every exercise."

Ricky Wayne, an IFBB Mr. World winner and Special Assignments Editor of *Muscle & Fitness* magazine, typifies bodybuilders who believe that Bench Presses are useless for building the chest muscles. "I did the movement for years," he recalls, "but I dropped it when I discovered I got nothing out of it. I also think that bench pressing injured my shoulders. As far as pectoral development goes, the Bench Press is a useless, or close to useless, movement.

"I've done all of the angles—inclines, declines, you name it—of Barbell Bench Presses, and I still feel that the movement is worthless. The Bench Press could be a good beginner's exercise, as long as the beginner doesn't look upon it as *the* solution to pectoral development. It's a great movement for building general upper body mass and power, and particularly for strengthening the shoulders and arms. It's a good basic exercise, as are Squats and Barbell Bent Rowing.

"I've interviewed most of the champs over the past 15 years, and they're generally down on the Bench Press. They've discovered that even though they thought that their pectoral development came from Bench Presses, they were also doing a lot of Dips, Flyes, and Crossovers, and that the development actually came from these movements."

In summary, the various champions have said that the Bench Press can be both a good and bad pectoral exercise, depending on an athlete's physical structure. Experiment with Bench Presses to see if they work well for you. Remember, in the final analysis, you must use the Weider Instinctive Training Principle to decide the value of Bench Presses and other movements for your own pectoral development.

PECTORAL-BUILDING STRATEGIES

The best bodybuilders seem to use a greater variety of exercises in their pectoral programs than they regularly perform for any other body part. Indeed, I recently checked out the full-body routines of 20 Weider-trained champions, and all but one of them did more exercises for his pecs than any other muscle group. The lone dissenter used a few more back movements than chest exercises, but his back has been a weak point for the past couple of years and he has been saturation bombing it to bring it up to par with the rest of his physique.

There's a good reason why champion bodybuilders do so many pectoral exercises: there are simply quite a large number of aspects to the pectorals, and no single exercise hits more than a couple of them. So, you will be forced to do a wider-than-normal variety of movements in your chest routine if you hope to ultimately develop complete-looking pecs.

For fully perfected pectoral muscles, you must do movements for the upper pecs, the pec-delt tie-ins, the middle pecs, the outer pecs, the inner pecs along the cleavage between the individual muscles, and the lower pecs. You must also do exercises that build pec mass, and other movements to create striations within the pectoral muscles themselves. Obviously, you have your work cut out for you when you train your pecs.

In the early stages of bodybuilding training, three or four total sets of Bench Presses will suffice as a pectoral workout. But as time goes on, your chest programs will grow more and more complex. You will next need to add Incline Presses to your routine to muscle up your upper pecs, and later some sort of lower-pectoral exercise, such as Decline Presses or Parallel Bar Dips.

I firmly believe that advanced bodybuilders and competitive athletes in an off-season cycle should train their chest twice a week on either a four-day or six-day split routine. They should do either three or four exercises for a total of 12–15 sets.

If you fall into the above category, you should concentrate primarily on basic exercises, such as Barbell Bench Presses, Bar-

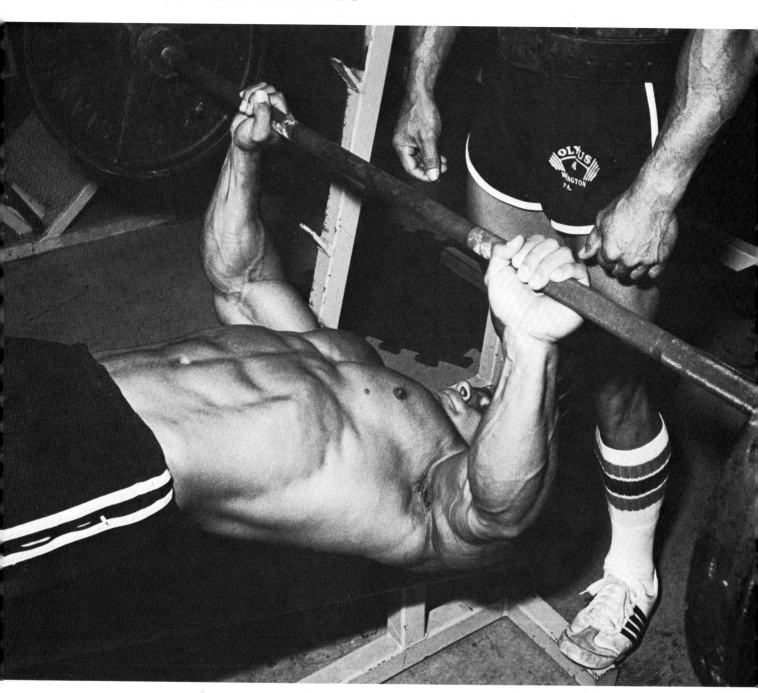

Decline Presses stress the lower pectoral muscles.

bell Inclines, Barbell Declines, weighted Parallel Bar Dips, and heavy Flyes. The off-season is a time for building pure muscle mass, so it would be senseless to do any isolation exercises during that cycle.

Train as heavy as you can in strict form for reps in the range of 5–8 on your basic exercises in the off-season. In order to have sufficient warm-up to prevent injury, pyramid your reps and poundages on the heaviest exercises. And, it is of paramount importance that you increase your exercise poundages as frequently as possible.

Concentrate on the weakest section of your pectorals during your off-season cycle. If, for example, your upper pecs lack thickness, bomb them into submission with a lot of heavy incline bench work. You might even profit from ignoring your more strongly developed lower pecs for a few months in order to devote more energy to your weak upper pecs. As you know, only a few weeks of intense lower-pec training will bring them back up to their former high level of development.

During your precontest cycle, you can pull out all of the stops by training your chest three days a week on either a six-day split routine or on a double-split routine. Increase your total sets of pec training to about 18–20, or even more if you feel that you need extra chest work. Many bodybuilders perform a total of 30–35 sets of pectoral work in their precontest chest routines.

Use more isolation movements, such as Cable Crossovers and Pec Deck Flyes, during your precontest cycle, but still do one or two basic movements to retain as much pectoral mass as possible. I also strongly recommend that you use plenty of peak contraction and continuous tension reps in your precontest chest workout. And you simply *must* make extensive use of the Weider Iso-Tension Training Principle to fully striate your pectorals.

Utilize the Weider Quality Training Principle to the maximum by reducing your average rest interval between sets to an absolute minimum. One of the best ways to accomplish this is to use the Weider Supersets Training Principle as much as possible. Most of the best bodybuilders use a lot of supersets in their chest workouts prior to competitions.

THE CHAMPS' PECTORAL EXERCISES

Following are 16 basic pectoral development exercises used at one time or another by all of the top IFBB bodybuilders. With variations on many of these movements, you will have more than 25 pectoral exercises to work with in your own chest-building routines.

Barbell Bench Press

Main Area of Emphasis—As mentioned earlier in this chapter, there is considerable debate over the value of Bench Presses in a bodybuilder's chest-building routine. Generally speaking, Bench Presses stress the entire pectoral muscle mass, particularly the lower and outer sections of the muscle.

Method of Performance—Lie back on a flat exercise bench with your loaded barbell resting on the rack at the end of the bench. Position your shoulders about six inches away from the uprights of the support rack. Take a grip on the barbell with your palms set about six inches wider on each side than the width of your shoulders. Your palms should be pointed toward your feet. Have a training partner give you a lift-off, so you can easily support the barbell at straight arms' length directly above your shoulder joints for the start of the movement. Slowly lower the barbell to lightly touch the middle of your chest, being certain that your upper arm bones travel as directly out to the sides away from your torso as possible. Slowly straighten your arms to push the barbell back to the starting point. Repeat the movement for the required number of repetitions.

Variations—Using a narrow grip (with your index fingers between six and eight inches apart) stresses the inner edges of the pectorals and the triceps much harder than the medium-grip Bench Press just described. Using a very wide grip places less stress on the triceps and more on the outer edges of the pectorals. You can also lower the barbell to the base of your neck, rather than to your chest. This type of movement allows you to stretch your pectorals more in the bottom position of the exercise.

Training Tips—Always have a spotter standing at the head end of the bench to rescue you if you fail to complete a repetition, or happen to pass out during a rep. Never hold your breath during a Bench Press repetition, since that can cause you to pass out. Be sure that your feet are set solidly on the floor on either side of the bench. Avoid arching your back to com-

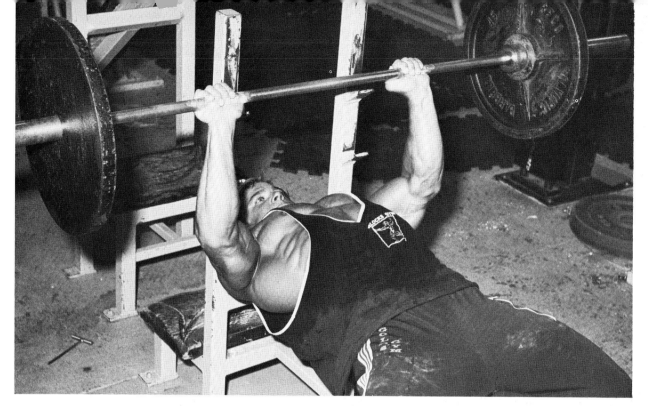

Bench Press with medium grip.

plete a repetition, since this cheating movement takes much of the stress off your upper pectorals. Never bounce a barbell off your chest to start a repetition. This could cause serious intrathoracic injuries. Avoid doing fewer than 3–4 repetitions on the Bench Press, since low reps increase the risk of injuries. Don't let your Bench Press become an "ego lift."

Barbell Incline Press

Main Area of Emphasis—All variations of the Incline Press stress the upper sections of the pectorals, plus the vital pec-delt tie-ins. There is also emphasis on the remainder of the pectoral muscle, the deltoids and the triceps.

Method of Performance—Lie back on an

Bench Press with narrow grip.

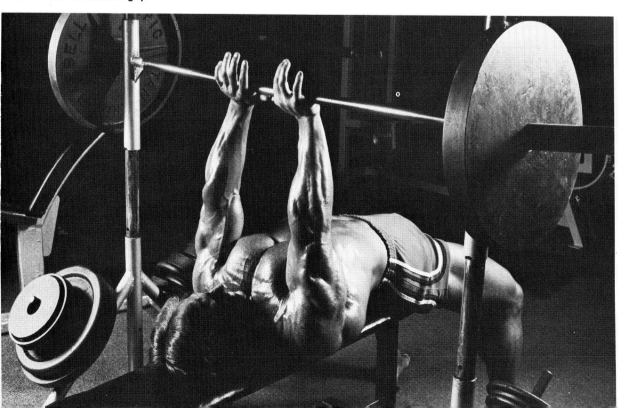

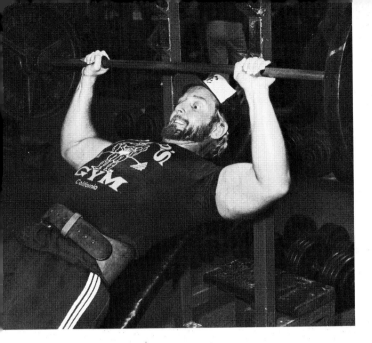

Incline Bench Press.

incline bench with your loaded barbell placed on the bench's support rack. Take the same grip on the barbell as for Barbell Bench Presses and have your training partner give you a lift-off, so you can easily get the barbell into the starting position at straight arms' length directly above your shoulder joints. Making sure that your upper arm bones travel directly out to the sides (or even a little to the rear if possible), bend your arms and slowly lower the barbell to touch your upper chest at the base of your neck. Slowly press the barbell back to the starting point, and repeat the movement for the required number of repetitions.

Variations—It's difficult to use a very narrow grip when doing Barbell Incline Presses, but a shoulder-width grip tends to stretch the pectorals a bit more in the bottom position of the movement. A wide grip will shift more emphasis to the outer sections of your upper pectorals. You can also experiment with different angles of your incline bench. Most commonly, variations of the Incline Press are done on a bench set at a 45-degree angle. Try a lower angle (e.g., a bench set at 30 degrees) to see how that affects your upper pectorals. Most bodybuilders feel that a bench set at a 30-degree angle places more stress on the upper pectorals and removes some from the front deltoids.

Training Tips—The type of incline bench with a seat that can be adjusted upward or downward is far better than one with either no seat or with a seat that is not adjustable. As with Barbell Bench Presses, be sure to have your training partner standing by to spot you in case you either fail a repetition or pass out while doing one. Again, don't hold your breath during the movement, particularly with limit weights, and don't do fewer than 3–4 reps in any set.

Barbell Decline Press

Main Area of Emphasis—Doing all variations of Bench Presses on a decline bench shifts stress primarily to the lower and outer sections of the pectorals.

Method of Performance—You will seldom see a decline bench with a support rack attached to it, so you must have your training partner lift the barbell up to the starting position of the movement for you. The best way to accomplish this is to lay the barbell on the floor behind your head and take the correct grip on it (the grip is the same as for Barbell Bench Presses). Then stiffen your arms and have your partner lift the barbell in a semicircular arc from the floor to the starting position where it is supported at straight arms' length directly above your shoulder joints. In pulling the

Decline Bench Press.

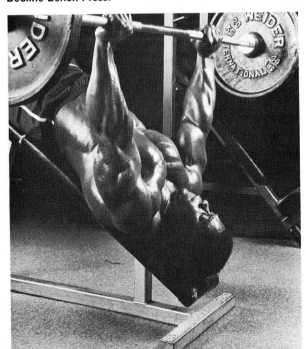

barbell to the starting position, your partner uses your arms to act as levers, with your shoulder joints as the hinge at one end of the levers.

Once you have the barbell in the correct starting position, slowly bend your arms and lower the barbell to touch the middle of your chest, being sure that your upper arms travel as directly out to the sides away from your torso as possible. After lightly touching your chest with the barbell, slowly straighten your arms and push it back to the starting point. Repeat the movement for the desired number of repetitions.

Variations—To achieve a greater degree of stress on the outer sections of your lower pectorals, you can use a wide grip on this movement. You can also lower it to the base of your neck to achieve a greater stretch in your pectorals at the bottom position of the movement.

Training Tips—The angle of your decline bench is most crucial in this exercise. You will get little or nothing from the movement if the bench is set at a decline greater than 30 degrees. The best effect will be felt in your lower pectorals when you do your Decline Presses on a bench set at an angle of 15–20 degrees. Be sure to use a spotter, don't hold your breath during the movement, and never do fewer than 4–5 repetitions of Barbell Decline Presses.

Dumbbell Bench Press

Main Area of Emphasis—This movement can be done on a flat bench (which affects the same muscles as a Barbell Bench Press), on an incline bench (which affects the same muscles as a Barbell Incline Press), or on a decline bench (which affects the same muscles as a Decline Barbell Press). The main advantage to using dumbbells in these movements is that they allow a longer range of motion. When you are using a barbell for Bench Presses, you can lower your hands only to a certain point and stretch your pectorals only to a certain degree before the barbell contacts your chest and terminates the movement. With

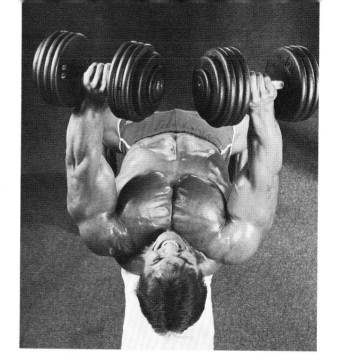

Dumbbell Bench Press.

dumbbells, you can lower your hands much more deeply and stretch your pectorals to a greater degree in the bottom position of the movement.

Method of Performance—Grasp the dumbbells and place them on-end on your knees. Then while leaning back onto the bench, heave them up to your shoulders and press them to straight arms' length directly above your shoulder joints. Your palms should be facing forward. Being sure that your upper arms travel directly out to the sides, slowly bend your elbows and lower the dumbbells as far below the level of your shoulders as possible. Slowly press them back to the starting point and repeat the movement for the desired number of repetitions.

Variations—You can use the same variations of bench angle as on Barbell Incline Presses and Barbell Decline Presses. The main variation when using dumbbells for various Bench Presses is to do the movement with your palms facing inward toward each other.

Training Tips—Try to force the dumbbells against each other at the top position of the movement to affect a greater contraction in your pectorals. On Dumbbell Bench Presses, your training partner can give you forced reps most conveniently by pulling up on your elbows just enough for you to

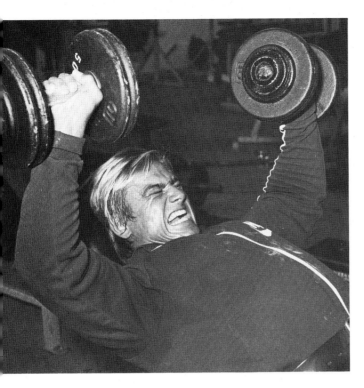

Dumbbell Bench Press on incline.

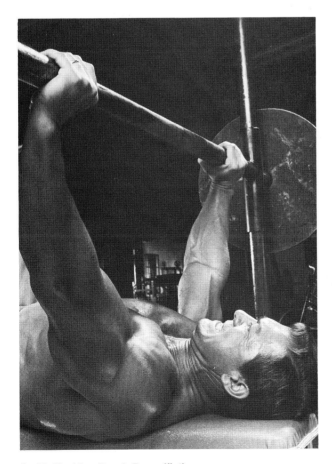

Smith Machine Bench Press (flat).

complete the repetition, rather than pulling up on the middle of the bar, as on all variations of the Barbell Bench Press. With dumbbells, there is no problem with being pinned under the weight, but your partner should be alert to you losing control of the dumbbells, because one of them could then hit you in the face.

Smith Machine Bench Press

Main Area of Emphasis—This exercise can be done on all three angled benches, the same as Barbell and Dumbbell Bench Presses. The angle of the bench determines the effect on your pectorals.

Method of Performance—Set the machine's sliding bar at a height just below where it would be with your arms straightened out at the end of a movement. You can set the bar by slightly rotating it and moving the hooks attached to the bar into position to catch over the short bars projecting at intervals out from the uprights. Select a bench angle (you can prop up one end with either a large block of wood, or with a small exercise bench). Then simply lie back on the bench with your shoulders positioned directly under the sliding bar, take your grip on the bar, straighten your arms and rotate the hooks out of the way, and do your Bench Presses in the usual manner.

Variations—You can use the same variations of grip width and bench angle on this machine as you use when doing Barbell Bench Presses.

Training Tips—If you get stuck near the bottom of the movement, you can rotate the bar slightly and catch a pair of the lower projecting bars. Then you can simply slide out from beneath the bar.

Universal Gyms Machine Bench Press

Main Areas of Emphasis—As with Barbell and Dumbbell Bench Presses, this movement can be done on a flat bench, incline bench and decline bench. The angle of the bench determines the effect on your pectorals.

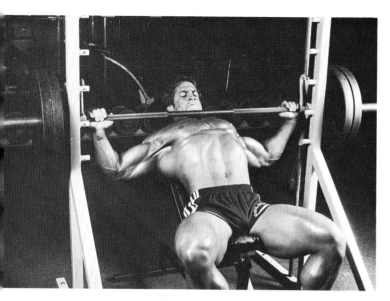

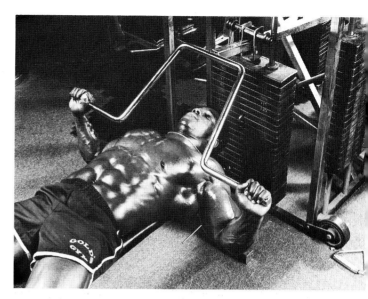

Smith Machine Bench Press on incline, above; on decline, below.

Universal Gyms Machine Bench Press above; on slight incline below.

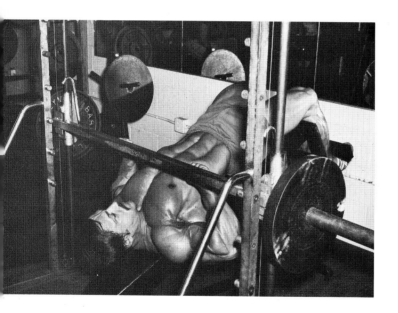

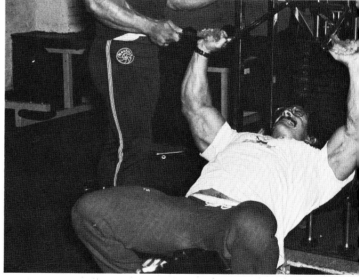

Method of Performance—Slide a flat, decline or short incline bench beneath the Bench Press station lever arm. If you have a normal incline bench, you can slide it under the Seated Pressing station lever arm instead. Regardless of angle, you may need to place blocks of wood under the legs of the bench to adjust it to a correct height. Lie back on the appropriate bench, take a grip on the pressing handles, and push the handles upward until your arms are completely straight. Then simply lower and raise the handles for the required number of repetitions.

Variations—The only real variation you can use on this movement is one of grip width, and even that is restricted by the relatively short length of the handles on each side of the lever arm. As with Barbell and Dumbbell Bench Presses, you can, of course, also play with various angles of the incline and decline benches.

Training Tips—This machine is very safe to use, since there is a gap between the pressing handles and it's impossible to be pinned beneath the weight. Your training partner can easily give you forced reps by pulling up on the lever arm of the machine.

Nautilus Bench Press

Main Area of Emphasis—This movement primarily stresses the lower and outer sections of the pectorals, much the same as does a Decline Barbell or Dumbbell Bench Press.

Method of Performance—You can adjust the height of the seat on the machine to whatever level you like, but this adjustment factor is more important for the Nautilus Flyes movement, which I will discuss a little later in this chapter. For Bench Presses, set the seat at a height so that your arms are approximately parallel to the floor when fully straight. Fasten the lap belt around your hips and place your feet on the large pedal directly in front of you. Push down with leg strength on that pedal to bring the handles of the pressing part of the machine forward into a position where you can grasp them with your palms facing inward. Push hard on the pedal to help fully straighten your arms. From that position, slowly bend your arms as fully as possible, making sure that your upper arm bones travel out at 90-degree angles from your torso. Slowly straighten your arms to push the pressing handles back to the starting position. Repeat the movement for the required number of repetitions.

Variations—The main variation that you can use on this machine is to utilize the foot pedal to push a much heavier weight than you can normally handle to straight arms' length. This way, you can do negative repetitions without anyone helping you. Some extremely powerful bodybuilders have done this movement one arm at a time, but I personally don't recommend this, since it puts an odd torque on your spine. If you can use more weight than provided by the machine's weight stack, simply use a longer stack pin to add barbell plates to the full stack.

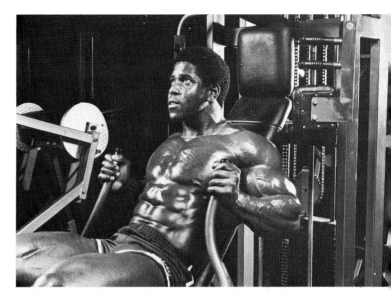

Nautilus Bench Press.

Flyes on a flat bench.

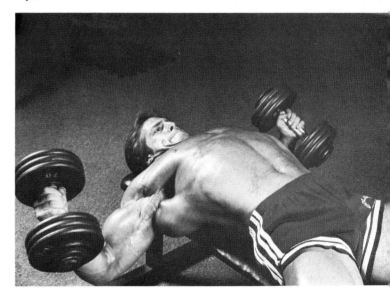

Training Tips—You can also give yourself forced reps using the foot pedal, but this isn't quite as efficient a method as having your training partner pull up on one side or the other of the pressing arms.

Flyes

Main Area of Emphasis—This movement can be done on a flat bench, incline bench or decline bench. The angle of the bench dictates the area of the pectorals that is most stressed by the exercise.

Method of Performance—I will describe how to do this movement on a flat bench, and you can from this description easily learn how to do Incline Flyes or Decline Flyes. Grasp two dumbbells and lie back on a flat bench. Place your feet flat on the floor on either side of the bench. Press the dumbbells to straight arms' length above your shoulder joints, being sure that your palms are facing toward each other. Touch the dumbbells together directly above the middle of your upper chest. Bend your arms about 10–15 degrees and maintain this degree of bend throughout the movement. Being sure that your upper arms travel directly out to the sides at 90-degree angles from your torso, slowly lower the dumbbells in semicircles outward and downward to as low a position as possible. Concentrate less on how low the dumbbells travel than on how low your elbows move, since the depth of descent of your elbows is what dictates the degree of stretch placed on your pectorals. Once you have reached the bottom position of the movement, slowly return the dumbbells back along the same arc to the starting point. Repeat the movement for the desired number of repetitions.

Variations—This movement is sometimes done with the arms held straight, but that usually puts an unnatural strain on the elbow joints. You can experiment with a wide variety of bench angles when you do Flyes.

Training Tips—Your training partner can easily give you forced reps by pulling up on your elbows just enough for you to finish a repetition. Some bodybuilders believe that they can achieve a better feel in their pectorals when doing Flat-Bench Flyes if they curl their legs up over their hips to isolate the legs from the movement.

Pec Deck Flyes

Main Area of Emphasis—This movement stresses the whole of the pectoral, but particularly the inner edges of the pecs where they attach to the sternum.

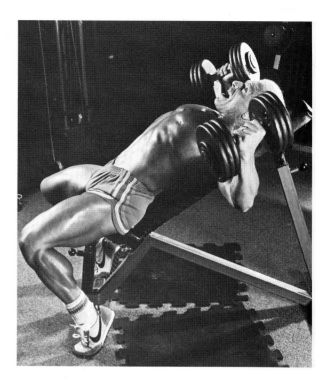

Flyes on an incline, above; on a decline, below.

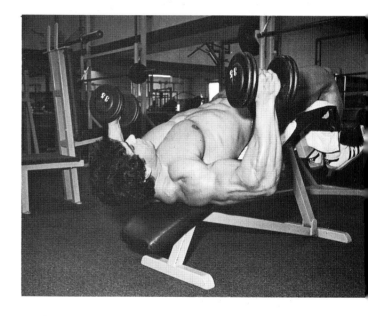

Method of Performance—Adjust the height of the seat so that your upper arms are parallel to the floor as you do the movement. Sit in the seat and force your forearms vertically against the movable pads of the machine and curl your fingers over the tops of the pads. Allow the pads to pull your elbows as far backward as possible to fully stretch the pectorals. Then slowly

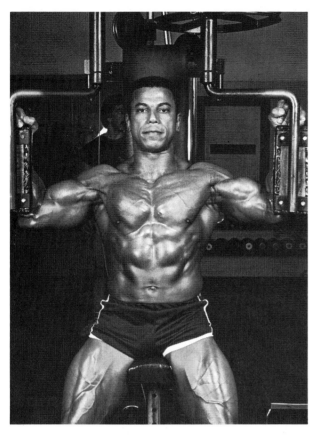

Pec Deck Flyes.

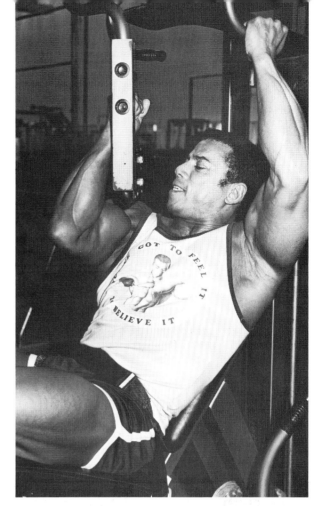

Nautilus Flyes with one arm.

force the pads together until they touch directly in front of the middle of your chest. Return the pads to the starting position and repeat the movement for the desired number of repetitions.

Variations—Experiment with different seat heights. Each new seat height will impart a little different "feel" to your pectorals.

Training Tips—Hold the position with the pads pressed together for three or four seconds for a peak contraction effect in your pectorals. If your training partner stands in front of you, he can help give you forced reps by pushing inward against the outsides of the movable pads just enough to allow you to complete a repetition.

Nautilus Flyes

Main Area of Emphasis—This movement stresses primarily the lower and inner sections of the pectoral muscles.

Method of Performance—Adjust the height of the machine's seat so that your upper arms are parallel to the floor as you perform the movement. Fasten the lap belt around your hips. Force your elbows against the movable pads of the machine and grasp one or the other set of gripping handles. Allow your elbows to travel as far to the rear as possible to fully stretch your pectorals. Then slowly force your elbows forward until the pads touch each other directly in front of your chest. Return the pads to the starting position and repeat the movement for the required number of repetitions.

Variations—As with Pec Deck Flyes, you can experiment with different seat heights. There is also a C-shaped handle above your shoulders as you lie in the machine that you can grasp with one hand, which then allows you to do Nautilus Flyes one arm at a time.

Training Tips—The best way to get

forced reps in this exercise is to have your training partner pull up on the weight stack just enough so you can finish each repetition. Doing this movement one arm at a time allows you to concentrate more on the action of the pectoral that is working. Splitting your attention on two working pecs gives you less of an effect on your chest muscles.

Parallel Bar Dips

Main Area of Emphasis—This is an excellent lower and outer pectoral exercise.

Method of Performance—Grasp the parallel bars with your palms facing each other and jump upward so you are supporting your body on straight arms above the bars. Bend your legs and cross your ankles. Place your chin on your chest and keep it there throughout the movement. Angle your upper body forward throughout the movement (doing Dips with your torso upright makes the movement more for the triceps). Allowing your elbows to move both backward and outward, slowly bend your arms and lower yourself as deeply between the bars as possible. Slowly push your body back to the starting position by straightening your arms.

Parallel Bar Dips.

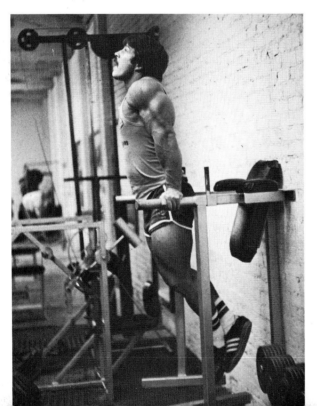

Variations—There are a variety of grip widths that you can use for this movement, and many gyms have parallel bar setups that are actually angled inward in a "V" at one end to allow for different grip widths. You can also use a rope to hang a dumbbell between your legs to add weight to the movement. And, there is a special Dipping machine on the market that uses a waist belt attached to a cable and weight stack that adds resistance to Parallel Bar Dips.

Training Tips—Your partner can help you to do forced reps in this movement by merely holding your feet in a stationary position. This way you can slightly straighten your thighs with just enough force to allow yourself to complete each forced repetition.

Weighted Dips Between Benches

Main Area of Emphasis—This movement stresses the entire pectoral mass, but particularly the lower and outer sections of the muscles.

Method of Performance—Place two flat exercise benches parallel to each other and about 2½ feet apart. Place a third one between the other two, but with the front end of it at the same plane as the back ends of the other two benches. Place your feet on the middle bench and your hands on the other two benches, your fingers facing forward. Stiffen both your body and both arms. Have your training partner place a heavy barbell plate on your upper back, and then bend your arms to sink as far down as possible. Your chest should be well below the level of the benches at the bottom position of the movement. Slowly straighten your arms to push your body back to the starting position. Repeat the movement for the desired number of repetitions.

Variations—You can do these Dips with your fingers pointed outward away from your body. You can also vary the distance between the benches on which you place your hands.

Training Tips—If you need to use more than one barbell plate on this movement,

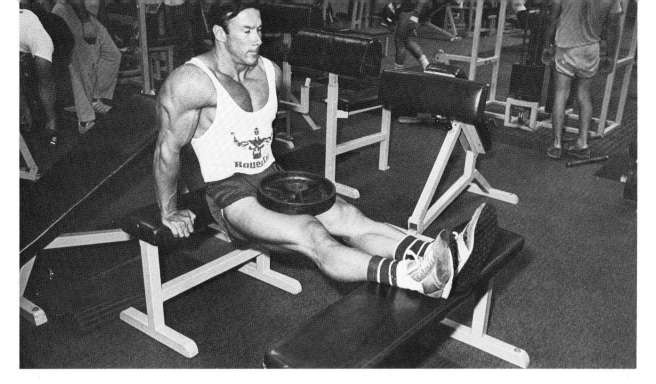

Weighted Dips Between Benches.

it's safest to have your training partner hold them on your back. Or, you can simply have your training partner push down on your back with an appropriate degree of pressure.

Straight-Arm Barbell Pullovers

Main Area of Emphasis—This movement stresses the whole of the pectoral muscles, and builds up the serratus muscles.

Method of Performance—This exercise is performed exactly like the Breathing Pullovers described earlier in this chapter, but it is done with heavier weights and is intended as a muscle-building movement rather than one to stretch the rib cage.

Variations—You can use a variety of grip widths on this movement.

Training Tips—It's better on this movement to do high reps with moderate poundages. Heavy low-rep sets can ultimately injure your shoulders.

Straight-Arm Barbell Pullover.

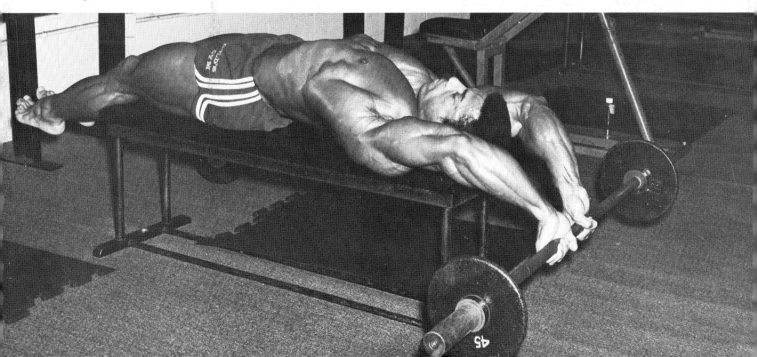

Bent-Arm Barbell Pullovers

Main Area of Emphasis—This movement emphasizes the same muscles as Straight-Arm Barbell Pullovers.

Method of Performance—Take the same grip in the middle of a barbell as you would for a Narrow-Grip Bench Press, and start the movement lying back on a flat exercise bench with the barbell resting on your chest, as at the bottom position of a Narrow-Grip Bench Press. Keeping your elbows bent at 90-degree angles, slowly lower the barbell backward over your face and behind your head to as low a position as possible. The barbell should move in roughly a semicircular arc from your chest to the finish position. Return the barbell back along this same arc to the starting point, and repeat the movement for the desired number of repetitions.

Variations—You can get different effects on your chest muscles by changing your head position from resting on the bench to hanging off the end of the bench.

Training Tips—It's very important as you do this movement that you keep your elbows as close together as possible. Incidentally, this exercise is also a very good lat-builder, making it one of the best of all upper body movements.

Cross-Bench Dumbbell Pullovers

Main Area of Emphasis—This movement emphasizes the same muscles as Straight-Arm Barbell Pullovers and Barbell Bent-Arm Pullovers.

Method of Performance—Place a moderately heavy dumbbell on end on the middle of a flat exercise bench. Lie on your back and shoulders across the bench next to the dumbbell, with your head hanging off one side and your feet set at shoulder width and your legs bent at 90-degree angles off the other side. Place your palms against the inside plate of the upper plates of the dumbbell and wrap your thumbs around the dumbbell bar. Pull the dumbbell up to a position where it is at straight arms' length directly above your chest. Simultaneously

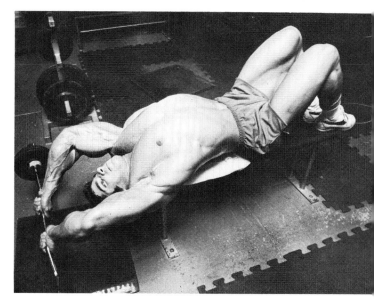

Bent-Arm Barbell Pullover.

Cross-Brench Dumbbell Pullover.

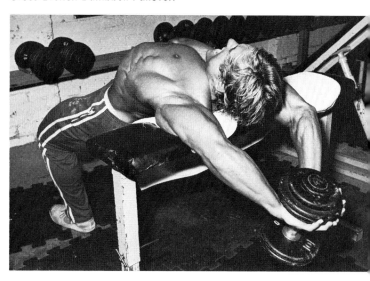

bend your arms slightly and lower the dumbbell in a semicircle backward to as low a position as possible. Return the dumbbell back along the same arc to the starting position, and repeat the movement.

Variations—You can experiment with various degrees of arm bend as you do this movement.

Training Tips—If you consciously lower your hips as the dumbbell descends behind your head, you can get a deeper stretch in your pectorals at the bottom position of the movement.

Cable Crossovers

Main Area of Emphasis—This movement affects primarily the outer, lower and inner pectorals. It is one of the best movements for carving striations across the pectoral muscles.

Method of Performance—Stand between the crossover pulleys, grasping one in each hand. Extend your arms upward in a "V" with your palms facing downward. Bend your arms slightly and keep them bent throughout the movement. Bend slightly forward at the waist and maintain this torso position throughout the movement. From this starting position, slowly pull the handles of the pulleys downward in semi-circles until your hands touch each other about six inches in front of your hips. Return the handles to the starting position and repeat the movement.

Variations—Some bodybuilders do this movement while kneeling on the floor, a variation that seems to make the exercise somewhat more strict, since the legs are isolated out. You can also do this exercise with one arm at a time.

Training Tips—When your hands come together at the bottom position of the movement, hold that position for a few seconds, fiercely contracting your pectorals. It is almost like doing a "Most Muscular" pose, and this technique is very effective in helping to etch striations across your pectorals.

CHAMPIONSHIP PECTORAL ROUTINES

In this section, I will present the pectoral training routines of 20 IFBB bodybuilding superstars. Keep in mind that these pec programs are of very high intensity and suitable only for advanced contest-level bodybuilders. If you are a relative beginner to bodybuilding, do only one or two sets of each recommended exercise, and perform no more than 6–8 total sets. Intermediates can do 10–12 total sets of pectoral exercise, and more advanced bodybuilders can profitably perform 12–15 total sets of pectoral work.

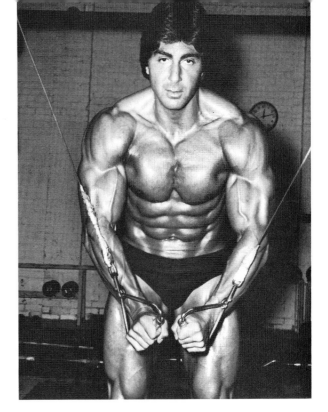

Cable Crossover.

One-Arm Cable Crossover.

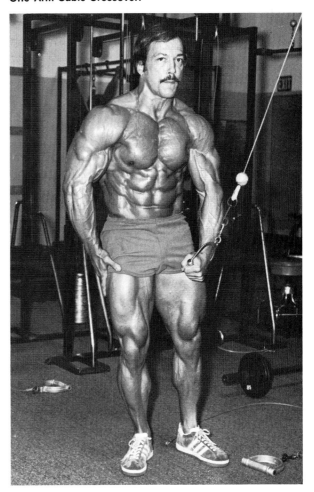

Arnold Schwarzenegger

Exercise	Sets	Reps
1. Incline Press	5	8–10
2. Bench Press	5	8–10
3. Flyes	5	8–10
4. Cable Crossovers	5	10–15

Lou Ferrigno

Exercise	Sets	Reps
1. Bench Press	5	6–10
2. Incline Press	5	6–10
3. Decline Press	5	6–10
4. Flyes	4	10–12
5. Cross-Bench Pullovers	3	15
6. Cable Crossovers	3	10–15

Note: Bracketed exercises are supersetted.

Casey Viator

Exercise	Sets	Reps
1. Barbell Incline Press	5–6	5–6
2. One-Arm Nautilus Flyes	4–5	6–8
3. Weighted Parallel Bar Dips	3–4	6–8
4. Incline Dumbbell Press	3–4	5–6
5. Flat-Bench Flyes	3–4	6–8
6. Cable Crossovers	3–4	10–12

Dr. Franco Columbu

Exercise	Sets	Reps
1. Bench Press	7	12–6
2. Barbell Incline Press	4	10–6
3. Flat-Bench Flyes	2–3	10–12
4. Parallel Bar Dips	2–3	10–15

Note: Bracketed exercises are supersetted.

Chris Dickerson

Exercise	Sets	Reps
1. Pec Deck Flyes	5	12
2. Incline Dumbbell Press	5	12–8
3. Dumbbell Bench Press	5	6–8
4. Cable Crossovers	5	12

Frank Zane

Exercise	Sets	Reps
1. Bench Press	5	12–6
2. Incline Dumbbell Press	3	15–6
3. Flyes (on slight decline)	3	10
4. Cross-Bench Dumbbell Pullovers	3	10

Albert Beckles

Exercise	Sets	Reps
1. Dumbbell Bench Press	5	10–12
2. Flyes	5	10–12
3. Weighted Parallel Bar Dips	5	10–15
4. Cross-Bench Dumbbell Pullovers	5	10–15

Jusup Wilkosz

Exercise	Sets	Reps
1. Incline Barbell Press	5	10–12
2. Narrow-Grip Bench Press	5	10–12
3. Parallel Bar Dips	5	10–12
4. Cable Crossovers	5	10–12

Bertil Fox

Exercise	Sets	Reps
1. Bench Press	6–8	15–4
2. Flyes	6–8	6–8
3. Parallel Bar Dips (weighted)	6–8	8–10
4. Incline Dumbbell Press	6–8	6–8

Boyer Coe

Exercise	Sets	Reps
1. Machine Incline Press	3–4	8
2. Pec Dec Flyes	3–4	8
3. Vertical Machine Bench Press	2–3	8
4. Incline Machine Flyes	2–3	8

Robby Robinson

Exercise	Sets	Reps
1. Incline Dumbbell Press	4	8–10
2. Flyes	4	8–10
3. Parallel Bar Dips (weighted)	4	8–10
4. Cross-Bench Dumbbell Pullovers	2–3	10–15
5. Cable Crossovers	2–3	10–15

Note: Bracketed exercises are supersetted.

Roy Callender

Exercise	Sets	Reps
1. Dumbbell Incline Press	4–6	8–12
2. Incline Flyes	4–6	10–12
3. Parallel Bar Dips	3–5	10–12
4. Cross-Bench Dumbbell Pullovers	3–5	10–15
5. Flat-Bench Flyes	3–5	10–12
6. Cable Crossovers	3–5	10–15

Note: Bracketed exercises are supersetted.

Ron Teufel

Exercise	Sets	Reps
{1. Bench Press	6–8	12–4
{2. Cross-Bench Dumbbell Pullovers	6–8	10–15
{3. Machine Incline Presses	5	8–10
{4. Dumbbell Decline Presses	5	8–10
{5. Barbell Decline Presses	5	8–10
{6. Cable Crossovers	5	8–10

Note: Bracketed exercises are supersetted.

Danny Padilla

Exercise	Sets	Reps
1. Bench Press	5	10–12
2. Flat-Bench Flyes	5	10–12
3. Barbell Incline Press	5	10–12
4. Barbell Decline Press	5	10–12
{5. Cross-Bench Dumbbell Pullovers	5	10–12
{6. Cable Crossovers	5	10–12

Note: Bracketed exercises are supersetted.

Ray Mentzer

Exercise	Sets	Reps
1. Barbell Incline Press	2–3	8–3
2. Pec Deck Flyes	2–3	6–8
3. Cable Crossovers	2–3	6–8
4. Flat-Bench Flyes	2–3	6–8

Samir Bannout

Exercise	Sets	Reps
1. Bench Press	4–5	12–5
2. Dumbbell Incline Press	3–4	8–10
3. Flat-Bench Flyes	3–4	8–10
{4. Parallel Bar Dips	3–4	10–15
{5. Cross-Bench Dumbbell Pullovers	3–4	10–15

Note: Bracketed exercises are supersetted.

Greg DeFerro

Exercise	Sets	Reps
{1. Incline Barbell Press	4–5	8–10
{2. Flat-Bench Flyes	4–5	8–10
{3. Universal Bench Press	4–5	8–10
{4. Cable Crossovers	4–5	8–10
5. Parallel Bar Dips	3–4	10–12
6. Cross-Bench Dumbbell Pullovers	3–4	10–15

Note: Bracketed exercises are supersetted.

Andreas Cahling

Exercise	Sets	Reps
1. Incline Barbell Press	2–3	8–12
2. Incline Flyes	2	10–12
3. Pec Deck Flyes	2	10–12
4. Parallel Bar Dips	2	10–15
{5. Cross-Bench Dumbbell Pullovers	2	10–15
{6. Cable Crossovers	2	10–15

Note: Bracketed exercises are supersetted.

Tom Platz

Exercise	Sets	Reps
1. Incline Dumbbell Press	4–5	12–6
2. Barbell Bench Press	4–5	12–6
3. Low-Incline Flyes	3–4	10–12
4. Parallel Bar Dips (weighted)	3–4	10–15
5. Cable Crossovers	3–4	10–15

Scott Wilson

Exercise	Sets	Reps
1. Machine Incline Press	4–5	8–5
2. Dumbbell Incline Press	4–5	8–5
3. Incline Flyes	4–5	6–8
4. Barbell Bench Press	4–5	8–5
5. Flat-Bench Flyes	4–5	6–8
6. Weighted Parallel Bar Dips	4–5	8–10

SUMMARY

In this chapter I have given you the chest training techniques that you need to know to build up your chest, plus 16 of the best pectoral exercises, and presented 20 proven pectoral-building exercise routines of IFBB superstar bodybuilders. I have also thoroughly discussed how to go about expanding the volume of your rib cage. I am confident that, using the information in this chapter, you can build a deep chest with thick and striated pectorals. Go for it!

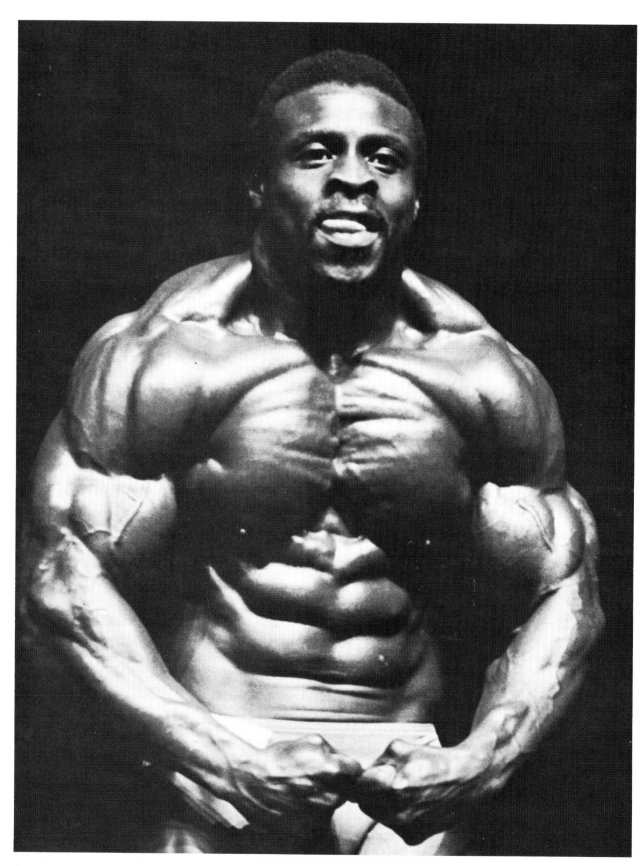

Roy Callender.

12

Cannonball Deltoid Development

The deltoid muscle group takes its name from the triangular-shaped Greek letter *delta*. Most champion bodybuilders consider the deltoids to be among the most important muscle groups of the body. Indeed, it has been said by many bodybuilding superstars that "You can't overdevelop the deltoids."

Along with the abdominals and calves, the deltoids are supremely important to competitive bodybuilders, because they can be seen from all angles—front, back, both sides, and every angle in between—and in virtually all poses. It is impossible to hide poorly developed deltoids, so you should make up your mind immediately to build them up to the max.

While you can do nothing to lengthen your clavicles (collarbones) and thus broaden the width of your shoulder skeletal structure, you *can* add several inches to the width of your shoulders by fully developing your deltoids. A good example of a bodybuilder who greatly broadened his shoulders in this manner is Larry Scott, one of my greatest pupils and winner of the first two Mr. Olympia competitions.

The Great Scott was not blessed with a wide-shoulder skeletal structure. In fact, his shoulders were quite narrow when he first took up hard bodybuilding training. But through intelligent deltoid training, particularly of the side section of the muscle complex, he was able to broaden his shoulders remarkably. Eventually, his cannonball deltoid development was the envy of millions of bodybuilding fans around the world.

All of the recent IFBB superstars have had superb deltoid development. Indeed, bodybuilding has progressed so rapidly as a sport in recent years that it's virtually impossible to win even a regional title without pronounced half-cantaloupe delts, standing semirelaxed in the prejudging lineup, and deltoids that striate into a hundred tiny fibers of muscle when standing under tension in a posing routine.

Some of the IFBB superstars with particularly good shoulder development include Arnold Schwarzenegger, Mike Mentzer, Albert Beckles, Pete Grymkowski, Chris Dickerson, Bertil Fox, Casey Viator, Dr. Franco Columbu, Dennis Tinerino, Roy Callender, Danny Padilla, Lou Ferrigno, Andreas Cahling, and Scott Wilson. And most of the other top bodybuilders have extremely good deltoid development as well.

DELTOID ANATOMY AND KINESIOLOGY

The deltoid muscle covers the point of the shoulder in the form of a cap. It originates at various points around the shoulder joint and attaches via a tendon to the outside of the humeris (upper arm bone). Primarily, the deltoid contracts to move the upper arm bone in various directions.

Each deltoid is formed from three lobes of muscle called *heads.* The anterior (front) deltoid head contracts to move the upper arm bone forward and upward, to move the upper arm forward horizontal to the floor, or any combination of these two functions. The medial (side) deltoid head contracts to move the upper arm bone laterally to the side when the palm is held down. And the posterior (rear) deltoid head moves the upper arm bone upward to the rear, or to the rear horizontal to the floor.

The deltoids, particularly the anterior and posterior heads, often act in concert with the pectorals and back muscles in various exercises. As an example, when you do Incline Presses, Decline Presses, Bench Presses and Parallel Bar Dips, you strongly stress the anterior deltoids, along with your pectorals. When you do Chins, Pulldowns or Bent Rows for your lats, you also strongly involve the posterior heads of your deltoids. And when you do Upright Rows for your trapezius muscles, you involve the whole deltoid, particularly the medial heads of your deltoids.

DELTOID EXERCISE VARIETY

There are three primary types of deltoid exercises: pressing movements, leverage exercises, and pulling movements. In general, the pressing movements are good mass builders, particularly of the front deltoids. Leverage exercises are primarily for shaping and striating the delts, particularly the medial and posterior heads. And pulling exercises such as Upright Rows are

The Deltoid Muscles.

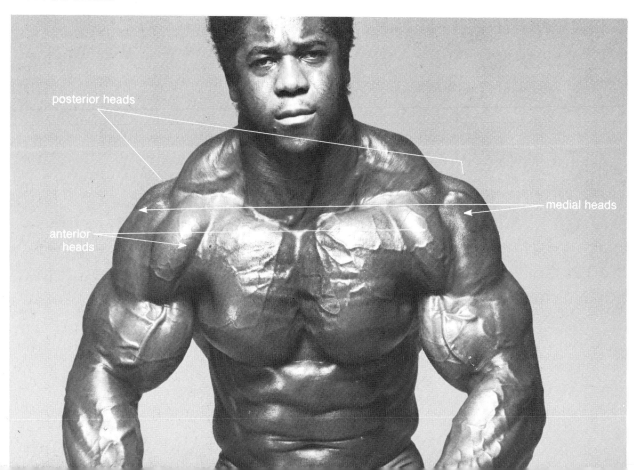

good for completing the deltoid-trapezius tie-ins.

I've seen bodybuilders develop very good deltoids exclusively through the use of the pressing movements, but they generally lack rear-delt impressiveness and good delt-trap tie-ins. To build complete-looking deltoids, with all three heads fully and proportionately developed, you will need to use pressing, leverage, *and* pulling exercises.

DELTOID PREEXHAUSTION

You can use preexhaustion quite efficiently when working your deltoid. Simply superset Dumbbell Side Laterals with any type of overhead pressing movement for a good preexhaustion combination. The Side Laterals prefatigue the deltoids, which are then temporarily weakened as you do the Presses. This way, your triceps muscles are proportionately stronger as you do the Presses, and they don't fatigue and fail before the front delts have been fully stimulated.

I have a good "quicky" deltoid program that you can use whenever you are too rushed to do a full delt workout. It consists of three trisets—or a total of nine sets—including a preexhaustion component. And it has exercises to stress all three heads of your deltoids.

Try this deltoid triset when you're short on workout time:

Exercise	Sets	Reps
1. Dumbbell Side Laterals	3	8–10
2. Standing Barbell Press Behind Neck	3	8–10
3. Dumbbell Bent Laterals	3	8–10

To optimally bomb your delts in approximately 10 minutes with this triset, you should have your weights loaded and set next to each other on the floor in front of you. As soon as you finish your Side Laterals, place the dumbbells on the floor, grasp the barbell, and clean it up to a position behind your neck for the Presses. And the second you finish your presses, bend over and push the barbell out of the way. Grasp

the original pair of dumbbells without even straightening up, and do your Bent Laterals with them.

Done quickly and with approximately 60–90 seconds' rest between trisets, you can get a terrific deltoid pump with this simple routine!

THE CHAMPS' DELTOID EXERCISES

In this section, you will find 15 deltoid exercises that are used by all of the champs. With variations on many of these movements, you will have something in the neighborhood of 25 deltoid movements with which you can work in making up your own shoulder-building programs.

Military Press

Main Area of Emphasis—This is primarily a front deltoid movement, although it also stresses the medial and posterior deltoids to a lesser degree. The triceps, upper pectorals, and upper back muscles are also stressed when doing Military Presses.

Method of Performance—Take an overgrip on a barbell with your hands set about six inches wider on each side than the width of your shoulders. Clean the barbell to your chest and rotate your elbows under the bar. From this starting position, and being careful not to bend your torso backward as you do the Presses, slowly push the barbell directly upward past your face until it is locked out at straight arms'

Military Press.

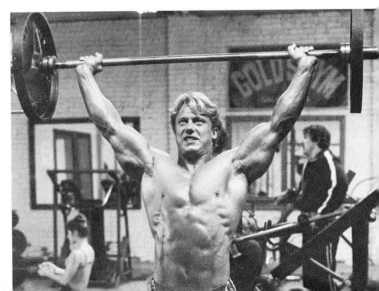

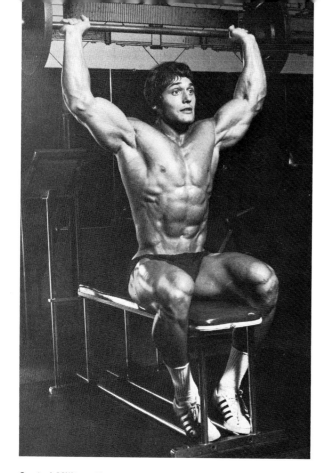

Seated Military Press.

used for Military Presses and rest the barbell across your shoulders behind your neck. Rotate your elbows directly beneath the bar and keep them there throughout the movement. From this basic starting position, press the weight slowly upward until your arms are locked out and the barbell is directly above your head. Slowly lower the barbell directly downward to the starting point and repeat the movement for the desired number of reps.

Variations—This exercise can be done both standing and seated on a flat exercise bench. You can experiment with various grip widths.

Training Tips—With very heavy weights, you can either take the barbell off a squat rack after placing your hands in the proper gripping position, or you can place your hands on the bar as it rests on a bench press rack, lean your head under the barbell to rest it across the base of your neck, then do the top part of a Hyperextension movement to get it into the proper position for a Seated Press Behind Neck.

length directly above your head. Slowly lower the barbell back to the starting point and repeat the movement for the desired number of repetitions.

Variations—This movement is often done seated on a flat bench, or seated on a bench with a vertical back rest attached. You can also experiment with varying degrees of grip widths.

Training Tips—Military Presses are the most basic of all deltoid exercises, so they should be done early in your workout. It's also important to pyramid your reps and training poundages on each succeeding set.

Press Behind Neck

Main Area of Emphasis—Like Military Presses, this is primarily a front deltoid exercise, although it tends to influence the other two heads of the delts a bit more strongly than do Militaries. Triceps and trapezius strength is also important.

Method of Performance—Take a grip on a barbell slightly wider than that which you

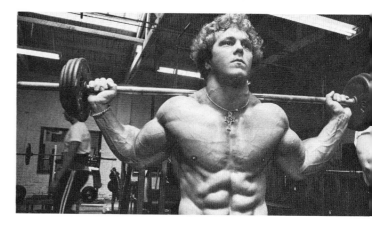

Press Behind Neck.

Seated Press Behind Neck.

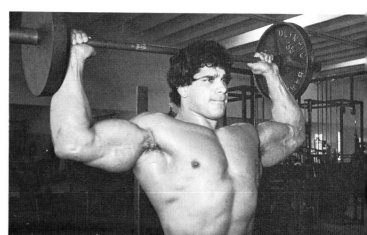

Dumbbell Press

Main Area of Emphasis—This movement stresses the same muscles as both a Military Press and Press Behind Neck, but usually over a longer range of motion. Also, when using dumbbells, it is impossible for a stronger arm to take over some of the weight in the movement.

Method of Performance—Grasp two moderately heavy dumbbells and clean them to your shoulders so that your palms are facing forward. Slowly press them directly upward from your shoulders until they touch in the middle directly above your head at straight arms' length. Slowly lower the dumbbells back to the starting position, and repeat the movement for the desired number of repetitions.

Dumbbell Press.

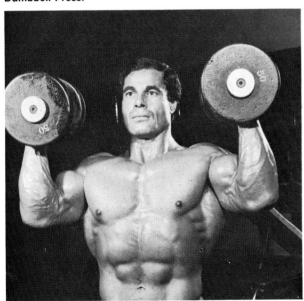

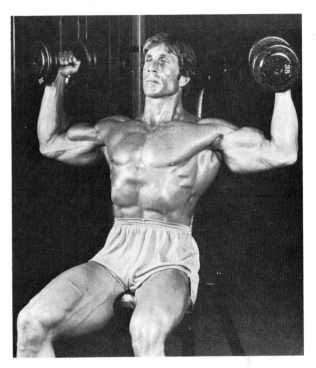

Seated Dumbbell Press.

Alternate Dumbbell Press.

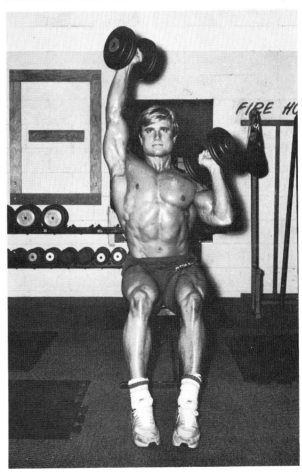

Variations—This movement can be done with the palms facing inward toward each other, in alternate fashion (with one dumbbell going upward as the other descends), or seated on a flat bench with all of the above variations. You can also press one dumbbell at a time while holding on to a solid vertical support with your free hand.

Training Tips—The key with Dumbbell Presses is to lower the dumbbells as far down at the bottom of the movement as possible to effect a longer range of motion to the movement.

"Arnold" Press

Main Area of Emphasis—This movement stresses the same muscle groups—although somewhat more intensely—as a normal Dumbbell Press.

Method of Performance—Begin with two moderately heavy dumbbells held in the finish position for a Dumbbell Curl. From there, stretch your hands downward as far as is comfortable and then begin to press the dumbbells upward. As you press the dumbbells upward, slowly rotate your hands so that your palms are forward during the midrange of the movement. Do not lock out your arms at the top of the movement, since this would take tension off your working deltoids. Slowly lower the weights back to the starting position. Repeat the movement for the required number of repetitions.

Comments—This exercise was originated and extensively used by the great Arnold Schwarzenegger. I don't feel that I need to give it any more of a recommendation.

Machine Press

Main Area of Emphasis—This exercise stresses the same muscle groups as Military Presses and Presses Behind Neck.

Method of Performance—This exercise can be performed on a Smith machine, a Nautilus Double-Shoulder machine, or on the pressing station of a Universal Gyms machine. Grasp the handles and seat yourself beneath the weight handles so that they will be slightly in front of your neck. From that position, slowly press the handles directly upward until your arms are locked out straight. Lower the weight back to the starting position and repeat the movement for the desired number of repetitions.

Variations—On the Universal Gyms machine, you can do Machine Presses either facing toward or facing away from the weight stack. On the Nautilus machine, you can move the seat upward or downward for a shorter or longer range of motion on the Presses. And on a Smith ma-

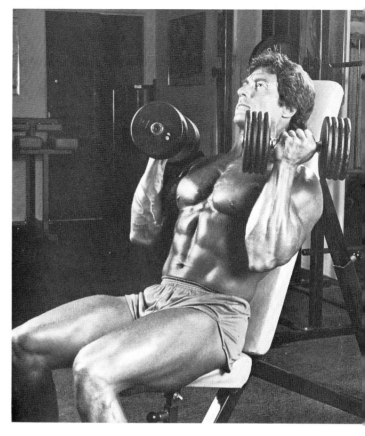

"Arnold" Press—start, above; finish, below.

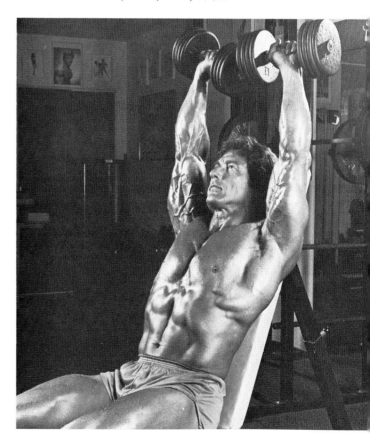

chine, you can do your Presses both behind the neck and with a variety of grip widths.

Dumbbell Side Lateral

Main Area of Emphasis—Side Laterals stress primarily the medial heads of the deltoids, with secondary emphasis placed on the anterior deltoids. There is also a small degree of stress placed on the trapezius muscles.

Method of Performance—Grasp two light dumbbells and stand erect with your feet set at about shoulder width. Bend over slightly at the waist and maintain that degree of torso inclination throughout the movement. With your palms facing each other, touch the dumbbells together four or five inches in front of your pelvis. Bend your arms slightly and keep them bent throughout the movement. From this basic starting position, slowly raise the dumbbells slightly forward and upward in semicircular arcs from the level of your pelvis

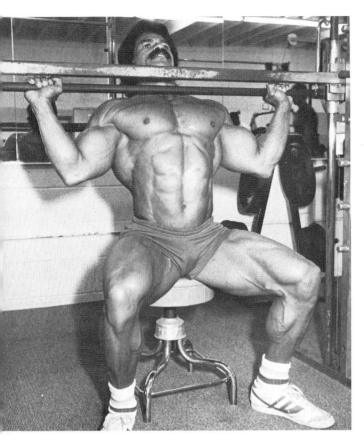

Smith Machine Press.

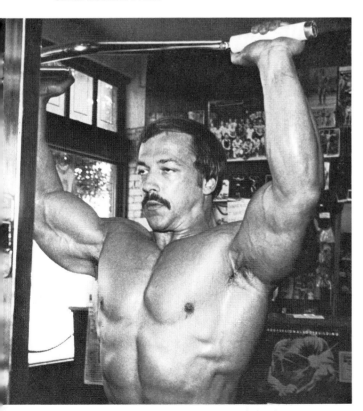

Universal Gyms Machine Press.

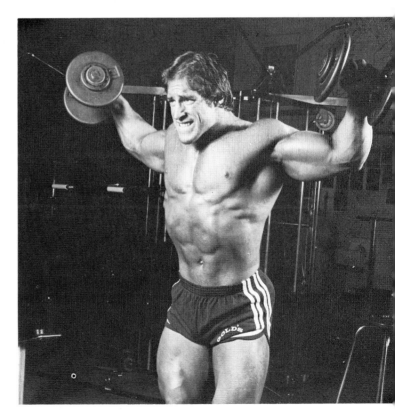

Dumbbell Side Lateral.

until they are above an imaginary line drawn through your shoulders. As you move the dumbbells upward, your palms should be facing downward at all times. Then, at the top of the movement, rotate your index fingers downward so that they are momentarily below the level of your little fingers, a movement which puts strong, direct stress on the medial heads of your deltoids. Hold this top position for a moment or two, then lower the dumbbells back along the same arcs until they are again touching each other in the starting position. Repeat the movement for the required number of repetitions.

Variations—This movement is occasionally done with one arm at a time, the free hand grasping a sturdy upright to steady the body in position throughout the exercise. This variation is a favorite of Boyer Coe's. When using either both arms at once or one arm at a time, you can begin the movement with the dumbbells behind your buttocks. Starting the exercise from this position places a little different stress on the deltoids.

Training Tips—The most common mistake made when doing Side Laterals is "swinging" the dumbbells upward with extraneous body movement. You should raise and lower the dumbbells rather slowly.

Cable Side Lateral

Main Area of Emphasis—This exercise has a slightly different "feel" from Dumbbell Side Laterals, but it stresses the same muscle groups. When using cables, you will probably feel more stress during the first half of the upward movement than you do when using dumbbells.

Method of Performance—This exercise is normally done with one arm at a time, which allows for better concentration on the working deltoid than when splitting your attention on two delts at once. Stand with your right foot about two feet away from a floor pulley with a loop handle attached to one end. Set your feet a comfortable distance apart and reach down to grasp the loop handle with your left hand. Stand erect with your left hand held in front of your pelvis and the cable running diagonally across your body down to the floor pulley. Bend your arm slightly and keep it bent throughout the movement. With your palm facing downward at all times, slowly raise your left hand in a semicircle from the starting position slightly forward and upward until it is above shoulder height. Slowly lower your hand back along the same arc to the starting point and repeat the movement. Be sure to

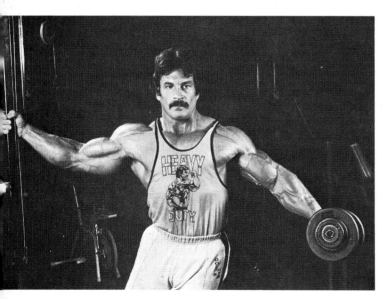

One-Arm Dumbbell Side Lateral.

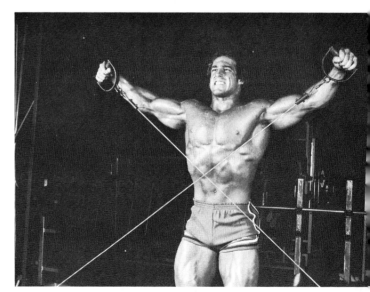

Cable Side Lateral.

do an equal number of sets and repetitions for both sides of your body.

Variations—You can do this exercise with the cable running behind your body rather than in front of it, a favorite alternative method at times of Andreas Cahling (Mr. International) and Bob Birdsong (IFBB Professional Mr. Universe). You can also do the movement one arm at a time without the cable running across your body. In this case, you would assume the same starting position as previously described, but grasp the loop handle in your right, rather than left, hand. Then you can do the movement almost as if raising a dumbbell, although it will give you a different "feel" than a dumbbell. A third variation of Cable Side Laterals can be done with both hands at one time, the cables crossing in front of your body. This variation is done bent slightly over at the waist, and it's a favorite of Lou Ferrigno (Mr. America, Mr. International, twice Mr. Universe, television and film star) and Larry Scott (Mr. America, Mr. Universe and winner of the first two Mr. Olympia titles).

Training Tips—When you do any movement with one arm or one leg at a time, such as in the normal method of performing Cable Side Laterals, you can concentrate more on the working muscle. If you use both arms at once, you must split your attention between two working muscles.

Nautilus Side Lateral

Main Area of Emphasis—This movement very strongly stresses the medial heads of the deltoids.

Method of Performance—Adjust the seat on the machine until you can sit in it with your shoulder joints on the same level as the pivot points of the lateral raise apparatus. Sit in the machine, buckle the lap belt around your waist, cross your ankles below the seat to isolate your legs from the movement, place the outsides of your wrists against the insides of the movable lateral raise pads, and grasp the handles just in front of these pads. From this basic starting position, use your deltoid strength to raise the pads outward and upward as

One-Arm Cable Side Lateral.

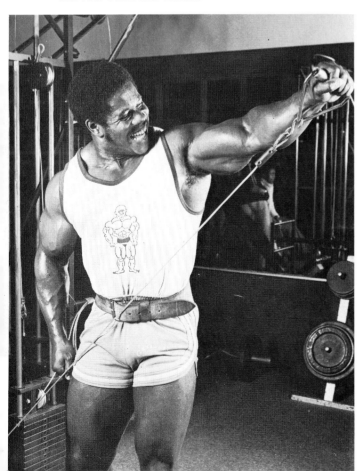

Nautilus Side Lateral.

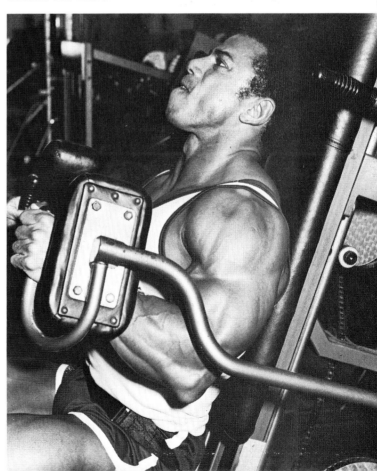

high as possible. Hold the top position of the movement for a moment, then lower the pads back to the starting point. Repeat the movement for the desired number of repetitions.

Variations—The main variation of this movement is to do it with one arm at a time. Very strong bodybuilders like Casey Viator can use the whole weight stack on the machine with one arm, so he must use longer stack pins to add barbell plates to the stack to make the weight heavy enough to tax his deltoids.

Training Tips—The real key to this movement is in how high you can move your elbows. I often see men in the various bodybuilding gyms here in Southern California who raise their hands very high in the movement, but who neglect to do the same thing with their elbows.

Prone Incline Dumbbell Laterals

Main Area of Emphasis—This exercise strongly stresses both the medial and posterior sections of the deltoids. As such, it is a very versatile movement.

Method of Performance—Grasp two light dumbbells and lie facedown on an incline bench with your arms dangling down from your shoulder joints. Your palms should be facing inward and your arms must be slightly bent throughout the movement. Touch the dumbbells together beneath the bench and then raise them slowly in semi-circular arcs out to the sides and slightly forward until they are above the level of your shoulders. Lower the dumbbells back along the same arc to the starting position, and repeat the movement.

Variations—You can use different angles of benches for this movement, and every

Prone Incline Dumbbell Lateral.

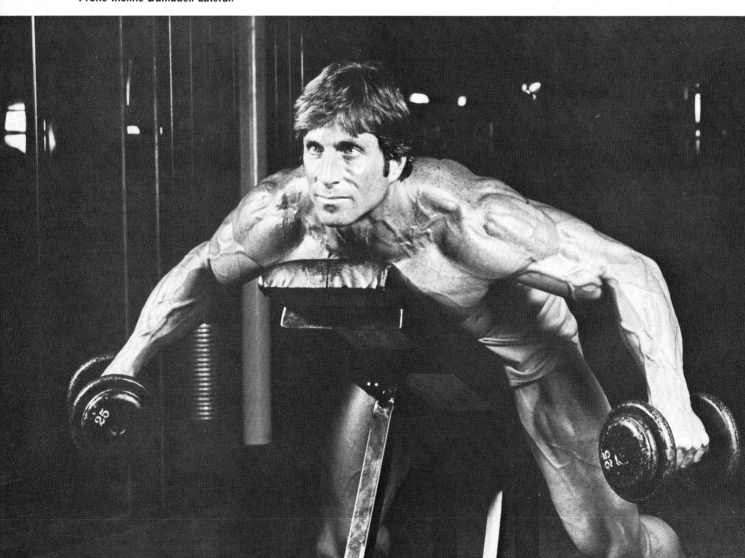

angle attacks a little different section of the deltoids. Most bodybuilders do this exercise on a 45-degree angled incline bench, and a few gyms have such benches with a "window" cut in them so that you won't smash your nose as you lie facedown on the bench. I feel that a 30-degree incline bench gives the best results in this movement, but Boyer Coe even does the movement lying facedown on a flat exercise bench, which directly stresses the posterior heads of his deltoids.

Training Tips—As with Dumbbell Side Laterals, you can rotate your index fingers downward at the top of the movement for a slightly different stress on your medial and posterior deltoids. You can also experiment with raising the dumbbells more or less forward as you are moving them upward to the finish position of the movement. Raising the dumbbells a little more forward also stresses the delts from a little different angle, and every different angle helps.

Incline Dumbbell Side Lateral Raise

Main Area of Emphasis—This type of Side Lateral Raise directly stresses the medial head of the deltoid.

Method of Performance—This exercise is usually done on an abdominal board set at a low incline, but it can be done on a low-angle incline bench. Lie on your right side and brace your body into a firm position with your legs and right hand, so that the body doesn't move during the performance of the exercise. Grasp a light dumbbell in your left hand and rest it on the padded abdominal board directly in front of your hip. Bend your left arm slightly, and keep it bent throughout the movement. From this basic starting position, raise the dumbbell in a semicircular arc until it is directly above the shoulder joint. Lower the dumbbell slowly back in the same arc to the starting point, and repeat the movement for the desired number of reps. Be sure to do an equal number of sets and repetitions for each arm.

Variations—Some bodybuilders start the dumbbell on its upward path from a position behind their buttocks, while others start the movement with the dumbbell resting on the side of their hip.

Training Tips—For different "feels" in your deltoids, you can vary the angle of the incline board or bench that you use. You can also do this movement while lying on the floor, although in my experience you won't feel it as much in your medial deltoid as when lying on your side on an incline abdominal board or incline bench.

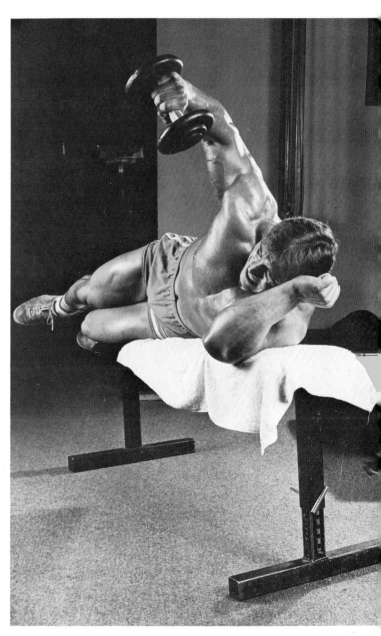

Incline Dumbbell Side Lateral Raise.

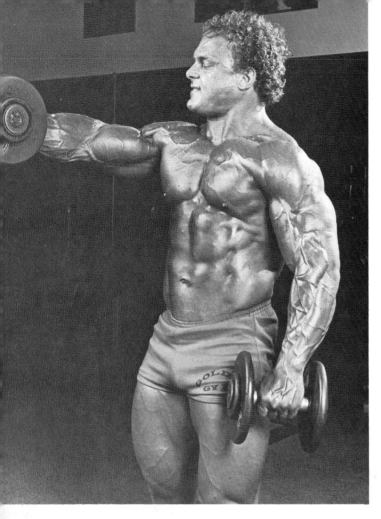
Alternate Front Dumbbell Raise.

Alternate Front Dumbbell Raise

Main Area of Emphasis—Front Dumbbell Raises stress primarily the anterior heads of the deltoids, although the medial heads of the delts come into play to a small degree in the movement.

Method of Performance—Grasp two light dumbbells in your hands and stand erect, with the dumbbells resting on the tops of your thighs. Your palms should be facing the floor throughout the movement, and your arms should be slightly bent at all times. Place your feet a comfortable distance apart. From this basic starting position, slowly raise the dumbbell in your right hand forward in a semicircular arc until it reaches shoulder level. Then as that dumbbell begins to descend, begin raising the dumbbell in your left hand. Continue like this in "see-saw" fashion until you have done the required number of repetitions with each arm.

Variations—Some bodybuilders do Forward Raises with a barbell held in both hands, taking various grips on the bar. The barbell can be raised either to shoulder level, or completely up to arms' length directly above your head. I have also seen top bodybuilders do this movement while holding a fairly heavy dumbbell in both hands. In such a case, it's a good idea to pad the dumbbell by wrapping a towel around it.

Training Tips—Lou Ferrigno has made a good suggestion regarding the method of performance of Alternate Front Dumbbell Raises. He feels that he gets more benefit from the movement if he raises the dumbbells either up the center line of his body, or even across this center line, than if he raises them along planes through his shoulders on each side.

Dumbbell Bent Lateral

Main Area of Emphasis—This is a direct posterior deltoid movement, but it also stresses most of the upper back muscles to some degree.

Method of Performance—Grasp two light dumbbells in your hands and place your feet a comfortable distance apart. Bend over at the waist until your torso is parallel to the floor and bend your knees slightly to take potential stress off your lower back. Hang your arms directly downward from your shoulder joints. Face your palms inward toward each other and maintain this hand position throughout the movement. You should also bend your arms slightly and maintain this arm position as you do the exercise. From this basic starting position, slowly raise the dumbbells directly out to the sides, or even slightly forward and outward, until they reach shoulder height. Hold the top position for a moment, then lower the dumbbells back along the same arc to the starting point. Repeat the movement for the required number of repetitions.

Variations—This movement can also be done while seated at the end of a flat exercise bench and with your torso resting on

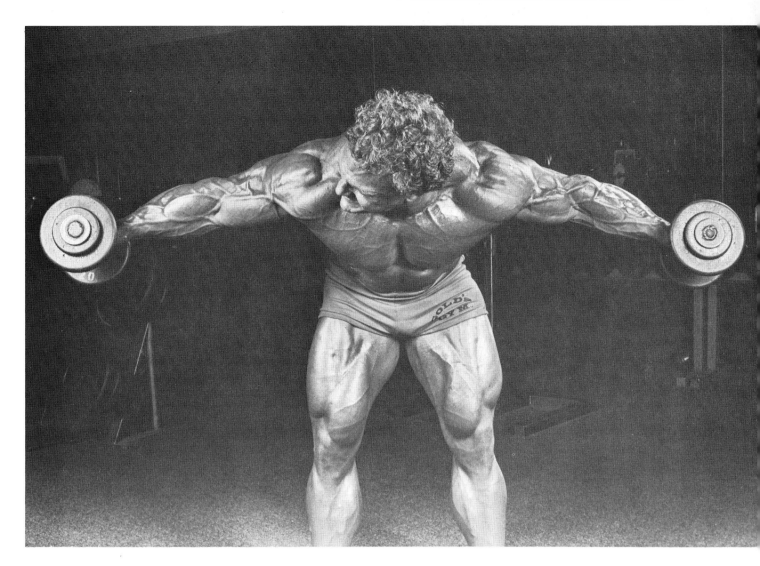

Dumbbell Bent Lateral.

Seated Bent Lateral.

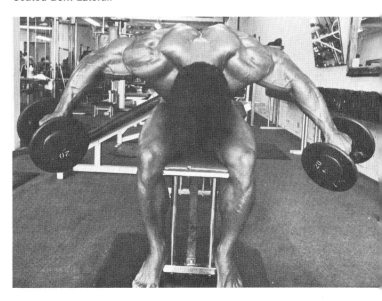

your thighs. That was a favorite method used by Arnold Schwarzenegger to work his rear deltoids. Jusup Wilkosz does a similar movement, except that he raises his torso slightly above the level of his legs, a position which makes the exercise somewhat like Prone Incline Dumbbell Laterals.

Training Tips—The main mistake that inexperienced bodybuilders make when doing this movement is raising the dumbbells somewhat to the rear. Doing this takes most of the stress off the rear delts and places it on the triceps and upper back muscles. Be sure to raise the dumbbells directly out to the sides, if not actually a little forward.

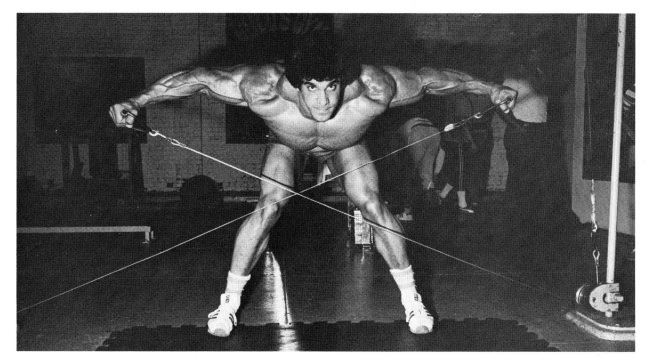

Cable Bent Lateral.

Cable Bent Lateral

Main Area of Emphasis—Like Dumbbell Bent Laterals, Cable Bent Laterals work primarily the posterior heads of the deltoids. Secondary emphasis is on all of the upper back muscles.

Method of Performance—This exercise is most often done with two arms simultaneously. Stand between a set of double low pulleys with loop handles attached to the cables. Reach with your right hand across your body and grasp the loop handle attached to the pulley on the left side of your body. Then grasp the loop handle attached to the right pulley with your left hand, so the cables will be crossed beneath your body as you do the movement. Bend over at the waist until your torso is parallel to the floor and slightly bend your knees to take potential stress off your lower back. Allow the weights on the pulleys to pull your arms across each other, your palms facing toward the floor during the movement and your arms bent slightly as you do the exercise. From this basic starting position, slowly raise your hands in semicircular arcs out to the sides and upward until they are slightly above shoulder height. Lower your hands back along the same arcs to the starting position. Repeat the movement for the desired number of repetitions.

Variations—This movement is often done one arm at a time, in order to allow for better concentration on the working posterior deltoid head. In such a case, the cable should run diagonally under your body, and your working arm should be against your torso at the beginning of the movement.

Training Tips—When you use cables for Bent Laterals, you achieve a longer range of motion. And you can also take advantage of the Weider Continuous Tension Training Principle more fully with cables than when using dumbbells.

Pec Deck Rear Delt Raise

Main Area of Emphasis—This movement strongly stresses the posterior deltoids and secondarily stresses the upper back muscles.

Method of Performance—Sit in the machine with your chest against the pad on

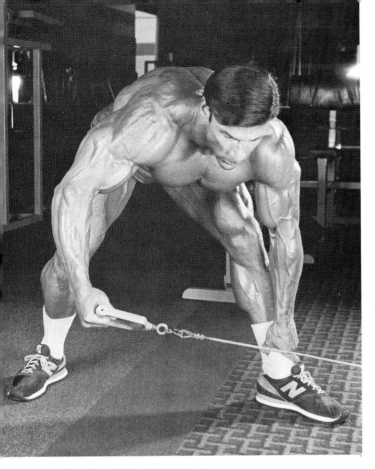

One-Arm Cable Bent Lateral.

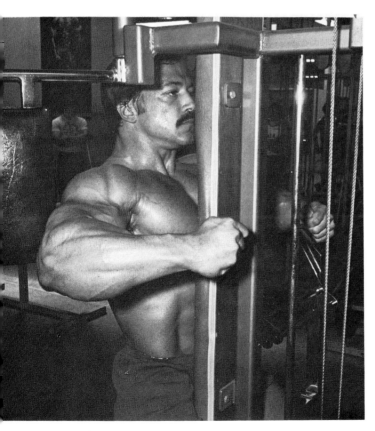

Pec Deck Rear Delt Raise.

which your back would normally rest. Place your elbows against the movable pads of the machine. Allow your elbows to move as far forward as possible, then force them as far to the rear as you can. Return to the starting point and repeat the movement for the required number of repetitions.

Variations—A similar exercise can be done on the Nautilus rowing machine. Instead of having your forearms horizontal to the floor as when doing the rowing movement, however, run them perpendicular to the floor and grasp the upright arms of the movable pads to stress the rear delts.

Training Tips—To maximize use of the Weider Peak Contraction Training Principle, hold the position of this movment with your elbows to the rear for a count of two before returning your elbows to the front position. This is a favorite technique of Mike Mentzer (Mr. America, Mr. Universe and the IFBB Professional Florida Grand Prix winner).

Upright Rowing

Main Area of Emphasis—This fine basic exercise stresses the trapezius and medial/-posterior deltoid groups most intensely. Secondary emphasis is placed on the biceps and the gripping muscles of the forearms.

Method of Performance—Take a narrow grip in the middle of a barbell (about six inches between your index fingers) with your palms facing your body at the start of the movement. Stand erect and hold your arms straight downward so the barbell and your hands rest across your upper thighs. From this basic starting position, slowly pull the barbell directly upward close to your body until it contacts the under part of your chin. As you are pulling the barbell upward, be sure to keep your elbows well above the level of your hands. It is particularly important to emphasize having your elbows high at the top point of the movement. Slowly lower the barbell back to the starting point, and repeat the movement for the desired number of repetitions.

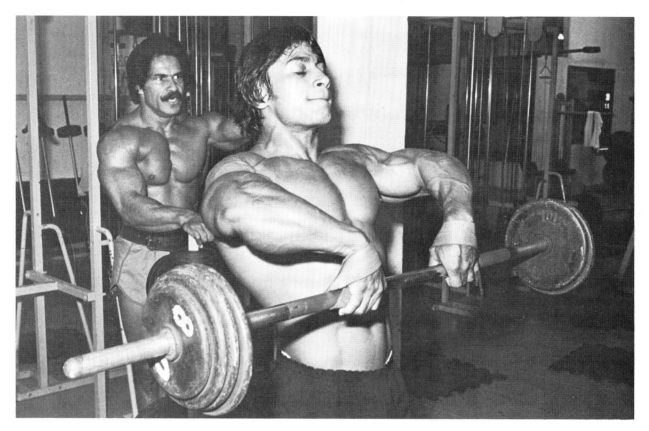

Upright Rowing.

Upright Cable Rowing.

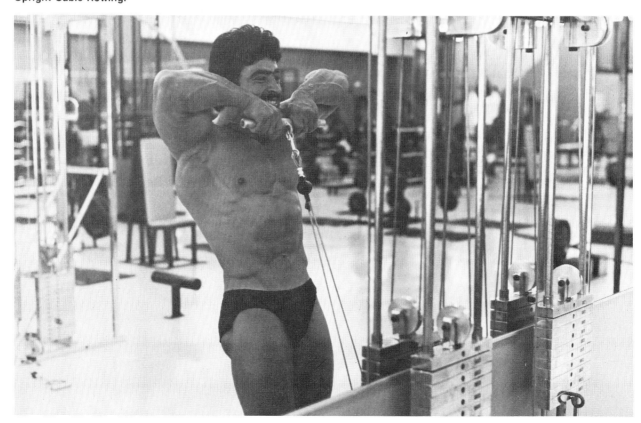

Variations—You can do this exercise using a floor pulley that has a short bar handle attached to it. You can also do the movement with two floor pulleys with loop handles attached to them. In either case, the use of pulleys is a good way to utilize the Weider Continuous Tension Training Principle.

Training Tips—Some bodybuilders seem to like doing Upright Rowing with a shoulder-width grip on the barbell, saying that it hits the deltoids more directly. In my vast experience, I believe that you will receive a much better trapezius-deltoid tie-in from doing Upright Rows in the manner I have just described them.

CHAMPIONSHIP DELTOID ROUTINES

In this section, I will present the deltoid training routines of 22 IFBB superstars. Keep in mind as you read these programs, however, that they are of very high intensity and suitable for use as written by only very advanced bodybuilders. If you are a relative beginner to bodybuilding, you should do only one or two sets of each listed exercise, and perform no more than 6–8 total sets. At the intermediate level of bodybuilding training, you can do 10–12 total sets of deltoid work, and more advanced bodybuilders can profitably perform 12–15 total sets of deltoid training.

Arnold Schwarzenegger

Exercise	Sets	Reps
1. Seated Press Behind Neck	4–5	8–10
2. "Arnold" Dumbbell Press	4–5	8–10
3. Dumbbell Side Laterals	4–5	8–10
4. Seated Dumbbell Bent Laterals	4–5	8–10
5. Cable Side Laterals	4–5	8–10

Albert Beckles

Exercise	Sets	Reps
1. Seated Dumbbell Press	4	10–12
2. Seated Press Behind Neck	4	10–12
3. Dumbbell Side Laterals	4	10–12
4. Dumbbell Bent Laterals	4	10–12
5. Barbell Upright Rowing	4	10–12

Pete Grymkowski

Exercise	Sets	Reps
1. Seated Front Barbell Press	8–10	12–4
2. Seated Dumbbell Press	4–6	12–6
3. Dumbbell Side Laterals	4–6	8–10
4. Seated Dumbbell Bent Laterals	4–6	8–10
5. Cable Side Laterals	4–6	8–10

Note: Bracketed exercises are supersetted.

Carlos Rodriguez

Exercise	Sets	Reps
1. Seated Machine Front Press	5	10
2. Dumbbell Bent Laterals	5	10
3. Seated Press Behind Neck	5	10
4. One-Arm Dumbbell Press	5	10
5. One-Arm Dumbbell Side Laterals	5	10
6. Seated Dumbbell Bent Laterals	5	10

Note: Bracketed exercises are supersetted.

Dennis Tinerino

Exercise	Sets	Reps
1. Machine Front Press	6	6–8
2. Rotating Dumbbell Shrug	4	10–12
3. Dumbbell Press	4	6–8
4. Cable Side Laterals	5	8–10
5. Dumbbell Bent Laterals	5	8–10

Joe Nazario

Exercise	Sets	Reps
1. Seated Press Behind Neck	5	8–10
2. Dumbbell Side Laterals	5	8–10
3. Dumbbell Presses	5	8–10
4. Dumbbell Alternate Front Raises	5	8–10
5. Nautilus Side Laterals	5	8–10
6. Dumbbell Bent Laterals	5	8–10

Note: Bracketed exercises are supersetted.

Ron Teufel

Exercise	Sets	Reps
1. Seated Barbell Front Press	5	12–5
2. Dumbbell Side Laterals	5	8
3. Seated Press Behind Neck	5	12–5
4. Dumbbell Side Laterals	5	8
5. Dumbbell Alternate Front Raises	5	8–10
6. Barbell Upright Rowing	5	8–10

Note: Bracketed exercises are supersetted.

Jusup Wilkosz

Exercise	Sets	Reps
1. Dumbbell Side Laterals	5	10–12
2. Seated Press Behind Neck	5	10–12
3. Dumbbell Bent Laterals	5	10–12
4. Barbell Upright Rowing	5	10–12
5. Cable Side Laterals	5	10–12

Note: Bracketed exercises are supersetted.

Mike Mentzer

Exercise	Sets	Reps
1. Nautilus Side Laterals	1–2	6
2. One-Arm Dumbbell Laterals	1	6
3. Universal Machine Press Behind Neck	1	6
4. Rear Delt Raise (Nautilus rowing machine)	2	6

Note: Approximately two forced reps are done on each set of exercises 1–4.

Tim Belknap

Exercise	Sets	Reps
1. Seated Press Behind Neck	3	8–12
2. Dumbbell Side Laterals	3	8–12
3. Cable Bent Laterals	3	8–12

Samir Bannout

Exercise	Sets	Reps
1. Seated Machine Press Behind Neck	4–5	6–8
2. Seated Bent Laterals	4–5	8–10
3. Seated Dumbbell Press	4–5	6–8
4. Standing Dumbbell Side Laterals	4–5	8–10
5. Cable Side Laterals	4–5	8–10

Note: Bracketed exercises are supersetted.

Scott Wilson

Exercise	Sets	Reps
1. Seated Machine Front Press	5	5–6
2. Seated Press Behind Neck	5	5–6
3. Seated Dumbbell Press	5	6–8
4. Dumbbell Side Laterals	5	6–8
5. Nautilus Side Laterals	5	6–8
6. Dumbbell Bent Laterals	5	6–8
7. Cable Bent Laterals	5	6–8

Jacques Neuville

Exercise	Sets	Reps
1. Seated Press Behind Neck	5	10–12
2. Seated Dumbbell Bent Laterals	5	10–12
3. Cable Side Laterals	5	10–12
4. Upright Rowing	5	10–12

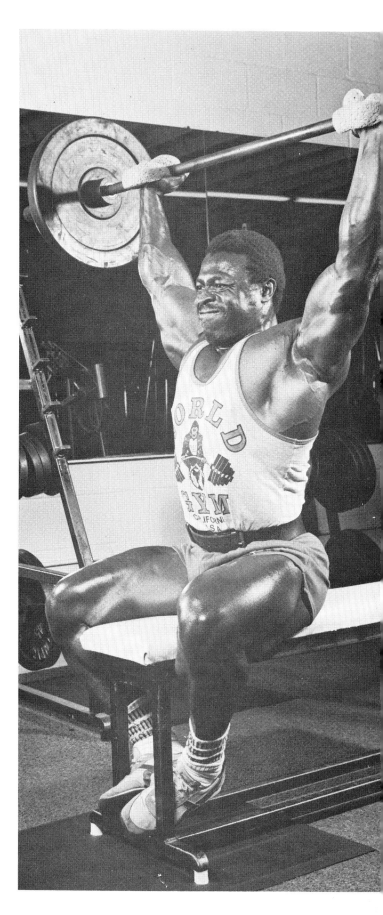

Boyer Coe

Exercise	Sets	Reps
1. One-Arm Cable Bent Laterals	2	10
2. Face-Down Lying Dumbbell Laterals	2	10
3. Seated Machine Front Press	4	8
4. One-Arm Dumbbell Side Laterals	2	10
5. Lateral Raise/Shrug with Dumbbells	2	15
6. Barbell Shrugs (in power rack)	4	10

Lou Ferrigno

Exercise	Sets	Reps
1. Seated Press Behind Neck	5	7–10
2. Seated Machine Front Press	5	10–12
3. Dumbbell Side Laterals	5	10–12
4. Dumbbell Bent Laterals	5	10–12
5. Dumbbell Alternate Front Raise	5	10–12

Larry Scott

Exercise	Sets	Reps
1. Dumbbell Press	5–6	6–8
2. Prone Incline Laterals	4–5	6–8
3. Cable Bent Laterals	4–5	6–8
4. One-Arm Dumbbell Side Laterals	5	6–8

Casey Viator

Exercise	Sets	Reps
1. One-Arm Nautilus Side Laterals	4–5	6–8
2. Seated Press Behind Neck	4–5	6–8
3. Universal Machine Seated Press	4–5	6–8
4. Pec Deck Rear Delt Raise	4–5	8–10
5. Upright Rowing	4–5	6–8
6. Cable Side Laterals	4–5	8–10

Note: Bracketed exercises are supersetted.

Dr. Franco Columbu

Exercise	Sets	Reps
1. Dumbbell Side Laterals	4	10
2. Dumbbell Bent Laterals	6	10
3. Seated Press Behind Neck	4	8
4. Dumbbell Alternate Front Raise	3	8
5. Cable Side Laterals	3	10

Chris Dickerson

Exercise	Sets	Reps
1. Seated Press Behind Neck	6	12–8
2. Dumbbell Side Laterals	6	8–10
3. Seated Dumbbell Press	6	8
4. Seated Dumbbell Bent Laterals	4	12–15
5. Barbell Upright Rowing	4	10–12

Andreas Cahling

Exercise	Sets	Reps
1. Seated Press Behind Neck	2–3	8–12
2. Dumbbell Side Laterals	2–3	8–12
3. Seated Dumbbell Bent Laterals	2–3	8–12
4. Barbell Front Raise	2–3	8–12
5. Cable Side Laterals	1–2	8–12

Bill Grant

Exercise	Sets	Reps
1. Dumbbell Side Laterals	5	10–12
2. Universal Machine Seated Press	5	8–10
3. Barbell Upright Rowing	5	10
4. Dumbbell Bent Laterals	5	10–12

Danny Padilla

Exercise	Sets	Reps
1. Seated Barbell Front Press	4	6–10
2. Seated Machine Press Behind Neck	4	6–10
3. Dumbbell Side Laterals	4	8–12
4. Cable Side Laterals	4	8–12
5. Seated Dumbbell Bent Laterals	4	8–12
6. Cable Bent Laterals	4	8–12

CONCLUSION

The contents of this chapter should give you considerable food for thought in terms of developing your own deltoids to superstar caliber. Adapt the routines of the champs to your own purposes and abilities, train consistently, use heavy weights in good form on all exercises, and you'll soon have a pair of your own cannonball delts!

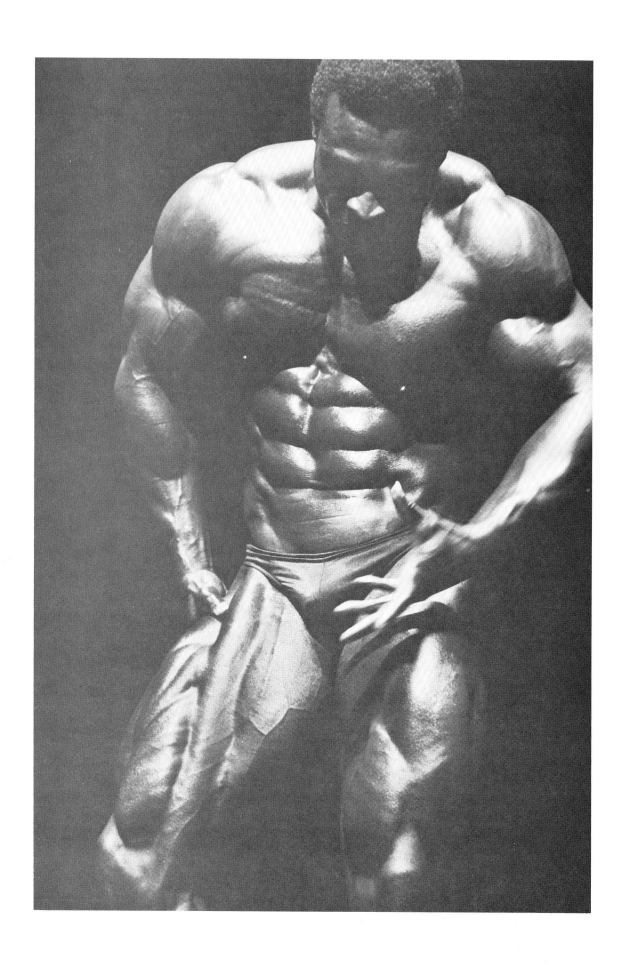

13

Tree-Trunk Thighs

Huge, fully muscled, and deeply grooved columns of thigh muscle are the hallmark of a powerfully developed Olympian physique. And Tom Platz (Mr. Universe) best epitomizes this type of thigh development among IFBB superstar bodybuilders. Not only does he have the most huge, well-shaped, and fully striated thighs in bodybuildingdom, but these columns of power are so strongly developed that he can routinely do 20 reps with 600 pounds and 10 repetitions with 700 pounds in the Squat when in heavy contest training.

The tree-trunk thighs of Tom Platz are most closely rivaled—if, indeed, they can be rivaled at all—by those of Tim Belknap, a new lion of the bodybuilding scene. Belknap won the 1981 Mr. America title, and he has also squatted 10 repetitions with 700 pounds. For the short length of time that Belknap has been training, his thighs are phenomenally developed. Indeed, they had gotten so huge that he has now turned to a lighter shaping and defining thigh-training program.

Arnold Schwarzenegger had terrific thighs, with very deep separations between the major muscle groups. Indeed, the grooves between his major thigh muscles were so deeply pronounced that you could probably have hidden a quarter in them. Other great Weider-trained champs with outstanding thigh development include Mike Mentzer, Casey Viator, Samir Bannout, Robby Robinson, Chris Dickerson, Boyer Coe, Frank Zane, Bertil Fox, Danny Padilla, Roy Callender, and Johnny Fuller.

Indeed, it is difficult to be an IFBB champ in this era without having tree-trunk thighs with tremendous shape and great cuts—even cross striations—in every muscle group. And in this chapter, I intend to tell you exactly how the Weider-trained champs have built their superb thighs.

THE SQUAT

Every champ that I've ever known who possessed superior thigh development was a consistently heavy squatter. And since the Squat involves such huge muscle groups—all of the thigh muscles, the buttocks and lower back—it involves tremendous energy expenditures to do Squats regularly. As a result, squatting *hurts* physiologically and you must steel yourself against this pain in order to develop tree-trunk thighs.

The best squatters—champs like Platz, Belknap, and Viator, who do 20 reps with 600+ pounds in every thigh workout—learn to love the movement. They love the heavy work of squatting, because when they are huffing and puffing like steam locomotives and their thighs feel like someone is playing a blowtorch over them, they *know* that they're having a great workout. And not only have they improved their thighs, but they've stimulated their entire body metabolism into a naturally anabolic state when they squat heavily.

Since bodybuilders do Squats with such heavy weights, all of them wrap their knees with elastic gauze bandages to protect those joints from injury. The "Superwraps" (available through ads in *Muscle & Fitness* magazine) that powerlifters wear are the best. All top bodybuilders also wear a Weider weightlifting belt while squatting in order to protect their lower backs and abdomens from injury.

A few lesser bodybuilders avoid doing Squats because they say that their knees hurt, and as a result they have birdlike legs. But don't tell that to Dennis Tinerino, who's won Mr. America, Mr. World and Mr. Universe titles. He squats heavily and has superb thigh development, even though his knees are disaster areas as a result of participation in youth and high school sports!

Dennis has developed a unique knee-protection method that you can try if your own knees are a bit painful. First Dennis slips a pair of neoprene rubber bands over his knees. These rubber knee bands add a little support to Dennis's knees, but mainly they hold the heat generated by his heavy thigh workouts in the knee area. And because every bodybuilder perspires profusely, this is a damp heat, which is very soothing and therapeutic. These rubber knee bands are available at many sporting goods stores or through ads in *Flex* and *Muscle & Fitness.*

Over his neoprene rubber bands, Dennis

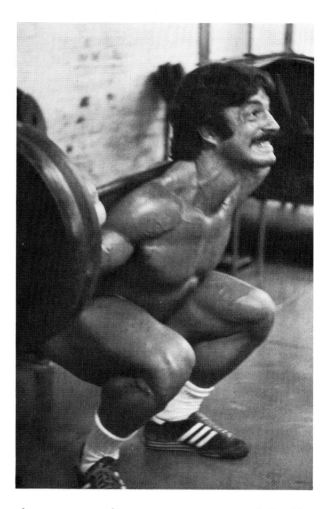

slips a pair of warmup pants. And finally he winds Superwraps securely around his knees *over* the sweat pants and neoprene bands. These elastic gauze wraps provide maximum support to Tinerino's knees. And after several sets of Leg Extensions and high-rep warm-up sets of Squats, his knees feel good enough to work up to well over 500 pounds in his Squat workout.

If Dennis Tinerino, with his extremely painful knees, can do Squats, there's no reason why you can't, too. And you won't build great thighs without doing heavy Squats!

Injuries from Squatting

In discussing Dennis Tinerino's knee difficulties, one could conclude that squatting is injurious to the knees. Indeed, back in the 1950s, athletic coaches widely condemned the Squat (to say nothing of weight training in general) on the premise that it stretched the knee ligaments and badly injured the knees.

Practically speaking, nothing could be further from the truth, as long as the Squat is done in proper form. Squat down slowly and *never* bounce at the bottom position of a Squat, and you'll never injure your knees doing the movement. In fact, properly performed Squats will actually strengthen your knees and make them less prone to athletic injuries. Indeed, athletic coaches worldwide now make extensive use of the Squat in the strength-conditioning programs of their athletes!

I think it's actually easier to injure the lower back while doing Squats. If bodybuilders or powerlifters bend over rather sharply at the waist to help cheat up a heavy Squat rep, they are likely candidates for a lower back injury, since this type of poor exercise form makes their lower backs very vulnerable to injury. But if you use proper biomechanical form by keeping your torso as upright as possible during the movement, you will never injure your lower back while squatting. Indeed, I've known very few champion bodybuilders who have injured their lower backs in this manner when using good form.

Vince Gironda and the Squat

During the 1960s, Vince Gironda developed several champion bodybuilders at his Vince's Gym in North Hollywood, California. Although Vince hasn't produced a champion for more than a decade, he still has very definite opinions of the Squat. Vince doesn't even have a squat rack in his gym, because he believes that Squats build "unaesthetically" large buttocks. Instead of Squats, he has his gym members perform lots of Hacks, Leg Extensions, and Sissy Squats.

I interviewed several champion bodybuilders on Vince Gironda's theory about Squats, and to a man they condemned it. "I've done Squats for as long as I've been a bodybuilder," said Arnold Schwarzenegger (winner of seven Mr. Olympia titles), "and I'd never have built my thighs up enough to win my Mr. Olympia titles without squatting. And besides, a herculean bodybuilder would look silly and incompletely developed if he hadn't also developed powerful-appearing hips and buttocks."

"You only have to look at the bodybuilders who come out of his gym to see how absurdly wrong Vince's theory is," Dr. Franco Columbu (twice a Mr. Olympia winner) noted. "No bodybuilder from Vince's Gym—and you can include Vince himself in his prime in this group—has ever had what most bodybuilders would call outstanding thigh development.

"Throughout my bodybuilding career, I've done plenty of heavy Squats in every thigh workout, often working up to over 600 pounds for reps. My thighs have grown from pencils to massive columns of power, primarily as a result of doing so much squatting. Are my hips wide as a result? Certainly not! And are my buttocks the size of those of a hippo? Certainly not! They are merely in powerful proportion with my thighs and the rest of my physique."

Boyer Coe (winner of 15 World Championships) concludes the argument against Vince Gironda's bias against Squats: "Up until after I had won the Mr. America title, the *only* thigh exercise I did was full Squats. I'd do 8–10 sets of 10–15 reps, and my thighs were massive, well-shaped and supermuscular from following this simple routine. And I certainly haven't developed a big butt from all of the Squats I've done over the years. In short, I think that Vince Gironda's theories on the Squat are pure bunk!"

THIGH ANATOMY AND KINESIOLOGY

With the back, the thighs (and their related hips and buttocks) have the most complicated anatomy and kinesiology of any muscle group in the human body. The front thigh complex is called the *quadriceps*, since it is composed of four main muscles—the *vastus lateralis, vastus medialis, rectus femoris,* and *sartorius.* All four of these muscles (particularly the first three named) function to fully straighten

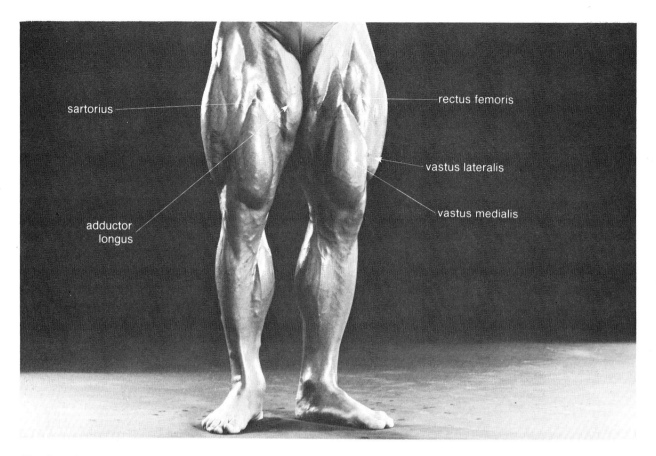

The Quadriceps Muscles.

the leg from a fully bent position. And each of the four quadriceps muscles works harder at certain points along the full range of motion of leg extension. Collectively, the quadriceps muscles are often called "thigh extensors."

The *sartorius* additionally functions to force the thighs together from a spread position. The *sartorius* is assisted in this function by the *adductor longus,* a long and potentially powerful muscle that runs vertically along the inside of the thigh. Collectively, the *sartorius* and *adductor longus* are called "thigh adductors," and adduction is the process of pulling the thighs together. Few bodybuilders work the thigh adductors, but they should do so in order to build thighs that have great width when viewed from both the front and back.

On the back of the thigh, there is one large two-headed muscle group called the *biceps femoris,* which acts to fully bend the

leg from a straight position. The *biceps femoris* is often called the "thigh biceps," and it gives great width to the thigh when seen from the side, such as in the case of Roy Callender (Amateur and Professional Mr. Universe). From the back, a well-defined thigh biceps, such as possessed by Boyer Coe, can have a very impressive appearance.

There are also two smaller muscle groups at the back of the thigh—the *semitendinosus* and *semimembranosus.* Both of these muscles assist the *biceps femoris* in fully bending the leg from a straight position. This collection of muscle groups is sometimes called "thigh flexors."

Tying in with the thigh flexors are the *gluteus maximus* and *gluteus medius,* which make up the buttocks, discussed earlier in relation to Vince Gironda's theories on the Squat. The buttocks act to move the torso and thighs into, and even past, a

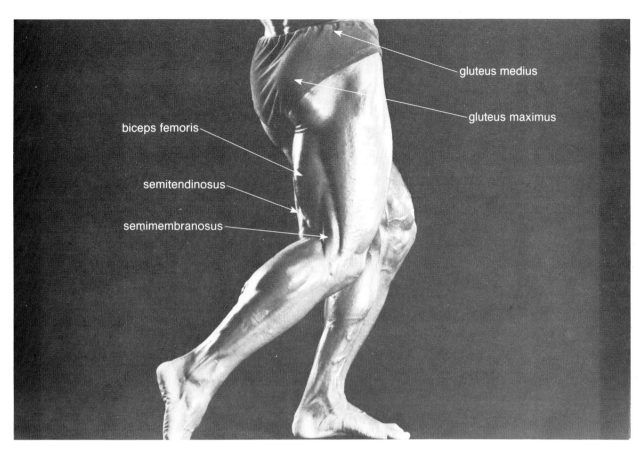

gluteus medius

gluteus maximus

biceps femoris

semitendinosus

semimembranosus

The Back Thigh Muscles.

straight line from a position with the torso fully bent forward and resting against the thighs.

From the foregoing discussion of thigh anatomy and kinesiology, you can easily see how complex this muscle group is. You should also understand that the thigh muscles grouped together make up the muscle group with the largest mass in the human body. And that is the reason why you must expend such huge quantities of energy to train your thighs. Many weak-willed bodybuilders shy away from the physiological fatigue pain associated with thigh training and thus fail to build championship thighs.

THE CHAMPS' THIGH EXERCISES

In this section, you will find 10 major thigh exercises that are used by all of the Weider-trained IFBB superstars. Counting variations of foot stance, type of machine used, methods of performance, etc., you have something in the neighborhood of 25 thigh movements with which you can experiment, using the Weider Instinctive Training Principle to make up your own thigh-building routines.

Squats

Main Area of Emphasis—This movement is called "The King of Lower Body Exercises" because it stresses all of the front thigh, hamstring, and buttocks muscles quite intensely. It also places secondary stress on the calves, abdomen, and lower back muscles.

Method of Performance—Place a loaded barbell on a squat rack and step under the bar to position it across your shoulders behind your neck. You will find holding the bar in this position to be fairly comfortable if you hump up your trapezius muscles to act as a pad for the bar. Or, you can wrap a towel around the bar as padding. Grasp the barbell out near the plates to steady it across your shoulders. Next, straighten your legs and lift the barbell free of the rack supports. Step backward one or two steps and set your feet at about shoulder width, your toes angled slightly outward. Tense all of the muscles of your back and keep them tensed throughout the movement. Keeping your torso as upright as possible during the movement, slowly bend your thighs and sink down into a fully squatting position. As you are squatting down, your thighs will spread slightly. Without bouncing at the bottom of the movement, slowly straighten your legs and return yourself to the starting position. Repeat the movement for the desired number of repetitions.

Variations—You can experiment with a wider or narrower foot stance as you do your Squats. You can also squat down to various depths, which is called doing Partial Squats. The most common forms of Partial Squats are Quarter Squats, Half Squats, Three-Quarter Squats, Parallel Squats and Bench Squats. In Bench Squats, you squat down to lightly touch your rump on a low bench or stool, but when doing so be sure not to bounce forcefully, since that could injure your back.

Training Tips—Always use one or two training partners as spotters when you are squatting with maximum or near maximum poundages, and always wear a weightlifting belt, even with your warmup weights. If you have difficulty balancing yourself in the bottom position of a Squat (which is usually a sign of ankle inflexibility), you can rest your heels on a 2 x 4-inch board to improve your balance.

Front Squat

Main Area of Emphasis—Front Squats work the same muscles as the regular Squat with a barbell held behind the neck, although a little less stress is placed on the buttocks muscles when doing Front Squats. You will also find that Front Squats tend to

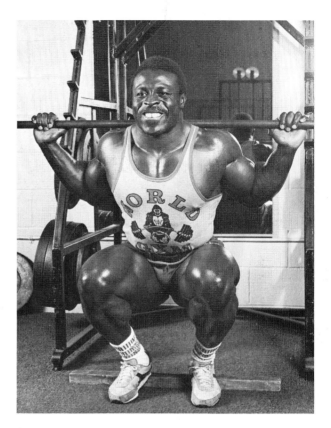

Squat.

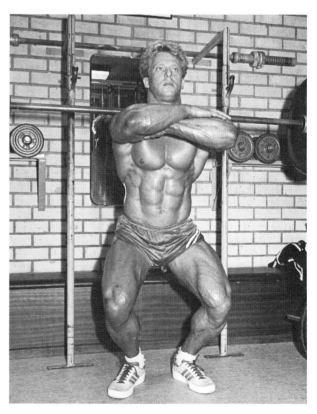

Front Squat.

stress the thigh muscles just above the knees a little more intensely than do regular Squats.

Method of Performance—Place a loaded barbell on a squat rack and step under the barbell with your arms extended directly out in front of your body parallel to the floor. Position the barbell across your deltoids and upper chest and cross your arms over the middle of the bar. As long as you hold your elbows up while maintaining this arm position for Front Squats, the bar will remain securely in position in front of your neck. Straighten your legs to lift the bar from the rack, step back a couple of steps and position your feet the same as for a normal back Squat. Keeping your torso perfectly upright (you will dump the weight off your shoulders if you allow your torso to lean forward), slowly squat down as fully as possible and then return to the starting point. Repeat the movement for the desired number of repetitions.

Variations—As with Squats, you can experiment with a variety of foot-stance widths, all of which will stress your thigh muscles a little differently. You can also hold the barbell at your shoulders like an Olympic-style weightlifter, if that arm position is more comfortable for you. This consists of grasping the barbell with a grip about four or five inches wider on each side than the width of your shoulders, then lifting your elbows high enough to maintain the bar in position across your shoulders as you do your Front Squats.

Training Tips—This is not a movement in which you should try to do maximum attempts, as in the regular back Squat. I would suggest doing no less than 6–8 reps a set on Front Squats. Be sure to wear a weightlifting belt, and if you have balance problems, stand with your heels on a 2 x 4-inch board, as in the Squat. You can also very comfortably and profitably do Front Squats in a Smith machine.

Hack Slide Squat

Main Area of Emphasis—This excellent movement strongly stresses the thigh mus-

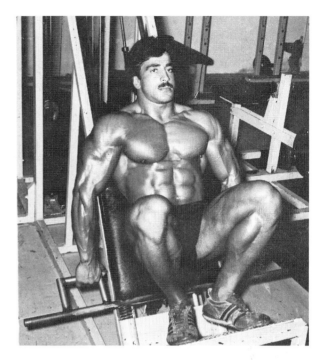

Hack Squat on slide platform.

cles, particularly those just above the knees. Most champion bodybuilders do Hack Squats in an effort to add cuts to their front thighs.

Method of Performance—Place your feet on the angled foot platform with your heels about eight inches apart and your toes angled outward at about 45 degrees on each side. Bend your legs fully, place your back against the sliding platform of the machine, and grasp the handles at the lower edges of the sliding platform. Fully straighten your legs. From the top position, slowly sink into a full squatting position, allowing your legs to spread so that your knees travel out over your feet as you squat down. At the bottom position of the movement, slowly straighten your legs and return to the top position. Repeat the movement for the desired number of repetitions.

Variations—There is another type of hack slide machine in common use in most larger gyms. Instead of a sliding platform, it has a pair of yokes that pass over your shoulders. Rotating stop handles at the sides of the yokes will release the machine for use in doing Hack Squats. Otherwise, the movement is identical to that described

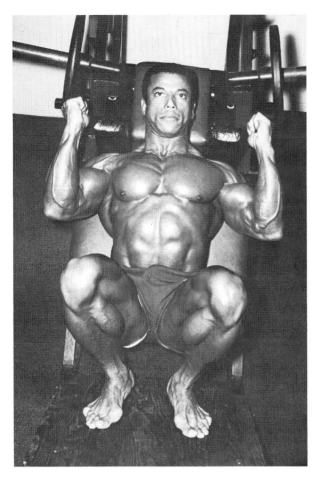

Hack Squat using yoke.

with the machine that has a sliding platform.

Training Tips—Experiment with various foot-stance widths when doing this movement. You can have a training partner help you with forced reps by pulling up on one of the handles of the machine just enough to allow you to force out an additional repetition or two.

Sissy Squat

Main Area of Emphasis—This movement directly stresses the front thigh muscles. Champion bodybuilders primarily do Sissy Squats close to a contest to cut up their front thighs.

Method of Performance—The easiest way to do this movement is to stand between a set of parallel bars and grasp the bars lightly to balance your body as you do the movement. Start with your feet parallel to each other and about six inches apart. From this position, simultaneously bend your legs, thrust your knees forward, rise up on your toes and lean backward until your torso is virtually parallel to the floor. It's easiest to get your torso parallel to the

Hack Squat using barbell.

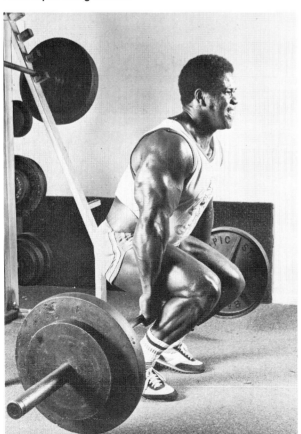

Sissy Squat.

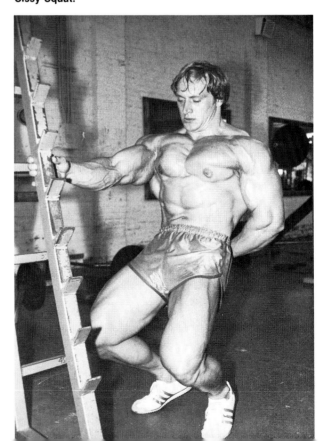

floor if you look up at the ceiling of the gym as you do the movement. If you have performed this movement correctly, you will feel a very strong stretching sensation in all of your front thigh muscles. Contract your thighs and reverse the lowering procedure to return to the starting position. Repeat the movement for the desired number of repetitions.

Variations—Some bodybuilders do this movement while grasping only one upright. When done in this fashion, you can hold a light dumbbell in your free hand to add resistance to the movement. In the variation done between parallel bars, you can wear a weight belt around your waist with a light dumbbell dangling from it.

Training Tips—The real key to using this movement effectively is in getting a strong stretch in your thighs at the bottom position of the exercise. If you don't get this stretch, you will receive little benefit from the movement.

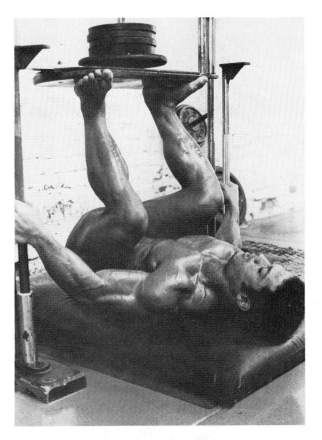

Leg Press on vertical machine.

Leg Press

Main Area of Emphasis—This movement strongly stresses the front thigh muscles and places secondary stress on the buttocks.

Method of Performance—Lie on your back beneath a vertical leg press machine with your hips positioned directly beneath the movable platform. You should be lying on a padded surface that is angled downward toward your head. Place your feet on the movable platform at about shoulder width, with your toes pointed slightly outward. Straighten your legs and rotate the machine's stop bars out of the way so that you can bend your legs and lower the platform as far as possible. As you lower the platform, it's best to spread your legs slightly so that your knees don't contact your chest. It's better for your knees to travel down on each side of your chest. From the bottom position, slowly straighten your legs and push the platform back to the starting position. Repeat the movement for the desired number of repeti-

tions. Be sure to replace the stop bars at the conclusion of your set.

Variations—This movement can be done on two machines in which you sit and push pedals horizontally—Nautilus and Universal Gyms machines. Both of these machines are missing stop bars, so you must push the pedals from the bottom position for the first repetition. They do, however, have adjustable seats so that you can control the range of motion over which you do the movement. And they have handles which you can grasp to steady your body in the seats provided during the movement. There is also a 45-degree angled machine with similar characteristics to that of a vertical machine, including stop bars. Many bodybuilders seem to favor this 45-degree angled machine in comparison to any of the other three types of leg press machines.

Training Tips—On all leg press machines, you can give yourself your own forced reps. Simply push on your knees

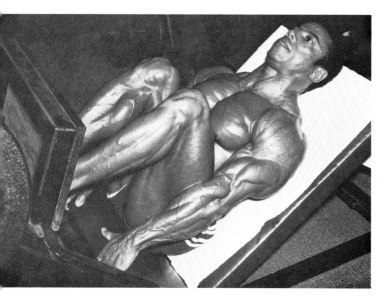

Leg Press on 45-degree-angled machine.

Training Tips—This is the best movement for utilizing the Weider Peak Contraction Training Principle for the front thighs. To get a good peak contraction in your quads, simply hold the top position of the movement for three or four seconds, strongly tensing your thigh muscles, before lowering back to the starting position of the movement.

Leg Extension.

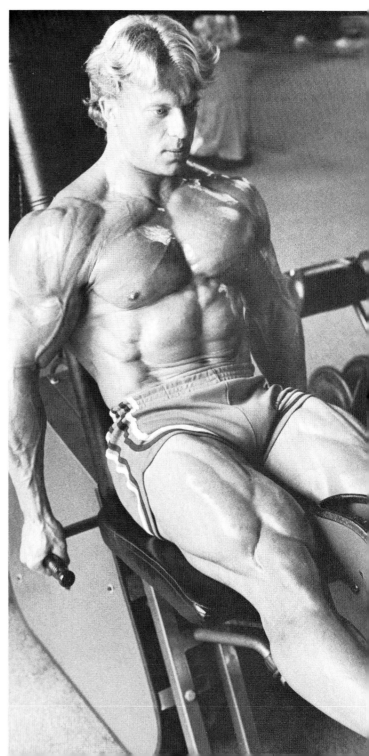

with your hands when you need a little assistance in completing a rep or two.

Leg Extension

Main Area of Emphasis—This fine movement isolates stress on the quadriceps muscles of the front thighs.

Method of Performance—Sit in a leg extension machine with the backs of your knees against the edge of the padded surface near the lever arm of the machine. Place your toes under the lower set of roller pads and grasp either the handles provided or the sides of the padded seating platform to steady your body in position throughout the movement. From this position, slowly straighten your legs. Hold them straight for a moment, and then bend them slowly to return your legs to the starting position. Repeat the movement for the desired number of repetitions.

Variations—This movement can be done on normal free-standing leg extension machines, the machines that come with Universal Gyms complexes, and on a Nautilus leg extension machine. A majority of top bodybuilders seem to prefer using the Nautilus leg extension machine. You can also do this movement one leg at a time if you wish.

Lying Leg Curl

Main Area of Emphasis—This movement directly stresses the thigh biceps muscles in isolation from the rest of the body.

Method of Performance—Lie facedown on a leg curl machine with your knees at the edge of the padded surface of the machine at the end with the machine's lever arm. Hook your heels under the set of padded rollers that are level with the surface of the machine. Grasp the handles provided with the machine or the sides of the padded surface of the machine to steady your body in position throughout the movement. From this basic starting position, slowly bend your legs as fully as possible. Hold the top position of the movement for a moment, then lower back to the starting point. Repeat the movement for the desired number of repetitions.

Variations—This exercise can be done on normal free-standing leg curl machines, the machines that come with Universal Gyms complexes, or on a Nautilus leg curl machine. A majority of top bodybuilders seem to prefer using the Nautilus leg curl machine. You can also do this movement with one leg at a time if you wish.

Training Tips—Be sure to keep your hips in contact with the padded surface of the machine throughout the movement, since lifting your hips will shorten the range of movement that you can attain in doing Leg Curls. Leg Curls are the best movement for utilizing the Weider Peak Contraction Training Principle for the thigh biceps. To get a good peak contraction effect in your thigh biceps, simply hold the top position of the movement for three or four seconds, strongly tensing your thigh biceps muscles, before lowering back to the starting position of the exercise.

Standing Leg Curl

Main Area of Emphasis—This movement strongly stresses the thigh biceps muscles one leg at a time in isolation from the rest of the body.

Method of Performance—Stand in the machine so that the backs of your lower

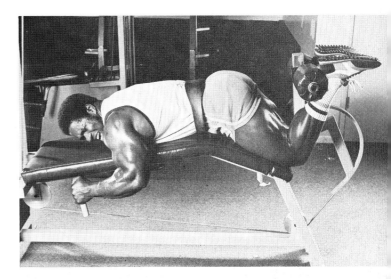

Lying Leg Curl.

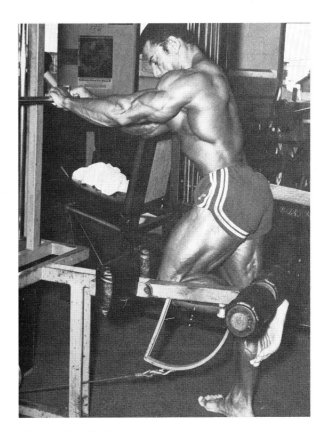

Standing Leg Curl.

legs are against the movable pads of the apparatus. Grasp the vertical uprights of the machine to balance your body in position throughout the movement. Starting with your left leg, bend your leg as fully as possible under the resistance of the machine. Pause for a second at the top of the movement and then return to the starting position. Repeat the movement for the desired number of repetitions. Be sure to do an equal number of sets and repetitions for both legs.

Variations—Other than the fact that there are several companies that manufacture slightly different versions of this machine, there are no real variations of methods of performing Standing Leg Curls.

Training Tips—As with Lying Leg Curls, this is an excellent movement in which to utilize the Weider Peak Contraction Training Principle to stress the thigh biceps. You will also notice that you can get a better contraction in your thigh biceps when you do one leg at a time, because then you don't need to split your attention between two legs. Many top bodybuilders do both Lying Leg Curls and Standing Leg Curls in the same leg workout.

Stiff-Leg Deadlifts

Comment—This movement is described and illustrated as a back exercise in Chapter 9, but it is a superb thigh biceps developer used by such champs as Ken Waller (Mr. America, Mr. Universe, and Mr. Olympia class winner). You should give it a try in your thigh biceps routine.

Stiff-Leg Deadlift.

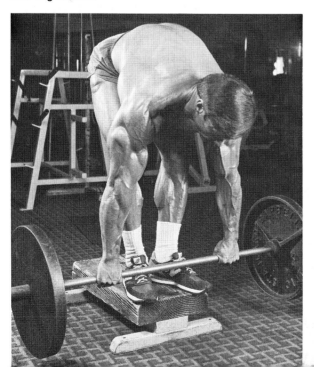

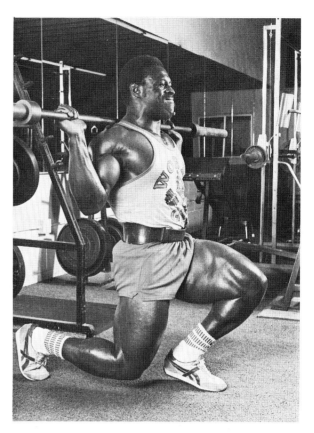

Lunge.

Lunges

Main Area of Emphasis—This movement stresses the front thighs and buttocks. Most champion bodybuilders use it for a few weeks prior to a competition to cut up their front thighs.

Method of Performance—Place a light barbell across your shoulders as though preparing to do a set of Squats. Your feet should be set about 12–14 inches apart and parallel to each other. Step 2½–3 feet forward with your left foot. Keeping your right leg as straight as possible, slowly bend your left leg as far as you can. You should actually bend your left leg far enough so that your knee is ahead of your ankle. At the bottom position of this movement, you should feel a strong stretching sensation in your right front thigh muscles. Push back to the starting position by straightening your left leg, and do your next repetition by stepping forward with your right foot. Continue alternating feet like this until you have done the full number of required repetitions with each leg.

Variations—Rather than holding a barbell across your neck, you can hold two dumbbells in your hands while you do Lunges. Some bodybuilders also like to lunge up onto the top of a flat exercise bench with their front foot when doing this movement.

Training Tips—The real key to cutting up your upper thighs with lunges is getting a good stretch in the front thigh muscles of your rear leg on each repetition.

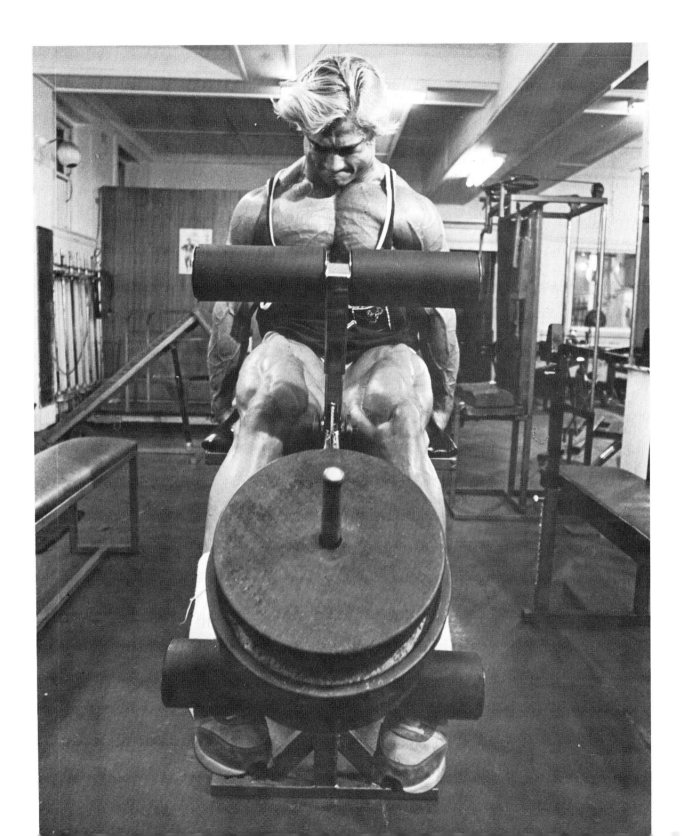

CHAMPIONSHIP THIGH ROUTINES

In this section, I will present the thigh training programs of 20 superstar bodybuilders. Bear in mind as you read these routines, however, that they are of very high intensity and suitable for use as written by only very advanced Olympian bodybuilders.

If you are a relative beginner to bodybuilding, you should do only one or two sets of each listed exercise, and perform no more than 8–10 total sets. At the intermediate level of bodybuilding training, you can do 12–15 total sets of thigh work, while more advanced bodybuilders can profitably perform up to 15–20 total sets of thigh training.

Tom Platz

Exercise	Sets	Reps
1. Squats	8–10	20–5
2. Hack Slide Squats	5	10–15
3. Leg Extensions	5–8	10–15
4. Leg Curls	6–10	10–15

Arnold Schwarzenegger

Exercise	Sets	Reps
1. Squats	7	12–8
2. Front Squats	4–5	12–8
{3. Leg Curls	4	8–12
{4. Lunges	4	10–15

Note: Bracketed exercises are supersetted.

Boyer Coe

Exercise	Sets	Reps
1. One-Leg Leg Extension	4	10
2. One-Leg Leg Curl	4	10
3. Leg Presses (45-degree machine)	3–4	15
4. Partial Leg Presses (45-degree machine)	3	15
5. Squats	1–2	20–30

Lou Ferrigno

Exercise	Sets	Reps
1. Front Squat	5–6	10–15
2. Hack Slide Squat	4–5	10–15
3. Leg Extension	4–5	10–15
4. Leg Curl	5–6	10–15
5. Lunges	3–4	10–15

Frank Zane

Exercise	Sets	Reps
1. Leg Curls	5	20–8
2. Leg Extensions	5	20–8
3. Squats	5	20–8

Note: During a precontest phase, Lunges (five sets of 10–15 reps) are substituted for Squats.

Dennis Tinerino

Exercise	Sets	Reps
1. Leg Extensions	4–5	6–8
2. Squats	8–10	20–6
3. Hack Slide Squats	4	6–8
4. Leg Curls	5	6–8
5. Lunges (during precontest cycle only)	4	20

Mohamed Makkawy

Exercise	Sets	Reps
1. Leg Extensions	5	10–15
2. Leg Curls	5	10–15
3. Hack Slide Squats	5	10–15

Note: Makkawy squatted extensively and heavily in his early years of training and built a high degree of thigh muscle mass. Nowadays, he's seeking thigh cuts, so he eschews the use of Squats in his thigh routine.

Jusup Wilkosz

Exercise	Sets	Reps
{1. Leg Extensions	4–6	15–8
{2. Squats	4–6	15–8
{3. Lunges	4–6	15–8
{4. Hack Slide Squats	4–6	15–8
5. Leg Curls	5	20–10

Note: Bracketed exercises are supersetted.

Samir Bannout

Exercise	Sets	Reps
1. Squats	5	20–8
2. Leg Extensions	4	15
3. Hack Slide Squats	4	10–15
4. Leg Curls	6	15–8

Chris Dickerson

Exercise	Sets	Reps
1. Leg Press (45-degree machine)	6–8	8–10
2. Hack Slide Squats	5–6	10–15
3. Squats	5–6	10–15
4. Leg Extensions	6–8	10–15
5. Standing Leg Curls	4–5	10–15
6. Lying Leg Curls	4–5	10–15

Tim Belknap

Exercise	Sets	Reps
1. Hack Slide Squats	4	12–15
2. Nautilus Leg Extensions	4	12–15
3. Nautilus Leg Curls	6	12–15

Note: As mentioned earlier in this chapter, Belknap squatted quite heavily in his earlier years of training. Now he seeks thigh shape and muscularity, so he doesn't do Squats.

Andreas Cahling

Exercise	Sets	Reps
1. Leg Extensions	4–6	8–12
2. Front Squats	2–3	8–12
3. Hack Slide Squats	2–3	8–12
4. Lunges	2–3	20–25
5. Leg Curls	4–5	8–12

Dr. Franco Columbu

Exercise	Sets	Reps
1. Squats	8–10	15–5
2. Leg Extensions	6–8	15–8
3. Leg Curls	5–6	10–12

Mike Mentzer

Exercise	Sets	Reps
1. Leg Extensions	1–2	6–8
2. Leg Presses	1	6–8
3. Squats	2	6–8
4. Leg Curls	1–2	6–8

Note: On exercises 1, 2, and 4, Mike does 2–3 forced reps at the end of each normal full-rep set.

Sergio Oliva

Exercise	Sets	Reps
1. Squats	8–10	15–2
2. Leg Extensions	5–6	10–15
3. Leg Curls	8–10	10–15
4. Lunges (during precontest phase only)	3–5	10–15

Johnny Fuller

Exercise	Sets	Reps
1. Leg Presses (45-degree machine)	10	15–20
2. Front Squats	5	10–15
3. Squats	5	10–15
4. Leg Extensions	5	10–15
5. Lunges (during precontest phase only)	5	15–20
6. Leg Curls	10	10–15

Casey Viator

Exercise	Sets	Reps
1. Squats	8–10	30–20
2. Leg Presses (45-degree machine)	8–10	30–20
3. Nautilus Leg Extensions	6–8	15–10
4. Nautilus Leg Curls	6–8	15–10
5. Nautilus Adduction Machine	6–8	15–10
6. Lunges	6–8	15–10

Robby Robinson

Exercise	Sets	Reps
1. Nautilus Leg Extensions	5–8	10–15
2. Nautilus Leg Curls	5–8	10–15
3. Hack Slide Squats	5–8	10–15
4. Standing Leg Curls	5–8	10–15
5. Squats (very narrow foot stance)	5–8	10–15
6. Lunges (precontest phase only)	5–8	10–15

Note: Bracketed exercises are supersetted.

Danny Padilla

Exercise	Sets	Reps
1. Squats	6–8	15–8
2. Hack Slide Squats	5	10
3. Front Squats	5	10
4. Nautilus Leg Extension	5	10
5. Nautilus Leg Curls	5	10
6. Standing Leg Curls	5	10

Bertil Fox

Exercise	Sets	Reps
1. Squats	6	15–8
2. Hack Squats	5	15–8
3. Leg Extensions	5	15–8
4. Leg Curls	5	15–8

Note: Bracketed exercises are supersetted.

CONCLUSION

The contents of this chapter will have given you considerable food for thought as you develop routines to build your own tree-trunk thighs. Adapt the routines of the champs to your own abilities and purposes, train consistently, use heavy weights in good form in all of your exercises, and you'll soon have a pair of your own tree-trunk thighs!

Index